I0044392

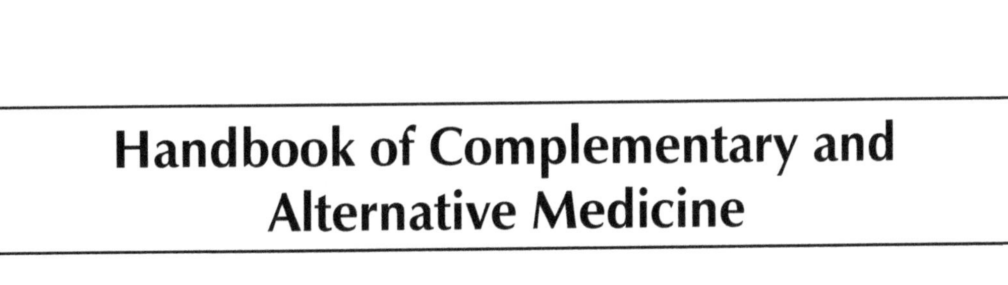

Handbook of Complementary and Alternative Medicine

Handbook of Complementary and Alternative Medicine

Editor: Penelope Higgins

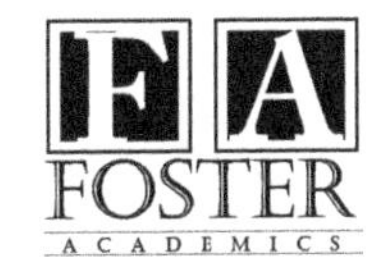

www.fosteracademics.com

www.fosteracademics.com

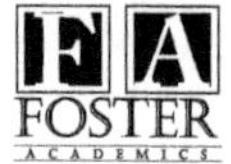

Cataloging-in-Publication Data

Handbook of complementary and alternative medicine / edited by Penelope Higgins.
p. cm.
Includes bibliographical references and index.
ISBN 978-1-63242-858-5
1. Alternative medicine. 2. Medicine. 3. Alternative medicine specialists. I. Higgins, Penelope.
R733 .H36 2019
615.5--dc23

Foster Academics,
118-35 Queens Blvd., Suite 400,
Forest Hills, NY 11375, USA

ISBN 978-1-63242-858-5 (Hardback)

Contents

Preface

Complementary medicine refers to the use of alternative medicine with functional medical treatment, for the purpose of improving the treatment effects. Alternative medicine involves the use of such practices, which are unproven to relieve the pain or to achieve other healing effects of medicine. Naturopathy and homeopathy are two of the most common forms of alternative medicine. Naturopathy is a natural and non-invasive therapeutic treatment method based on the belief that the body heals on its own by using a vital energy, which guides the bodily processes. The belief, that the substances, which cause the symptoms of a disease in healthy people, cure similar symptoms in sick people, forms the roots of homeopathy. The various advancements in complementary and alternative medicine are glanced at and their applications as well as ramifications are looked at in detail in this book. Different approaches, evaluations, methodologies and advanced studies on alternative practices have been included in it. Those in search of information to further their knowledge will be greatly assisted by this book.

After months of intensive research and writing, this book is the end result of all who devoted their time and efforts in the initiation and progress of this book. It will surely be a source of reference in enhancing the required knowledge of the new developments in the area. During the course of developing this book, certain measures such as accuracy, authenticity and research focused analytical studies were given preference in order to produce a comprehensive book in the area of study.

This book would not have been possible without the efforts of the authors and the publisher. I extend my sincere thanks to them. Secondly, I express my gratitude to my family and well-wishers. And most importantly, I thank my students for constantly expressing their willingness and curiosity in enhancing their knowledge in the field, which encourages me to take up further research projects for the advancement of the area.

Editor

1

Molecular evaluation of anti-inflammatory activity of phenolic lipid extracted from cashew nut shell liquid (CNSL)

Marilen Queiroz de Souza[1,5], Isabella Márcia Soares Nogueira Teotônio[1,5], Fernanda Coutinho de Almeida[1,5], Gabriella Simões Heyn[2], Priscilla Souza Alves[2], Luiz Antônio Soares Romeiro[2,3], Riccardo Pratesi[1,5], Yanna Karla de Medeiros Nóbrega[2,4,5] and Claudia B. Pratesi[1,4*]

Abstract

Background: *Anacardium occidentale L* phenolic lipid (LDT11) is used in traditional medicine as anti-inflammatory, astringent, antidiarrheal, anti-asthmatic and depurative. Phenolic derivatives, such as anacardic acid, extracted from cashew nut shell liquid (CNSL) have demonstrated biological and pharmacological properties, and its profile makes it a candidate for the development of new anti-inflammatory agents.

The objective of the present study was to evaluate the anti-inflammatory profile of a derivative, synthesized from LDT11, on an in vitro cellular model.

Methods: Organic synthesis of the phenolic derivative of CNSL that results in the hemi-synthetic compound LDT11. The cytotoxicity of the planned compound, LDT11, was analyzed in murine macrophages cell line, RAW264.7. The cells were previously treated with LDT11, and then, the inflammation was stimulated with lipopolysaccharide (LPS), in intervals of 6 h and 24 h. The analysis of the gene expression of inflammatory markers (*TNFα, iNOS, COX-2, NF-κB, IL-1β* and *IL-6*), nitric oxide (NO) dosage, and cytokine IL-6 were realized.

Results: The results showed that the phenolic derivative, LDT11, influenced the modulatory gene expression. The relative gene transcripts quantification demonstrated that the LDT11 disclosed an immunoprotective effect against inflammation by decreasing genes expression when compared with cells stimulated with LPS in the control group. The NO and IL-6 dosages confirmed the results found in gene expression.

Discussion: The present study evaluated the immunoprotective effect of LDT11. In addition to a significant reduction in the expression of inflammatory genes, LDT11 also had a faster and superior anti-inflammatory action than the commercial products, and its response was already evident in the test carried out six hours after the treatment of the cells.

Conclusion: This study demonstrated LDT11 is potentially valuable as a rapid immunoprotective anti-inflammatory agent. Treatment with LDT11 decreased the gene expression of inflammatory markers, and the NO, and IL-6 production. When compared to commercial drugs, LDT11 showed a superior anti-inflammatory action.

Keywords: Fenolic lipid, Anacardic acid, Gene expression, Cashew nut shell liquid, CNSL, Anti-inflammatory activity

* Correspondence: cpprates@eckerd.edu
[1]Interdisciplinary Laboratory of Biosciences and Celiac Disease Research Center, School of Medicine, University of Brasilia, Asa Norte – CEP 70910900, Brasilia, DF, Brazil
[4]Post-graduate Program in Health Sciences, Faculty of Health Sciences, University of Brasilia, Brasilia, DF, Brazil
Full list of author information is available at the end of the article

Background

Cashew nut shells are considered a residue of the cashew nut processing by the agribusiness. However, for those in search of useful substances from renewable sources it has proven to be valuable bio-based material. The cashew nut shell contains a liquid (CNSL) that is a caustic, viscous oil comprising 25% of the fruit weight *in natura.* CNSL extracted by the cashew processing industry, which separates the almond and the oil, is one of the most abundant sources of non-isoprenoid phenolic lipid, such as anacardic acid, cardol, cardanol and methylcardol (Fig. 1) [1]. The CNSL components, in addition to an aromatic nucleus and several distinct functional groups, has an acyclic side chain containing multiple instabilities in the aliphatic chain, which results in an amphipathic behavior. From a synthetic point of view, CNSL properties characterize it as an extremely versatile material [2].

Nations in South America, Africa, and Asia have for decades use *Anacardium occidentale L.* phenolic lipid, extract from CNSL, in traditional medicine [3–5]. In folk medicine, CNSL is used as anti-inflammatory, astringent, antidiarrheal, anti-asthmatic, depurative and tonic medication. It is also used as diabetes medication [4, 6, 7] and wounds and wart treatment [8–10].

Past research has confirmed that phenolic and semi-synthetic derivatives of CNSL have biological properties [11], such as antibacterial, anti-inflammatory [12–14], and antioxidant activity [15]. Additionally, pharmacological properties included enzymatic inhibition [16, 17] and antiproliferative activity [16, 18]. A recent review by Hemshekhar et al. [19] reinforced anacardic acid multi-target pharmacological profile and its potentiality for the development of new anti-inflammatory drugs.

Inflammation is part of the complex biological response by body tissue to harmful stimuli, caused by infections, injuries or trauma. It is a complicated process regulated by several pro-inflammatory mediators, such as TNF-α, COX-2, iNOS, NF-kB, IL-1β, and IL-6 [20]. The rapid release of pro-inflammatory cytokines by activated macrophages plays a crucial role in triggering local immune response [21]. However, excessive production of inflammatory mediators may be more damaging than the event that triggered the immune response and may be associated with autoimmune diseases, diabetes, sepsis, diffuse intravascular coagulation, tissue injury, hypotension, and death [22]. The inhibition of these inflammatory mediators employing pharmacological modulators has been used as an effective therapeutic strategy to reduce inflammatory reactions [23].

Considering that biosynthetic molecules derived from CNSL have been tested in cellular models in vitro [24, 25], the present work proposes to evaluate the anti-inflammatory profile of *Anacardium occidentale L.* phenolic lipid (LDT11, Fig. 2), in the cellular model. Results of this analysis may offer alternative therapeutic strategies for the treatment of inflammation.

Methods

The production of inflammatory mediators was analyzed on RAW 264.7- TIB-71 murine macrophages cell culture (American Type Culture Collection - ATCC), previously treated with LDT11. Cells were purchased from the cell bank of the Adolf Lutz Institute (São Paulo, Brazil), and cultured according to the ATCC criteria.

Synthesis and characterization of LDT11 as a potential anti-inflammatory agent

LDT11 is a derivative designed from cashew nut shell liquid (CNSL) phenolic lipid. Compounds from library of the Laboratory of Development of Therapeutic Innovations (LDT), part of the University of Brasília (Brazil) were used in this research. LDT11 synthesis was performed as follows: to a solution of the mixture of anacardic acids (5 g, 14.5 mmol for average molecular wt 344) in ethanol (50.0 mL) was added 10% palladium-carbon (0.2 g) and shaken in a Parr apparatus (Parr Instrument Company©, Moline, IL, USA), under hydrogen atmosphere (4 atm, 60 psi) at room temperature. After six hours, the mixture was filtered and the solvent was evaporated under reduced pressure. The residue was recrystallized from hexane to afford a saturated anacardic acid (LDT11) as a white solid (4,55 g, 90%, mp 81 °C–83 °C, Rf 0.48 – Hex:AcOEt 4:1). IR (KBr) $\nu_{máx}$ cm^{-1}: 3326 (ν_{OH}); 2954 (ν_{asCH3}); 2920

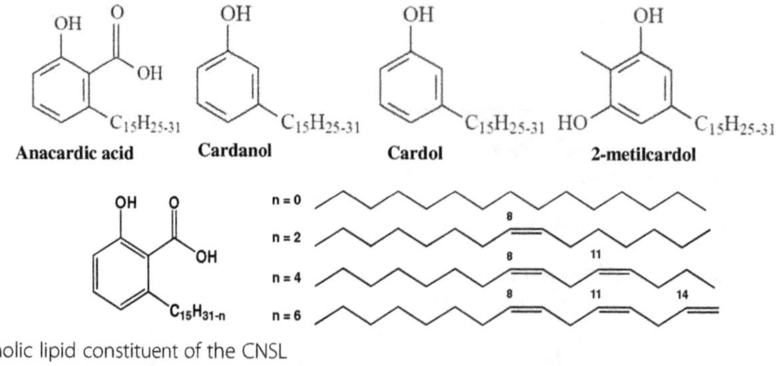

Fig. 1 Non-isoprenoid phenolic lipid constituent of the CNSL

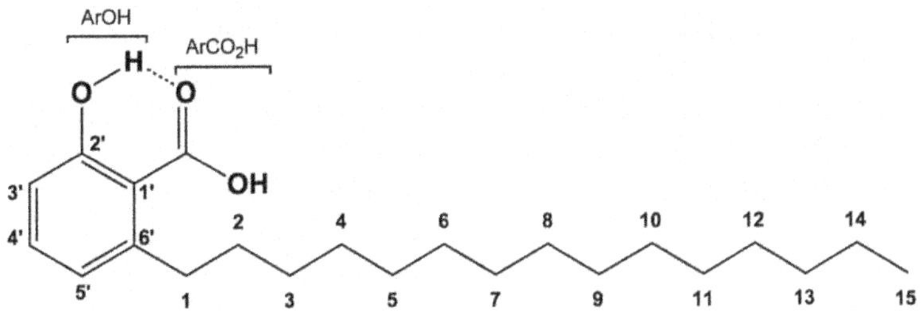

Fig. 2 Chemical structure of LDT11 molecule

(ν_{asCH2}); 2850 (ν_{sCH2}); 1610 ($\nu_{C=O}$); 1560, 1542, 1498 e 1466 ($\nu_{C=C}$); 1287(ν_{asC-O}); 1086 (ν_{sC-O}); ^1H NMR (300 MHz, $CDCl_3$): δ 0.89 (t, J = 6.5 Hz, 3H, 15); 1.26 (m, 24H, 3–14); 1.60 (qi, J = 6.6 Hz, 2H, 2); 3.00 (t, J = 7.7 Hz, 2H, 1); 6.79 (d, J = 7.4 Hz, 1H, 3′); 6.89 (d, J = 8.0 Hz, 1H, 5′); 7.37 (t, J = 7.9 Hz, 1H, 4′); 10.72 (s, ArOH); ^{13}C NMR (75 MHz, $CDCl_3$): δ 14.3 (CH_3, 15); 22.9 (CH_2, 14); 29.6–30.0 (CH_2, 3–12); 32.1 (CH_2, 13); 32.2 (CH_2, 2); 36.7 (CH_2, 1); 110.6 (C, 1′); 116.1 (CH, 3′); 123.0 (CH, 5′); 135.6 (CH, 4′); 148.1 (C, 6′); 163.8 (C, 2′); 176.5 ($Ar\underline{C}O_2H$).

The characterization of the molecule was carried out by the analysis of nuclear magnetic resonance (300 MHz Bruker Avance DRX NMR) of hydrogen and carbon-13, and by the infrared spectra (Spectrum BX, Perkin Elmer, Waltham, MA, USA). LDT11 was used for immunoprotective tests for inflammation in vitro. LDT11's biological activity was compared to two commercial drugs: acetylsalicylic acid (ASA) (Sedalive, Vitamedic, Brazil), which has a similar chemical structure to LDT11, and corticosteroid dexamethasone (DEX) (Decadron, Aché Laboratórios Farmacêuticos S.A, Brazil).

Quantitation of viable cell number - WST-8 assay

The cytotoxicity of the macrophages treated with synthetic phenolic derivatives was determined using the WST-8 assay (Cell Counting kit-8, Sigma-Aldrich, St. Louis, MO, USA). Cells were grown in complete Dulbecco's Modified Eagle's Medium (DMEM) at a concentration of 1×10^5 in 96-well plates and incubated at 37 °C in an atmosphere of 5% CO_2 for 48 h. The culture medium was subsequently exchanged for 100 μL of DMEM supplemented with 5% colorless fetal bovine serum (FBS), and 100 μL of LDT11 was added to the wells at concentrations of 25 μM, 50 μM, 75 μM, 100 μM, 125 μM, 150 μM, totaling a volume of 200 μL per well. After that, the plate was once more incubated under the previously described conditions.

The assay was performed using samples and controls in triplicate. After 48 h, the medium was discarded, and 100 μL of colorless DMEM, supplemented with 5% FBS was added, followed by the addition of 10 μL of WST-8 to each well. Non-stimulated cells were used as positive controls. Cell death control was performed using cells treated with 10 μL of 1% Triton-X. After an incubation of four hours with WST-8, the absorbance of the samples was measured in a TP-Reader microplate spectrophotometer (Thermoplate, Palm City, FL, USA) using a 450 nm wavelength filter.

Neutral red uptake assay

The Neutral red uptake assay was performed following the protocol described by Tanner et al. [26], with some modifications. The assay was carried out under the same conditions as the WST-8 assay. After 48 h of incubation with the LDT11, the medium was discarded, the cells were washed twice with phosphate buffered saline solution (1X PBS, pH 7.4), and 100 μl of DMEM supplemented, and 50 μg/mL of neutral red was added to the wells. The plate was incubated under the conditions described in the item 2.2. The medium was then discarded, and the cells were washed five times with 1X PBS to remove the excess of dye; which was followed by the addition of 100 μl of alcohol-acid solution (50% ethanol, 1% acetic acid and 49% distilled water) to each well to fix the neutral red to the cells. The plate was shaken for 10 min, and the absorbance of the samples was read in a TP-Reader microplate spectrophotometer (Thermoplate, Palm City, FL, USA) with a 492 nm filter. The results were expressed as a percentage, the value obtained for the positive control (untreated cells), being considered as 100% viability. The equation used was: viability (%) = (number of viable cells / total number of untreated cells) × 100.

Analysis of gene expression

To evaluate the influence of LDT11 on RAW 264.7 gene expression, after stimulation with LPS, quantitative real-time polymerase chain reaction (qPCR) was performed. The RNA from cells was extracted, purified and quantified, and the resulting complementary DNA was prepared for the qPCR reaction, as follow: RAW 264.7 cells were cultured in six well plates at a concentration of 5×10^6 cells/well, each containing 3 mL 10% complete DMEM medium. The plates were incubated (approximately 24 h) until an estimated confluence of 90% was obtained. The medium was discarded, and 3 mL of colorless DMEM medium without FBS supplementation was added in order restrain the cells growth rate. The immune-protective properties of LDT11 were analyzed in: (a) untreated cells (NT); (b) cells stimulated exclusively with LPS; (c) cells treated with LDT11, and subsequently exposed to LPS; (d) cells treated with ASA, and then exposed to LPS; (e) cells treated with DEX, and exposed to LPS.

Extraction, purification, quantification of RNA and cDNA synthesis

For the extraction and purification of RNA, Direct-zol ™ RNA Miniprep Kit (R2051, Zymo Research, Orange, CA, USA), was used following the manufacturer's recommendations. The quantification of extracted RNA was determined by using the NanoDrop 2000 spectrophotometer (Thermo Fisher Scientific, Waltham, MA, USA). The cDNA synthesis was performed using High-Capacity cDNA Reverse Transcription Kit (Applied Biosystems, Waltham, MA, USA), according to manufacturer's instructions.

Gene analysis and characterization

Genes involved in the inflammatory response were selected to test the biological activity of LDT11. Seven primers synthesized by Integrated DNA Technologies (Skokie, IL, USA) were used, as described in Table 1. The design of the primer pairs was performed using the Primer Express Program (Applied Biosystems, Waltham, MA, USA) based on sequences obtained from the Mouse Transcriptome Database (http://www.informatics.jax.org).

Quantitative real-time polymerase chain reaction

The Quantitative Real-Time Polymerase Chain Reaction (qPCR) was performed in triplicates, using SYBR Green system (Absolute qPCR SYBR Green Rox Mix - Thermo Fisher Scientific Inc., Vilnius, Lithuania, USA) in a solution containing 50 ng of cDNA, 5 pmol of each primer forward and reverse and QSP of ultrapure water, totalizing 20 μL. Amplification assays were performed on a StepOnePlus Real-Time PCR System (Applied Biosystems, Carlsbad, CA, USA) under the following conditions: initial denaturation temperature at 95 °C for 10 min, 40 cycles of denaturation at 95 °C for 15 s, annealing and extension at 60 °C for 1 min and 72 °C for 30 s. All reactions were performed three times for each gene, and *GAPDH* gene was used both as endogenous control and normalizing gene. Water was used as negative control substituting cDNA.

The result, expressed in CT value, refers to the number of cycles in qPCR required for the fluorescent signal to reach the threshold detection. The analysis of the gene expression of the inflammatory markers was obtained by the relative quantification of their transcripts by the Delta-Delta Ct (ΔΔCt) method, which allows a relative comparison with the group that did not receive treatment (NT) and cells stimulated with LPS. The melting curve was used as quality control of amplification products.

For the data analysis, the values found for the control group, LPS- stimulated cells, were considered 100% inflamed. The other tests, with their respective treatments (LDT11, ASA and DEX) were analyzed comparing with the inflamed group.

Nitric oxide quantification

For the analysis of Nitric Oxide (NO), was used the Griess method, by adding 100 μL of Griess reagent (1% [*w*/*v*] sulfanilamide, in a 5% phosphoric acid, and 0.1% [w / v] N-1- naphthyl-ethylenediamide dihydrochloride (NEED) in water). Samples of culture supernatants were analyzed by microplate reader (TP-Reader microplate spectrophotometer, Thermoplate, Palm City, FL, USA), using the spectrum 450 nm, and the results expressed in

Table 1 RAW 264.7 macrophages genes analyzed in the study. Primers Description Sequences Mt.*

Primers	Description	Sequences	Mt*
GAPDH	Glyceraldehyde-3-phosphate dehydrogenase	5'-CCGGTGCTGAGTATGTCG-3' 5'-CCCTGTTGCTGTAGCCGTA-3'	85,72
COX-2	Cyclooxygenase 2	5'-TGAGTACCGCAAACGCTTCTC-3' 5'-TGGACGAGGTTTTTCCACCAG-3'	80,35
IL-1β	Interleukin 1 beta	5'-TGAAATGCCACCTTTTGACAG-3' 5'-CCACAGCCACAATGAGTGATA-3'	54,80
IL-6	Interleukin 6	5'-GCTACCAAACTGGATATAATCAGGA-3' 5'-CAGGTAGCTATGGTACTCCAGAA-3'	73,48
iNOS	Induced nitric oxide synthase	5'-GGCAGCCTGTGAGACCTTTG-3' 5'-GCATTGGAAGTGAAGCGTTTC-3'	77,81
NF-κB	Nuclear Factor kappa b	5'-AGCCAGCTTCCGTGTTTGTT-3' 5'-AGGGTTTCGGTTCACTAGTTTCC-3'	77,81
TNF-α	Tumor necrosis factor alpha	5'-TCTTCTCATTCCTGCTTGTGG-3' 5'-GGTCTGGGCCATAGAACTGA-3'	81,70

**Mt* Melting temperature (°C)

μmol/L of NO - comparing the optical density (OD) obtained with a standard curve of NO - ranging from 1.56 μM to 100.0 μM.

IL-6 quantification

The quantification of Interleukin-6 (IL-6) was performed by applying the competitive immunoenzymatic assay, as established in the manufacturer's kit (#27768 Mouse IL-6 Kit – Immuno-Biological Laboratories Co., Ltda, Hamburg, Germany). The same treatment used in the gene expression assessment was applied in this assay, using the supernatants of RAW 264.7 cells treated with the synthetic phenolic derivative LDT11 at 50 μM concentration.

Statistical analysis

Statistical analysis was performed using the Analysis of Variance (ANOVA) test, followed by Post-Hoc tests (Bonferoni, Dunnett and t-test) when applicable, according to GraphPad Prism version 4.0 (GraphPad Software, San Diego, USA). Statistically significant differences were considered when $p < 0.05$.

Results

Cytotoxicity analysis and quantitation of viable cell number

The determination of the cytotoxic effect of LDT11 by the WST-8 and Neutral Red methods was performed using the following concentrations: 25 μM, 50 μM, 75 μM, 100 μM, 125 μM, and 150 μM.

WST-8 assay

LDT11 showed approximately 100% cell viability in a concentration of 25 μM. The cell viability declined to 90% with a LDT11 concentration of 50 μM. Concentrations equal or over 75 μM ensued a cell viability equal or lower than 60% and were considered cytotoxic (Fig. 3).

Neutral red uptake assay

Neutral Red Uptake Assay was performed to confirm the cell viability obtained by the WST-8 assay on the RAW264.7 cell line, using similar LDT11 concentrations. The assay showed results similar to those found by the WST-8 method (Fig. 4).

From the results of the cell viability assays, toxic concentrations of LDT11 were excluded from the study. The standardized concentration for the other tests was 50 μM. For further comparison, the following assays with ASA and DEX were also made using the same concentration established for LDT11, 50 μM.

Modulation and relative quantification of transcripts of inflammatory genes

Gene modulation of the inflammatory process was analyzed after interaction with the CNSL derivative, LDT11. Gene expression was evaluated by the relative quantification of *TNF-α, COX-2, iNOS, NF-kB, IL-1β* and *IL-6* genes in RAW264.7 cells. Inflammation was induced with 1 μg/mL LPS, both in control cells and in LDT11 treated cells. The analysis of the results was carried out 6 and 24 h post- treatment.

As seen in Fig. 5, the gene expression of *TNF-α*, six hours after interaction with LDT11, showed an eight-fold decrease (88%) in comparison with the gene expression disclosed by the control cells (LPS). The results obtained from the interaction with ASA and dexamethasone (DEX) were respectively one and a half times lower (33%) for ASA and two times lower (50%) for DEX (Fig. 5a). The results obtained 24 h after treatment were similar with those obtained after six hours. Both had a decrease in gene expression in all treatments analyzed. Cells treated with LDT11 disclosed 10 times (91%) less gene expression than the positive control, while cells treated with ASA and DEX respectively showed a gene expression two and three times lower (55 and 64%) than control cells, Fig. 5b.

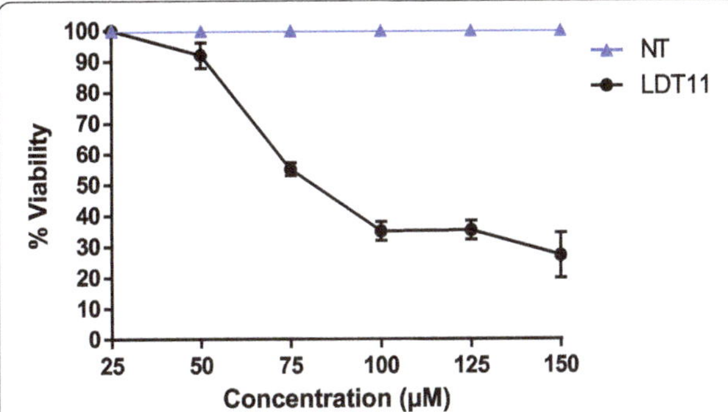

Fig. 3 Cell viability by the WST-8 method in RAW264.7 cell line, using different concentrations of the phenolic acid derivative LDT11. NT - untreated cells. LDT11 - cells treated with LDT11 and then with LPS

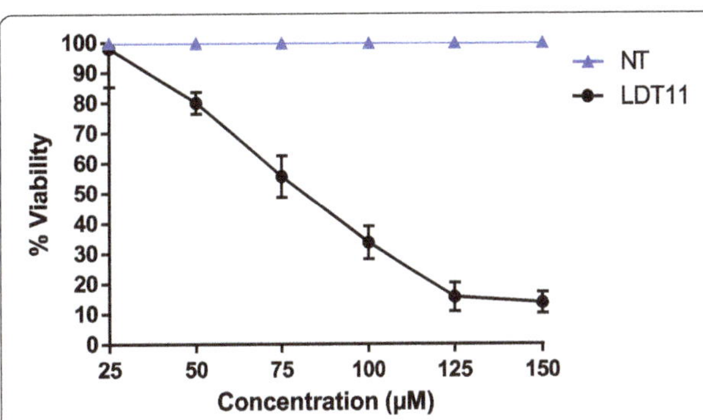

Fig. 4 Cell viability test by the Neutral Red Uptake Assay in RAW264.7 cell line, using different concentrations of the phenolic derivative, LDT11. NT - untreated cells. LDT11 - cells treated with LDT11 and then with LPS

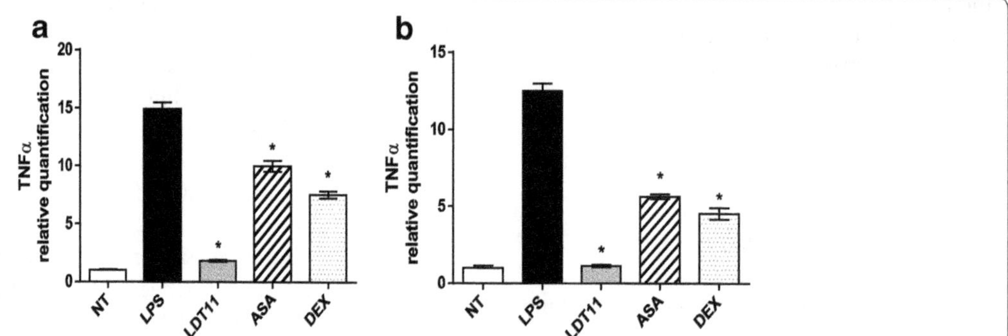

Fig. 5 Determination of the relative amount of *TNF-α* gene transcripts in RAW 264.7 cell line for the evaluation of inflammatory response at 6 (**a**) and 24 h (**b**) post-stimulus. NT- untreated cells; LPS - LPS-stimulated cells; LDT11 - cells treated with LDT11 and then with LPS; AAS - cells treated with commercial acetylsalicylic acid and then with LPS; DEX - cells treated with the commercial anti-inflammatory Dexamethasone and then with LPS. All data are from at least three independent experiments, *$p < 0.05$, statistically different compared with cells LPS-stimulated

COX-2 was the second gene analyzed (Fig. 6). After six hours of treatment with LDT11, *COX-2* gene expression decreased more than five-fold (81%) when compared to control cells (Fig. 6a). Cells treated with ASA did not show a significant difference, and those treated with DEX showed a four-fold decrease (74%) in gene expression when compared to control cells. After 24 h of interaction with LTD11 (Fig. 6b), the gene expression disclosed a six-fold decrease (84%) in treated cells than in control cells. The reduction in gene expression caused by both ASA and DEX was approximately 2-fold higher (30%) than that observed in control cells.

After six hours of LTD11 treatment, the expression of the *iNOS* gene, (Fig. 7) showed a 200 times decrease (100%) comparing with control cells. Treatment with ASA resulted 20-fold (99%) decreased expression, while cells treated with DEX showed a 60-fold (98%) gene suppression (Fig. 7a). After 24 h (Fig. 7b), both LDT11 and DEX treated cells showed approximately a 2-fold decreased gene expression (50%) while a threefold decrease (68%) was observed in ASA-treated cells.

The action of LTD11 on the *NF-kB* gene expression can be seen in Fig. 8. In comparison with control group, cells treated with LTD11 resulted an eight-fold (88%) decrease in *NF-kB* gene expression. The treatment of the cells with ASA and DEX produced respectively a decrease in gene expression equivalent to 1.5-fold (33%) for the first and two-fold (50%) for the second drug (Fig. 8a). In the treatment performed after 24 h (Fig. 8b), both LDT11 and ASA treated cells showed a decrease of about two-fold (55%) in the *NF-kB* gene expression. On the other hand, cells treated with DEX failed to show any significant difference when compared to the control cells.

The *IL-1β* gene also showed decreased expression in most of the assays (Fig. 9). After a six-hour interaction with LDT11, *IL-1β* gene expression decreased more than 14-fold (93%). Treatment with ASA did not cause a significant decrease in its expression whereas DEX led to a three-fold reduction (69%) when compared to control cells (Fig. 9a). After 24 h (Fig. 9b), when compared with control cells, those treated with LDT11 showed an approximately six-fold decrease (83%) in gene expression, whereas ASA and DEX caused respectively a two-fold (39%) and five-fold (75%) decline.

After six hours of treatment with LDT11 there was a 65-fold (98%) decrease in the gene expression of *IL-6*, in

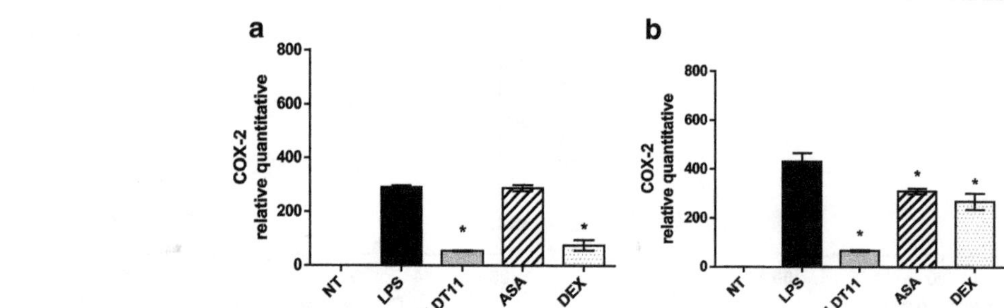

Fig. 6 Determination of the relative amount of *COX-2* gene transcripts in RAW 264.7 cell line for the evaluation of inflammatory response at 6 (**a**) and 24 h (**b**) post-stimulus. NT- untreated cells; LPS - LPS-stimulated cells; LDT11 - cells treated with LDT11 and then with LPS; AAS - cells treated with commercial acetylsalicylic acid and then with LPS; DEX - cells treated with the commercial anti-inflammatory Dexamethasone and then with LPS. All data are from at least three independent experiments, *$p < 0.05$, statistically different compared with cells LPS-stimulated

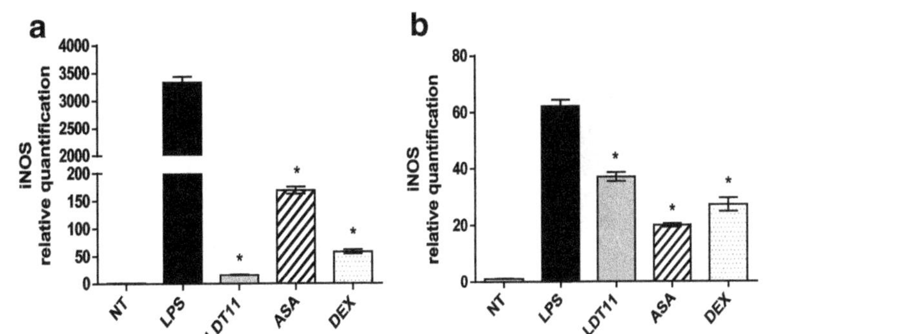

Fig. 7 Determination of the relative amount of *iNOS* gene transcripts in RAW 264.7 cell line for the evaluation of inflammatory response at 6 (**a**) and 24 h (**b**) post-stimulus. NT- untreated cells; LPS - LPS-stimulated cells; LDT11 - cells treated with LDT11 and then with LPS; AAS - cells treated with commercial acetylsalicylic acid and then with LPS; DEX - cells treated with the commercial anti-inflammatory Dexamethasone and then with LPS. All data are from at least three independent experiments, $*p < 0.05$, statistically different compared with cells LPS-stimulated

comparison with the control cells. Gene expression of *IL-6* decreased respectively 8-fold (88%) in ASA-treated cells and 27-fold (96%) in DEX-treated cells (Fig. 10a). After 24 h (Fig. 10b) the gene expression decreased 5-fold (79%) in the cells treated with LDT11 while the decrease was respectively two-fold (45%) in the cells treated with ASA and three-fold (65%) in the cells treated with DEX.

Assessment of nitric oxide and cytosine IL-6

Nitric oxide, resulting from the presence of oxygen and nitrogen reactive metabolites produced during the inflammatory process, causes an increase in the oxidative stress of the cells. The presence of NO in the supernatant of RAW 264.7 cells was measured to confirm the influence of LDT11 on anti-inflammatory activity. The following assays were performed with the same timing (six and 24 h) of the previous analysis. The LDT11 was able to protect RAW264.7 cells against oxidative stress by reducing NO production by about eight times (95%) after six hours, and about 15 times (100%) after 24 h (Fig. 11).

Additionally, to confirm the results obtained in the analysis of gene expression, the cytosine *IL-6* was also assayed. The pre-treatment of the cells with LTD11 resulted in a significant protective effect against inflammation, reducing *IL-6* production by more than 1700-fold (76%) after six hours (Fig. 12a) and more than 1400-fold (60%) after 24 h (Fig. 12b). Cells treated with ASA reduced *IL-6* production respectively by more than 120-fold (52%), after six hours and by more than 400 (17%) after 24 h. Treatment with DEX reduced the *IL-6* production at about 1000-fold (42%) after six hours and at about 1400-fold (60%) after 24 h.

Discussion

The present study evaluated the immunoprotective effect of LDT11; a compound synthesized from the anacardic acid extracted from the CNSL. This evaluation was performed through the quantification of gene transcripts involved in the inflammatory response, and the measurement of NO and IL-6 production in RAW 264.7 murine macrophages. The murine macrophages culture was firstly treated with LDT11 and posteriorly stimulated with LPS that mimicked the inflammatory response and induced high production cytosine and oxidative stress [27–29]. Overproduction of pro-inflammatory mediators such as TNF-α, COX-2, iNOS, NF-κB, IL-1β and NO has been implicated in several

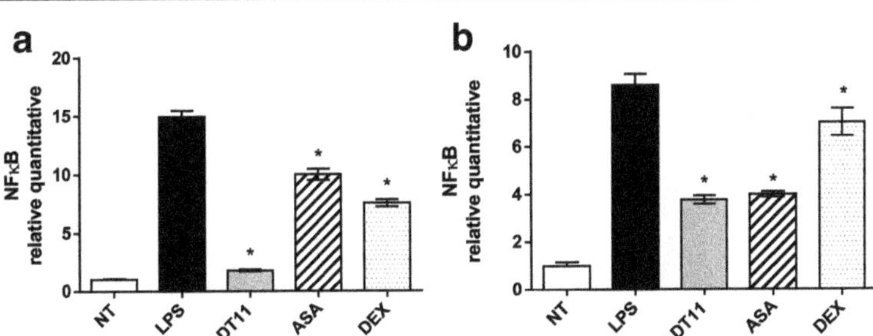

Fig. 8 Determination of the relative amount of *NF-kB* gene transcripts in RAW 264.7 cell line for the evaluation of inflammatory response at 6 (**a**) and 24 h (**b**) post-stimulus. NT- untreated cells; LPS - LPS-stimulated cells; LDT11 - cells treated with LDT11 and then with LPS; AAS - cells treated with commercial acetylsalicylic acid and then with LPS; DEX - cells treated with the commercial anti-inflammatory Dexamethasone and then with LPS. All data are from at least three independent experiments, $*p < 0.05$, statistically different compared with cells LPS-stimulated

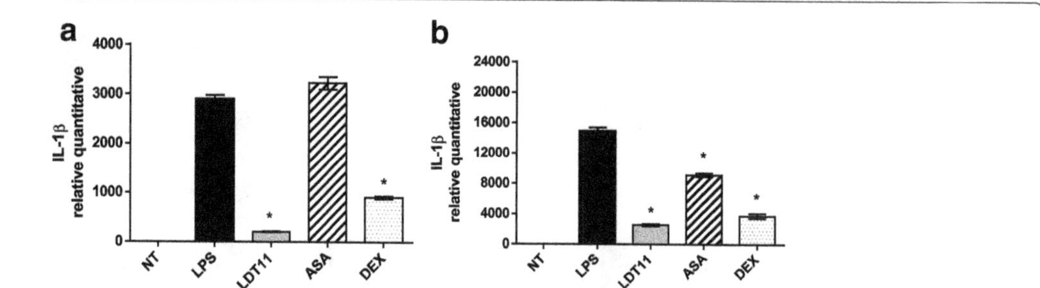

Fig. 9 Determination of the relative amount of *IL-1β* gene transcripts in RAW 264.7 cell line for the evaluation of inflammatory response at 6 (**a**) and 24 h (**b**) post-stimulus. NT- untreated cells; LPS - LPS-stimulated cells; LDT11 - cells treated with LDT11 and then with LPS; AAS - cells treated with commercial acetylsalicylic acid and then with LPS; DEX - cells treated with the commercial anti-inflammatory Dexamethasone and then with LPS. All data are from at least three independente experiments, *$p < 0.05$, statistically different compared with cells LPS-stimulated

inflammatory diseases [27, 29, 30]. Therefore, an agent that prevents the release of these mediators or downregulates the expression of these cytokines may be an valuable therapeutic strategy for preventing inflammatory reaction [27, 28], turning LDT11 a potential candidate for the formulation of new drugs.

In this study, two different colorimetric methods, the WST-8 assay, and the neutral red uptake test, were performed to evaluate if the LDT11 used in the experiments would show some degree of cytotoxicity. The analysis of its in vitro cytotoxicity allowed the determination of the concentrations needed to obtain the best performance of its biological activity without compromising the cellular viability. Viability and cytotoxicity results were similar for both tests at all concentrations used (25 μM, 50 μM, 75 μM, 100 μM, 125 μM, and 150 μM). At concentrations of 25 μM and 50 μM, cell viability was greater than 80%. However, the increase of the concentrations to 75 μM, 100 μM, 125 μM and 150 μM caused more than 60% decrease in cell viability, being consequently considered cytotoxic. Others studies found that the assay shows cytotoxic activity when cell death exceeds 50% [18, 31]. In the present research values above 60% were considered citotoxic. Therefore, the concentration chosen to continue the experiments of gene expression analysis was 50 μM of LDT11.

The *TNF-α* gene has the main physiological effect of promoting the inflammatory immune response through the recruitment and activation of neutrophils and monocytes. Consequently, TNF-α is responsible for a several effects on the body, promoting vasodilation and acting on endothelial cells, stimulating the secretion of a group of cytokines that have chemotactic action on leukocytes. TNF-α is also the cytokine responsible for septic shock, in addition to inhibiting the appetite and inducing fever through the release of the adrenocorticotrophic hormone (ACTH) [30, 32]. Additionally, it is also a major inducer of the transcription factor NF-κB, and degrades the inhibitor of NF-κB (IκB). Degradation of IκB allows NF-κB to be translocated to the nucleus. [21, 33]. Pretreatment with LDT11 showed suppression of the *TNF-α* gene in LPS-stimulated cells greater than the suppression observed in cells treated with commercial anti-inflammatory drugs. Consequently, a similar suppression was observed in *NF-κB* and *TNF-α*, being greater in LDT11-treated cells than in the cells treated with commercial drugs.

NF-κB is responsible for the transcription of innumerable genes related to pro-inflammatory activity, such as *IL-1, IL-6, iNOS, COX-2* [34–36]. Consequently, a decrease in the gene expression of these inflammatory mediators was also observed. Compared with LPS-stimulated cells, the

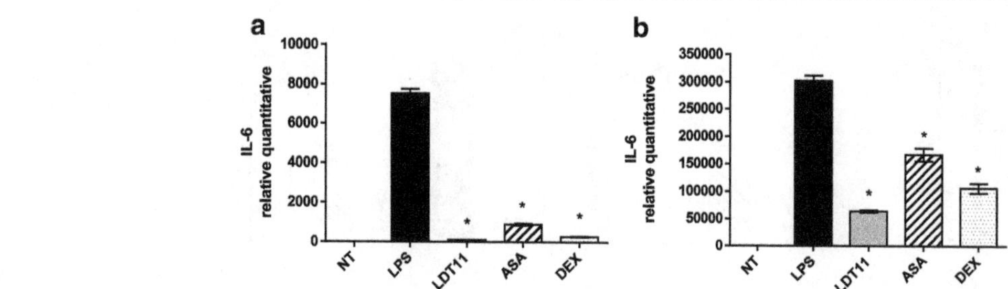

Fig. 10 Determination of the relative amount of *IL-6* gene transcripts in RAW 264.7 cell line for the evaluation of inflammatory response at 6 (**a**) and 24 h (**b**) post-stimulus. NT- untreated cells; LPS - LPS-stimulated cells; LDT11 - cells treated with LDT11 and then with LPS; AAS - cells treated with commercial acetylsalicylic acid and then with LPS; DEX - cells treated with the commercial anti-inflammatory Dexamethasone and then with LPS. All data are from at least three independente experiments, *$p < 0.05$, statistically different compared with cells LPS-stimulated

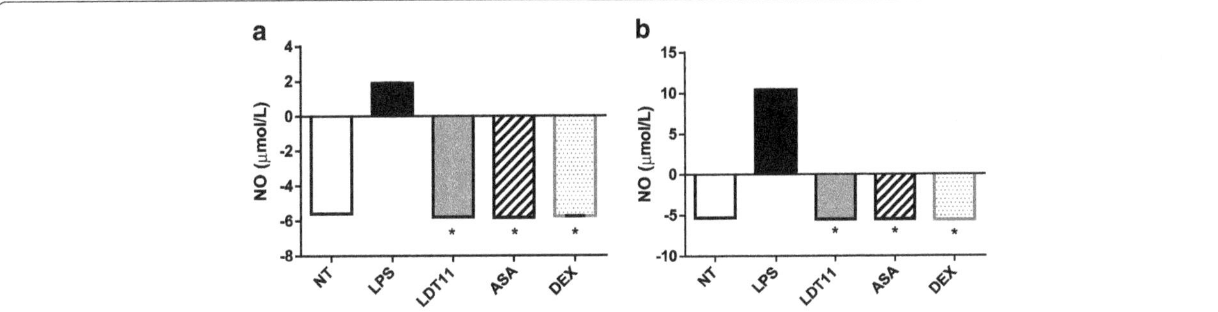

Fig. 11 Evaluation of the potential immunoprotective effect of the CNSL derivatives by measuring the levels of nitric oxide production in the supernatant at 6 h (**a**) and 24 h (**b**) post-stimulus. NT- untreated cells; LPS - LPS-stimulated cells; LDT11 - cells treated with LDT11 and then with LPS; AAS - cells treated with commercial acetylsalicylic acid and then with LPS; DEX - cells treated with the commercial anti-inflammatory Dexamethasone and then with LPS. All data are from at least three independente experiments, *$p < 0.05$, statistically different compared with cells LPS-stimulated

COX-2 and *IL-1β* genes showed more than 80% gene suppression after treatment with LDT11. The suppression of *iNOS* and *IL-6* genes was practically total in LDT11 pre-treated cells.

The evaluation of the treatment after 24 h showed that the relative amount of *iNOS* decreased in all the tests performed, including in the LPS treated cells. Consequently, the gene suppression was less expressive than that observed in experiments conducted after six hours. Gene expression of *iNOS* after 24 h was the only outcome in which treatment with LDT11 was inferior to the results obtained with the commercial drugs. Although, treatment with LDT11 was also capable of reducing the *iNOS* gene expression when compared to LPS treated cells.

Nitric oxide (NO), an important molecule produced in the process of oxidative stress, is synthesized by the enzyme nitric oxide synthetase, that is a product of the *iNOS* gene. It acts as a biological mediator similar to neurotransmitters and can regulate the tonus of blood vessels. On the other hand, it is an oxygen free radical that can function as a cytotoxic agent in pathological processes, especially in inflammatory diseases [37–39].

Interleukin-6 (IL-6) is one of the leading mediators of the acute phase of inflammation, with a crucial activity on eosinophil chemotaxis to the inflammation site, and has a vital role on coagulation [20, 40]. IL-6 is known as a multifunctional cytokine, which in addition to its pro-inflammatory and sclerosing functions, also affects the activity of neoplastic cells [30, 41]. In addition to its critical local effects, this cytokine has systemic activity, which contributes to the defense of the organism. One of these effects is the elevation of body temperature, causing fever from an endogenous source [21].

Therefore, NO and IL-6 were measured to confirm the results found with the analysis of the transcripts obtained by qPCR. The assays were performed using the supernatants of cell cultures submitted to the treatment already described on 2.4 item. The potential immune-protective activity of LDT11 was evidenced by the results obtained, both at 6 LPS treated and at 24 h post-treatment, which

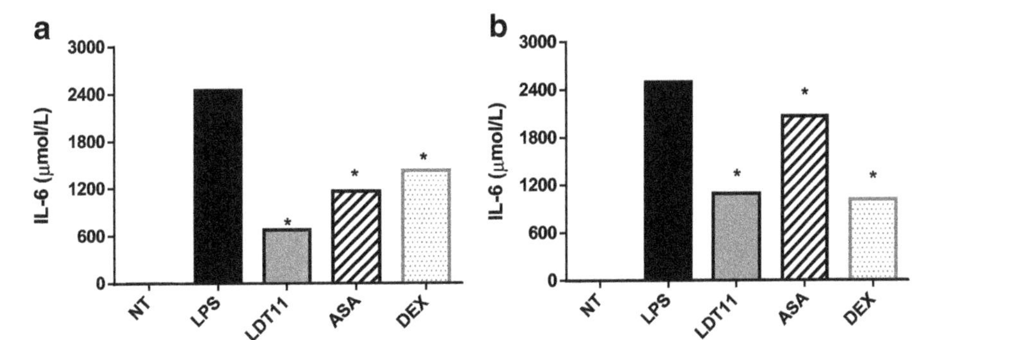

Fig. 12 Evaluation of the potential immunoprotective effect of the CNSL derivatives by measuring the levels of cytosine *IL-6* production in the supernatant at 6 h (**a**) and 24 h (**b**) post-stimulus. NT- untreated cells; LPS - LPS-stimulated cells; LDT11 - cells treated with LDT11 and then with LPS; AAS - cells treated with commercial acetylsalicylic acid and then with LPS; DEX - cells treated with the commercial anti-inflammatory Dexamethasone and then with LPS. All data are from at least three independent experiments, *$p < 0.05$, statistically different compared with cells LPS-stimulated

demonstrated a significant reduction in the production of NO and IL-6 when compared to LPS treated cells.

The evaluation of expression of the genes *TNF-α, COX-2, iNOS, NF-κB, IL-1β* and *IL-6* at 6 and 24 h after treatment of the cells with LDT11, makes evident that the LDT11 was most effective in protecting against the inflammation when compared with results obtained with the use of commercial drugs.

In addition to a significant reduction in the expression of inflammatory genes, LDT11 also had a faster and superior anti-inflammatory action than the commercial products, and its response was already evident in the test carried out six hours after the treatment of the cells, suggesting that this molecule can be used as an anti-inflammatory drug.

Conclusion

LDT11, a phenolic derivative of CNSL, showed potential immunoprotective and anti-inflammatory properties, having a rapid and effective activity. Treatment with LDT11 decreased the expression of the *TNF-α, COX-2, iNOS, NF-κB, IL-1β* and *IL-6* inflammatory genes. Additionally, LDT11 protective effect on inflammation was confirmed by the decreased of NO and IL-6 production. The anti-inflammatory activity of LDT11 was superior to commercial drugs, ASA and DEX.

Abbreviations

ANOVA: Analysis of variance; ASA: acid acetylsalicilic; ATCC: American Type Culture Collection; cDNA: complementary DNA sequence; CNSL: cashew nut shell liquid; CO_2: Carbon dioxide; COX-2: cyclooxygenase isoform 2; CT: Crossing threshold; DEX: Dexamethasone; DMEM: Dulbecco's Modified Eagle Medium; DMSO: Dimethyl Suffoxide; DNA: Deoxyribonucleic acid; DNAse: Deoxyribonuclease; dNTP: Deoxynucleotides 5'-triphosphate; ELISA: Enzyme Linked Immuno Sorbent Assay; FC: Fold-change; GAPDH: Glyceraldehyde-3-phosphate dehydrogenase; IL-1β: Interleukin-1β; IL-6: Interleukin-6; iNOS: Nitric oxide synthase induced; LDT11: semisynthetic molecule 11 - of the Laboratory of Development of Therapeutic Strategies; LDT13: semisynthetic molecule 13 - of the Laboratory of Development of Therapeutic Strategies; LPS: Lipopolysaccharide; NEED: N- (1-Naphthyl) ethyl-enedinamine; NF-κB: Nuclear transcription factor κB; NO: Nitric oxide; OD.: Optical Density; p: statistical significance; PBS: Phosphate buffered saline; pH: Hydrogen ionic potential; PMN: Polymorphonuclear; RNA: Ribonucleic acid; RNAse: Ribonuclease; RT: Reverse Transcription; SBF: Fetal bovine sérum; SYBR Green or SyBrgreen: Fluorescent dye that attaches to DNA tape; Tm: Melting temperature or dissociation temperature; TNF-α: Tumor Necrosis Factor alpha (α); WST-8: 5-(2,4-disulfophenyl)-3-(2-methoxy-4-nitrophenyl)-2-(4-nitrophenyl)-2H-tetrazolium, inner salt, monosodium salt

Funding

I gratefully acknowledge the funding received towards my Ph.D. from CAPES, Coordination for the Improvement of Higher Education Personnel.

Authors' contributions

MQS: responsible for the gene expression tests and NO and IL-6 dosages. IMSNT: accountable for the primers efficiency tests used in the study for evaluation of gene expression. FCA: Responsible for cell culture and cytotoxicity testing. RP: Advisor responsible concept for the project. GSH: Responsible for the purification and organic modification for the synthesis of LDT11. LASR: Coordinator of the Laboratory of Therapeutic Strategies Development, where LDT11 was obtained for this research. YKMN: Coordinated the project, responsible analysis of gene expression data. CBP: Assisted in the conceptualization of the study, revised the protocol, corresponding author. All authors read and approved the final version of the manuscript.

Competing interests

The authors have declared that there are no conflict of interest or competing interests to declare.

Author details

[1]Interdisciplinary Laboratory of Biosciences and Celiac Disease Research Center, School of Medicine, University of Brasilia, Asa Norte – CEP 70910900, Brasilia, DF, Brazil. [2]Department of Pharmacy, Faculty of Health Sciences, University of Brasilia, Brasilia, DF, Brazil. [3]Post-graduate Program in Pharmaceutical Sciences, Faculty of Health Sciences, University of Brasilia, Brasilia, DF, Brazil. [4]Post-graduate Program in Health Sciences, Faculty of Health Sciences, University of Brasilia, Brasilia, DF, Brazil. [5]Post-graduate Program in Medical Sciences, School of Medicine, University of Brasilia, Brasilia, DF, Brazil.

References

1. Mazzetto SE, Lomonaco D, Mele G. Cashew nut oil: opportunities and challenges in the context of sustainable industrial development. Quim Nova. 2009;32:732–41.
2. Hamad F, Mubofu E. Potential biological applications of bio-based Anacardic acids and their derivatives. Int J Mol Sci. 2015;16:8569–90.
3. Ayyanar M, Ignacimuthu S. Herbal medicines for wound healing among tribal people in southern India: ethnobotanical and scientific evidences. Int J Appl Res Nat Prod. 2009;2:29–42.
4. da Silva DPB, Florentino IF, da Silva Moreira LK, Brito AF, Carvalho W, Vasconcelos GA, et al. Chemical characterization and pharmacological assessment of cashew gum extract (*Anacardium occidentale* L .), polysaccharide free. J Ethnopharmacol [Internet]. 2017 [cited 2017 Nov 29]; Available from: http://linkinghub.elsevier.com/retrieve/pii/S0378874117327034
5. Kudi AC, Umoh JU, Eduvie LO, Gefu J. Screening of some Nigerian medicinal plants for antibacterial activity. J Ethnopharmacol. 1999;67:225–8.
6. Debrito E, Pessanhadearaujo M, Lin L, Harnly J. Determination of the flavonoid components of cashew apple (Anacardium occidentale) by LC-DAD-ESI/MS. Food Chem. 2007;105:1112–8.
7. Tédong L, Dzeufiet PDD, Dimo T, Asongalem EA, Sokeng SD, Flejou J-F, et al. Acute and subchronic toxicity of Anacardium occidentale Linn (Anacardiaceae) leaves hexane extract in mice. Afr J Tradit Complement Altern Med. 2007;4:140–7.
8. Mbatchou VC, Kosoono I. Aphrodisiac activity of oils from Anacardium occidentale L seeds and seed shells. Phytopharmacology. 2012;2:81–9.
9. Santos ABN, AraúJo MP, Sousa RS, Lemos JR. Plantas medicinais conhecidas na zona urbana de Cajueiro da Praia, Piauí, Nordeste do Brasil. Rev Bras Plantas Med. 2016;18:442–50.
10. Schirato GV, Monteiro FMF, de Oliveira Silva F, de Lima Filho JL, Leão AM dos AC, Porto ALF. O polissacarídeo do Anacardium occidentale L. na fase inflamatória do processo cicatricial de lesões cutâneas. Ciênc Rural. 2006;36:149–54.
11. Stasiuk M, Kozubek A. Biological activity of phenolic lipid. Cell Mol Life Sci. 2010;67:841–60.
12. Green IR, Tocoli FE, Lee SH, Nihei K, Kubo I. Molecular design of anti-MRSA agents based on the anacardic acid scaffold. Bioorg Med Chem. 2007;15:6236–41.
13. Green IR, Tocoli FE, Lee SH, Nihei K, Kubo I. Design and evaluation of anacardic acid derivatives as anticavity agents. Eur J Med Chem. 2008;43:1315–20.
14. Sung B, Pandey MK, Ahn KS, Yi T, Chaturvedi MM, Liu M, et al. Anacardic acid (6-nonadecyl salicylic acid), an inhibitor of histone acetyltransferase, suppresses expression of nuclear factor- B-regulated gene products involved in cell survival, proliferation, invasion, and inflammation through inhibition of the inhibitory subunit of nuclear factor- B kinase, leading to potentiation of apoptosis. Blood. 2008;111:4880–91.

15. Trevisan MTS, Pfundstein B, Haubner R, Würtele G, Spiegelhalder B, Bartsch H, et al. Characterization of alkyl phenols in cashew (Anacardium occidentale) products and assay of their antioxidant capacity. Food Chem Toxicol. 2006;44:188–97.
16. Paramashivappa R, Phani Kumar P, Subba Rao PV, Srinivasa Rao A. Synthesis of sildenafil analogues from Anacardic acid and their Phosphodiesterase-5 inhibition. J Agric Food Chem. 2002;50:7709–13.
17. Stasiuk M, Bartosiewicz D, Kozubek A. Inhibitory effect of some natural and semisynthetic phenolic lipid upon acetylcholinesterase activity. Food Chem. 2008;108:996–1001.
18. Chandregowda V, Kush A, Reddy GC. Synthesis of benzamide derivatives of anacardic acid and their cytotoxic activity. Eur J Med Chem. 2009;44:2711–9.
19. Hemshekhar M, Sebastin Santhosh M, Kemparaju K, Girish KS. Emerging Roles of Anacardic acid and ITS derivatives: a PHARMACOLOGICAL overview: PHARMACOLOGICAL ROLES OF AA AND ITS DERIVATIVES. Basic Clin Pharmacol Toxicol. 2012;110:122–32.
20. Volp ACP, Alfenas R de CG, Costa NMB, Minim VPR, Stringueta PC, Bressan J. Capacidade dos biomarcadores inflamatórios em predizer a síndrome metabólica: inflammation biomarkers capacity in predicting the metabolic syndrome. Arq Bras Endocrinol Metabol. 2008;52:537–49.
21. Hotamisligil GS. Inflammation, metaflammation and immunometabolic disorders. Nature. 2017;542:177–85.
22. Tall AR, Yvan-Charvet L. Cholesterol, inflammation and innate immunity. Nat Rev Immunol. 2015;15:104–16.
23. Malcangio M, Clark AK, Old EA. Neuropathic pain and cytokines: current perspectives. J Pain Res. 2013:803.
24. Osmari MP, de Matos LF, Salab BL, Diaz TG, Giotto FM. Líquido da casca da castanha de caju: características e aplicabilidades na produção animal. PUBVET. 2015;9:101–57.
25. Watanabe Y, Suzuki R, Koike S, Nagashima K, Mochizuki M, Forster RJ, et al. In vitro evaluation of cashew nut shell liquid as a methane-inhibiting and propionate-enhancing agent for ruminants. J Dairy Sci. 2010;93:5258–67.
26. Tanner NA, Zhang Y, Evans TC. Visual detection of isothermal nucleic acid amplification using pH-sensitive dyes. BioTechniques [Internet]. 2015 [cited 2017 Nov 7];58. Available from: https://www.future-science.com/doi/pdf/10.2144/000114253.
27. Hong Y-H, Weng L-W, Chang C-C, Hsu H-F, Wang C-P, Wang S-W, et al. Anti-inflammatory effects of *Siegesbeckia orientalis* ethanol extract in *In Vitro* and *In Vivo* models. Biomed Res Int. 2014;2014:1–10.
28. Jung HW, Yoon C-H, Park KM, Han HS, Park Y-K. Hexane fraction of Zingiberis Rhizoma Crudus extract inhibits the production of nitric oxide and proinflammatory cytokines in LPS-stimulated BV2 microglial cells via the NF-kappaB pathway. Food Chem Toxicol. 2009;47:1190–7.
29. Lee M-Y, Lee J-A, Seo C-S, Ha H, Lee H, Son J-K, et al. Anti-inflammatory activity of Angelica dahurica ethanolic extract on RAW264.7 cells via upregulation of heme oxygenase-1. Food Chem Toxicol. 2011;49:1047–55.
30. Griffin GK, Newton G, Tarrio ML, Bu D -x, Maganto-Garcia E, Azcutia V, et al. IL-17 and TNF- sustain neutrophil recruitment during inflammation through synergistic effects on endothelial activation. J Immunol. 2012;188:6287–99.
31. Sebaugh JL. Guidelines for accurate EC50/IC50 estimation. Pharm Stat. 2011; 10:128–34.
32. Vitale RF. Ribeiro F de AQ. Section: Artigo de Revisão Pages: 123 to. 2007:127.
33. Schütze S, Wiegmann K, Machleidt T, Krönke M. TNF-induced activation of NF-κB. Immunobiology. 1995;193:193–203.
34. Rothschild DE, McDaniel DK, Ringel-Scaia VM, Allen IC. Modulating inflammation through the negative regulation of NF-κB signaling. J Leukoc Biol [Internet]. 2018 [cited 2018 Feb 28]; Available from: http://doi.wiley.com/10.1002/JLB.3MIR0817-346RRR
35. Xiao W. Advances in NF-kappaB signaling transduction and transcription. Cell Mol Immunol. 2004;1:425–35.
36. Yamamoto Y, Gaynor RB. IκB kinases: key regulators of the NF-κB pathway. Trends Biochem Sci. 2004;29:72–9.
37. Aktan F. iNOS-mediated nitric oxide production and its regulation. Life Sci. 2004;75:639–53.
38. Coleman JW. Nitric oxide in immunity and inflammation. Int Immunopharmacol. 2001;1:1397–406.
39. Robinson MA, Baumgardner JE, Otto CM. Oxygen-dependent regulation of nitric oxide production by inducible nitric oxide synthase. Free Radic Biol Med. 2011;51:1952–65.
40. Varella PP, Forte WCN. Citocinas: revisão. Rev Bras Alerg E Imunopatol. 2001; 24:146–54.
41. Teotônio IMSN. Efeitos anti-inflamatórios de espécies de Pouteria spp. sobre macrófagos murinos RAW 264.7 estimulados com LPS. 2016;

2

In vitro pro-inflammatory enzyme inhibition and anti-oxidant potential of selected Sri Lankan medicinal plants

Hettiarachchige Dona Sachindra Melshandi Perera[1], Jayanetti Koralalage Ramani Radhika Samarasekera[1*], Shiroma Mangalika Handunnetti[2], Ovitigala Vithanage Don Sisira Jagathpriya Weerasena[2], Hasitha Dhananjaya Weeratunga[1], Almas Jabeen[3] and Muhammad Iqbal Choudhary[4]

Abstract

Background: The extracts of the ten selected Sri Lankan medicinal plants have been traditionally used in the treatment of inflammatory mediated diseases. The extracts were investigated for anti-inflammatory and anti-oxidant potential in vitro to identify bio-active extracts for further chemical characterization.

Methods: In vitro anti-inflammatory activities of total ethanol extracts were investigated measuring the inhibitory activities of four pro-inflammatory enzymes, arachidonate-5- lipoxygenase (A5-LOX), hyaluronidase (HYL), xanthine oxidase (XO) and inducible nitric oxide (iNO) synthase. Cytotoxicity of extracts were determined by MTT assay. Oxidative burst inhibition (OBI) on human whole blood (WB) and isolated polymorphoneutrophils (PMNs) was carried out for a selected bio-active extract. Anti- oxidant activities of the extracts were determined by 2,2-diphenyl-1-picrylhydrazyl (DPPH) free radical scavenging, ferric reducing antioxidant power (FRAP), ferrous ion chelation (FIC) and oxygen radical absorbance capacity (ORAC) assays. Total polyphenol and total Flavonoid contents of the extracts were also determined. The most active plant extract was analysed using Gas chromatography-Mass spectrometry (GC-MS) and High Performance Liquid Chromatography (HPLC).

Results: The ethanol bark extract of *Flacourtia indica* showed the highest A5-LOX (IC_{50}: 22.75 ± 1.94 g/mL), XO (70.46 ± 0.18%; 250 μg/mL) and iNOs inhibitory activities on LPS- activated raw 264.7 macrophage cells (38.07 ± 0.93%; 500 μg/mL) with promising OBI both on WB (IC_{50}: 47.64 2.32 μg/mL) and PMNs (IC_{50}: 5.02 0.38 μg/mL). The highest HYL inhibitory activity was showed by the leaf extracts of *Barathranthus nodiflorus* (42.31 ± 2.00%; 500 μg/mL) and *Diospyros ebenum* (41.60 ± 1.18%; 500 μg/mL). The bark and leaf extracts of *Callophyllum innophyllum* (IC_{50}: 6.99 ± 0.02 μg/mL) and *Symplocus cochinchinesis* (IC_{50}: 9.85 ± 0.28 μg/mL) showed promising DPPH free radical scavenging activities. The GC-MS analysis of ethanol bark extract of *F. indica* showed the presence of two major bio-active compounds linoleic acid ethyl ester and hexadecanoic acid, ethyl ester (> 2% peak area). The HPLC analysis showed the presence polyphenolic compounds.

Conclusion: The ethanol bark extract of *F. indica* can be identified as a potential candidate for the development of anti-inflammatory agents, which deserves further investigations. The bio-active plant extracts may be effectively used in the applications of cosmetic and health care industry.

Keywords: Anti-inflammatory, Enzyme inhibition, Anti-oxidant, Medicinal plants, *F. indica*, Gas chromatography-mass spectrometry, High performance liquid chromatography

* Correspondence: radhika@iti.lk
[1]Industrial Technology Institute (ITI), 363, Bauddhaloka Mawatha, Colombo 07, Sri Lanka
Full list of author information is available at the end of the article

Background

In Sri Lanka, medicinal plants have always been used and still remain a major source in the treatment of number of diseases including inflammatory and oxidative-stress associated chronic diseases. Free radicals can be either beneficial or deleterious to the body depending on the level. The excess levels of free radicals will cause damage to most cellular macromolecules such as proteins (enzymes), lipids and DNA leading to a condition called oxidative stress [1]. Oxidative stress has been recognized as a key factor in the pathogenesis of many diseases including inflammatory diseases [2]. The excess of reactive oxygen species (ROS) generated will lead to inflammation by stimulating cytokines and activation of pro-inflammatory enzymes such as lipoxygenase, hyaluronidase, inducible nitric oxide synthase and xanthine oxidase [3]. Lipoxygenases are capable of generating lipid mediators such as leukotrines and prostaglandins, which can provoke several inflammatory diseases such as bronchial asthma, allergic rhinitis, cardiovascular diseases, rheumatoid arthritis and certain types of cancer [4]. Hyaluronidase will lead to degranulation of mast cells and release inflammatory mediators leading to several pathological conditions including rheumatoid arthritis [5]. Upon activation of inflammatory cells, inducible nitric oxide synthase (iNOs) will generate excessive amount of nitric oxide (NO), which can cause inflammation [6]. Xanthine oxidases also play a major role in the metabolic disease called gout, which is closely associated with inflammation and some other inflammatory mediated diseases due to the formation of free radicals during the catalytic function of the enzyme. It is evident that these pro-inflammatory enzymes play an important role in the pathogenesis of inflammation via different pathways. Hence, inhibition of these enzymes is considered as targets for the management of diseases associated with oxidative stress and inflammation [7].

Oxidative burst is characterized by the production and rapid release of reactive oxygen species (ROS) from immune cells, mainly by neutrophils. Though it is considered to play an important role as a defense mechanism in phagocytosis, the higher levels of ROS released during the oxidative burst has been identified to cause severe tissue injury and inflammation. Therefore inhibition of oxidative burst has been recognized as an interesting strategy in the research arena of anti-inflammatory drug research [8]. Anti-oxidants also play an important role in the management of inflammation. The efficacy of antioxidants and anti-inflammatory drugs derived from medicinal plants in the management of inflammatory diseases has been extensively documented. In this concern, medicinal plants are considered as valuable sources of potential therapeutic agents. A number of modern drugs have been isolated from medicinal plants based on the traditional use. There is an emerging interest in the use of natural products mainly those derived from medicinal plants in therapeutic applications [9]. In Sri Lanka, the practice of Ayurveda and traditional system of medicine has been implemented systematically for more than two thousand years to treat various diseases including inflammatory mediated diseases. Around 1414 of plant species including several endemic species have been used for the treatment and prevention of diseases. Among them, around 200 species are in general use and of them, nearly 50 species have been identified as heavily used plant species in Ayurveda and traditional system of medicine. With the estimated annual consumption of 2.2 million Kg, the potential for commercial exploitation of medicinal plants has risen high [10]. In the existing scenario of emerging global interest for natural products of high therapeutic potential, exploring bio-activities of Sri Lankan medicinal plants is of great importance and high demand to support traditional claims as well as to discover unexploited bio-active properties. Moreover, the bio-assay guided isolation of bio-active compounds from identified bio-active medicinal plant extracts may come up with more effective and safer therapeutic agents against various diseases including inflammatory diseases and other oxidative stress associated chronic diseases. Also the bioactive ingredients are of high commercial potential in health care and pharmaceutical industries.

Based on this rationale, we investigated A5-LOX, hyaluronidase, xanthine oxidase, nitric oxide production and oxidative burst inhibitory properties along with anti-oxidant capacities of ten selected Sri Lankan medicinal plants, which have been used in the traditional system of medicine in the management of diseases, associated with inflammation (Table 1).

Methods

Chemicals and equipment

A5-LOX (soybean), linoleic acid, baicalein, hyaluronic acid potassium salt (human umbilical cord), hyaluronidase (bovine testes), calcium chloride, sodium hydroxide, p-Dimethylaminobenzaldehyde (PDMAB), sodium borate, tannic acid, xanthine oxidase (bovine milk), xanthine, allopurinol, Dulbecco's modified Eagle's medium (DMEM), fetal calf serum (FCS), bacterial lipopolysaccharide (LPS), trypsin, 3-(4,5-dimethylthiazol-2-yl)-2,5-diphenyltetrazoliumbromide (MTT), NG-Monomethyl-L-argininep-dimethylamino benzaldehyde (NMMA), $HBSS^{++}$ (Hanks Balanced Salt Solution, containing calcium chloride and magnesium chloride) [Sigma, St. Louis, USA], serum opsonized zymosan (SOZ) [Fluka, Buchs, Switzerland], $HBSS^{--}$ (Hanks Balanced Salt Solution without calcium chloride and magnesium chloride),folin-ciocalteu reagent, gallic acid, quercetin, ethylenediaminetetraacetic acid disodium salt (EDTA-Na_2), dimethylsulfoxide (DMSO),

Table 1 Traditional uses of ten Sri Lankan medicinal plants

Plant name/(FAMILY)	Local name/English name	Part used in the study/ Voucher specimen No.	Traditional uses
Sphaeranthus indicus L. (Asteraceae)	Mudumahana/East India Globe Thistle	Leaf/SEL/15/11	Swelling in the neck, acute laryngitis and bronchitis, piles [42].
Acronychiapedunculata L. (Rutaceae)	Ankenda/Claw flowered laurel.	Leaf/APL/15/15	Skin diseases, rheumatism, ulcers asthma [43].
Calophyllum innophyllum Linn.(Clusiaceae)	Domba/Alexandrian laurel	Bark/CIB/15/21	Skin diseases, piles, sore eyes, migraine [44].
Symplocos cochinchinesis (Lour.) S. Moore. (Symplocaceae)	Sewalabombu/Lodh tree	Bark/SCB/15/27	Leprosy, tumors, menorrhagia, inflammation and uterine problems [45].
Tinospora cordifolia (Willd.) (Menispermaceae)	Rasakinda/heartleaf moonseed	Bark/TCB/15/32	Skin diseases, Jaundice, Diabetes, rheumatic pain, syphilis [46].
Flacourtia indica (Burm.f. Merr.) (Flacourica)	Uguressa/Governor's Plum	Bark/FIB/15/34	Rheumatoid arthritis, gout, intermittent fever [40, 47].
Leucus zeylanica L. (Lamiaceae)	Gata thumba/Ceylon slitwort	Leaf/LZL/15/41	Jaundice, scorpion, snake bite [48].
Barathranthus nodiflorus Thw. (Loranthaceae)	Pilila	Leaf/BNL/15/44	Bone fractures [49].
Diospyros ebenum J.Koenig ex Retz (Ebenaceae)	Kaluwara/Ceylon ebony	Leaf/DEL/15/47	Snake bite, diarrhoea, ulcers, biliousness [32].
Argyreia populifolia Choisy (Convolvulaceae)	Elephant creeper	Leaf/APL/15/48	Swellings [50].

2,2-diphenyl-2-picryl-hydrazyl (DPPH), 6-hydroxy-2-5-7-8-tetramethylchroman-2-carboxylic acid (trolox), potassium persulphate,2,2-azobis (2-amidinopropane) dihydrochloride (AAPH), sodium fluorescein, 2,4,6-tripyridyl-s-triazine (TPTZ) and 4,4′-disulfonic acid sodium salt (ferrozine) were purchased from Sigma-Aldrich (USA). All chemicals and reagents used in the experiment were of analytical grade. The bio-assays were performed using high throughput micro-plate readers (Spectra Max Plus384, Molecular Devices, USA and Spectra Max-Gemini EM, Molecular Devices Inc., USA).

Plant material collection and preparation of extracts

Fresh plant materials, leaves of *Sphaeranthus indicus* L.(Asteraceae), leaves of *Acronychia pedunculata* L (Rutaceae), bark of *Calophyllum innophyllum* Linn. (Clusiaceae), bark of *Symplocos cochinchinesis* (Lour.) S. Moore. (Symplocaceae), bark of *Tinospora cordifolia* (Willd.) (Menispermaceae), bark of *Flacourtia indica* (Burm.f. Merr.) (Salicaceae), leaves of *Leucus zeylanica* L. (Lamiaceae), leaves of *Barathranthus nodiflorus* Thw. (Loranthaceae), leaves of *Diospyros ebenum* J.Koenig ex Retz (Ebenaceae) and leaves of *Argyreia populifolia* Choisy (Convolvulaceae) were collected from Gampaha, Sri Lanka.

Plants were identified by Ms. S. Sugathadasa and voucher specimens were deposited at Herbal Technology Section, Industrial Technology Institute, Sri Lanka (leaves of *Sphaeranthus indicus* L: SEL/15/11, leaves of *Acronychia pedunculata* L: APL/15/15, bark of *Calophyllum innophyllum* Linn.: CIL/15/21, bark of *Symplocos cochinchinesis* (Lour.) S. Moore.: SCB/15/27, bark of *Tinospora cordifolia* (Willd): TCB/15/32, bark of *Flacourtia indica* (Burm.f. Merr.): FIB/15/34, leaves of *Leucus zeylanica* L.: LZL/15/41, leaves of *Barathranthus nodiflorus* Thw.: BNL/15/44, leaves of *Diospyros ebenum* J.Koenig ex Retz: DEL/15/47 and leaves of *Argyreia populifolia* Choisy: APL/15/48) Plant materials were shade-dried under well-ventilated conditions (Relative humidity: 65–75%), at room temperature (25 ± 2 °C) for 72 h and ground to make coarse powder using a mechanical grinder [11, 12]. Powdered plant materials (100 g) were soaked in ethanol (500 mL) overnight and stirred for 1 h using a mechanical stirrer at room temperature (25 ± 2 °C) followed by suction filtration through a celite bed, packed in a sintered funnel. The filtrates were concentrated under reduced pressure at 40 °C using a rotary evaporator to obtain the ethanol extracts [11]. The solvent free extracts were stored in air-tight glass containers at – 20 °C until used [13].

Enzyme inhibitory activity

Arachidonate 5-lipoxygenase (A5-LOX) inhibitory assay

A5-LOX inhibitory activity of plant extracts was determined by a modified spectrometric method [14]. Plant extracts were assayed within the concentration range of 10–1000 μg/mL. Briefly, sodium phosphate buffer (110 μL,100 mM, pH 8.0), plant extracts dissolved in methanol (10 μL), and A5-LOX solution (55 μL) were incubated for 10 min at 25 °C followed by the addition of linoleic acid solution (25 μL, 0.08 mM). Absorbance was measured at $\lambda = 234$ nm for 10 min at 25 °C.

Percentage inhibition of A5-LOX was determined by comparison of reaction rates of extracts relative to control using the formula $(E - S)/E \times 100$, where E and S are activities of the enzyme with and without extracts, respectively. IC_{50} values were determined. Baicalein was used as the reference standard.

Hyaluronidase inhibitory assay

Hyaluronidase inhibitory activity of plant extracts was evaluated by a spectrometric method with modifications [15]. Extracts were assayed at the concentrations of 100 and 500 µg/mL. Extracts (50 µL) were incubated with hyaluronidase enzyme solution (10 µL) at 37 °C for 10 min followed by the addition of calcium chloride (12.5 mM, 20 µL) and re-incubation at 37 °C for 10 min. Sodium hyaluronate (50 µL) was added to the reaction mixture and incubated at 37 °C for 40 min followed by the addition of Sodium hydroxide (0.9 M, 10 µL) and Sodium borate (0.2 M, 20 µL) and incubation at 100 °C for 3 min. p-Dimethylaminobenzaldehyde (PDMAB), (50 µL, 67 mM) was added to the reaction mixture and incubated at 37 °C for 10 min. Absorbance was measured at $\lambda = 585$ nm. Percent enzyme inhibition was calculated as given below, compared to the control. Tannic acid was used as the reference standard.

Inhibition (%) = [(Abs. control − Abs. sample)/Abs. control] × 100.

Xanthine oxidase inhibitory activity

Xanthine oxidase inhibitory activity of plant extracts was determined by a kinetic method [16] with slight modifications. Extracts were tested at the assay concentration of 250 µg/mL. Briefly, sodium phosphate buffer (150 µL, 50 mM, pH 7.4), extracts (10 µL) and xanthine oxidase solution (10 µL) were incubated at 25 °C for 10 min. The reaction was then initiated with the addition of xanthine solution (0.1 mM). Absorbance was monitored with the change of absorbance at $\lambda = 295$ nm for 15 min at 25 °C. Percentage inhibition of xanthine oxidase was calculated using the formula $(E - S)/E \times 100$, where E is the activity of enzyme without extracts and S is the activity of enzyme with extracts. Allopurinol was used as the reference standard.

Nitric oxide production inhibitory activity and viability of LPS-activated RAW 264.7 macrophages

Cell culture Murine macrophage (RAW 264.7) cell lines were purchased from ATCC, VA, USA. The RAW 264.7 cells were cultured and maintained in DMEM, supplemented with streptomycin sulfate (100 µg/mL), penicillin G sodium (100 units/mL), amphotericin B (0.25 µg/mL) and 10% fetal bovine serum (FBS) (Humidified atmosphere, 5% CO_2, 37 °C). Cells were split twice a week.

Monolayer cells were plated in 96-well micro-plates at a density of 1×10^5 cells/well followed by the incubation (humidified atmosphere, 5% CO_2, 37 °C) for 24 h. The plated cells were treated with extracts (500 µg/mL) and incubated for 30 min (humidified atmosphere, 5% CO_2, 37 °C), followed by the incubation with bacterial lipopolysaccharide (LPS, 1 µg/mL) for 24 h [17].

Nitric oxide production inhibition The inhibition of nitric oxide production was determined using the Griess assay [6]. After 24 h incubation with LPS, cell culture supernatants (100 µL) were reacted with Griess reagent (100 µL) and incubated for 10 min at room temperature and absorbance was measured at $\lambda = 540$ nm. The nitrite concentration was determined using a standard curve of sodium nitrite ($y = 0.012x + 0.036$, $R^2 = 0.999$). Percentage inhibition of nitric oxide formation by extracts was calculated [18].

Cell viability The cytotoxicity of the extracts on RAW 264.7 cells was determined by MTT assay [19]. Cells were initially incubated (humidified atmosphere, 5% CO_2, 37 °C) for 6 h and with plant extracts (500 µg/mL) for 30 min. The cells were treated with LPS (1 µg/mL) and incubated for 24 h. MTT solution (20 µL, 5 mg/mL in PBS) and FBS free DMEM (180 µL) were added to the cells and incubated (humidified atmosphere with 5% CO_2 at 37 °C) for 4 h. DMSO (100 µL) was added to dissolve the formed formazan salt and absorbance was measured at $\lambda = 570$ nm. Percentage cell viability was determined [18].

Oxidative burst inhibition Oxidative burst inhibition assay was conducted at Dr. Panjwani Center for Molecular Medicine and Drug Research, International Centre for Chemical and Biological Sciences, University of Karachi, Pakistan. The institute has obtained the ethical clearance for studies on human blood from independent ethics committee, ICCBS, UoK. No: ICCBS/IEC-008-BC-2015/Protocol/1.0.

Isolation of human polymorphoneutrophils (PMNs) Venous blood was collected from a healthy adult male volunteer (25–30 years age) to a heparinized tube and density gradient centrifugation was carried out to isolate neutrophils [20]. Briefly, whole blood (10 mL), $HBSS^{-}$ (10 mL) and lympho separation medium (LSM, 10 mL) were mixed and kept at room temperature for 45 min for serum separation. The separated serum was centrifuged at 400 g for 20 min and sedimented cells were re-centrifuged with an equal volume of LSM at 300 g,

4 °C for 10 min. The cells were re-suspended in $HBSS^{--}$ and cell count was adjusted to 1 x 10 ^{6} cells/ mL.

Chemiluminescence assay Luminol-enhanced chemiluminescence assay was performed according to a kinetic method [21] with modifications. Briefly, 25 μL of diluted whole blood in $HBSS^{++}$ was incubated with the plant extract (25 μL) at 37 °C for 15 min and 25 μL of serum opsonized zymosan (SOZ) and 25 μL of luminol were added into each well, except blank wells. The level of the ROS was recorded and inhibition of ROS production (%) was calculated. IC_{50} values were determined. Ibuprofen was used as the reference standard.

Antioxidant activity

2,2-diphenyl-2-picryl-hydrazyl (DPPH) free radical scavenging activity

The DPPH free radical scavenging activity of plant extracts was determined using a spectrophotometric method with modifications [22]. Extracts were assayed within the concentration range of 10–500 μg/mL. Extracts (100 μL) were incubated with DPPH solution (40 μg/mL, 200 μL) at room temperature (25 ± 2 °C) in dark for 10 min and absorbance was measured at 517 nm. The DPPH free radical scavenging activity was calculated using the following equation and IC_{50} values were determined. Trolox was used as the reference standard.

Scavenging activity (%) = [(Abs. control – Abs. sample)/ Abs. control] × 100.

Ferric reducing antioxidant power (FRAP)

The assay was performed according to a spectrophotometric method [23] with slight modifications. Extracts were tested within the assay concentration range of 25–500 μg/ mL. Extracts (50 μL) were incubated with freshly prepared FRAP reagent (Acetate buffer of 300 mM and pH 3.6, TPTZ in 10 mM in 40 mM HCl, and 20 mM ferric chloride hexahydrate solution mixed at 10:1:1, *v*/v/v) (150 μL) at room temperature (25 ± 2 °C) for 8 min. Absorbance was recorded at λ = 593 nm. FRAP of extracts was expressed as mg trolox equivalents (TE)/g of extract using a standard curve of trolox ($y = 0.008x + 0.046$, $R^2 = 0.996$).

Ferrous ion chelating (FIC) activity

Ferrous ion chelating activity was determined according to a spectrophotometric method [24] with modifications. Plant extracts were assayed in the assay concentration range of 100–5000 μg/mL. Extracts (140 μL) were incubated with ferrous sulfate solution (1 mM, 20 μL) at room temperature (25 ± 2 °C) for 10 min. After the incubation, ferrozine (40 μL) was added to the reaction mixture and re-incubated at room temperature (25 ± 2 °C) for 10 min. Absorbance was measured at 562 nm. Percentage chelating effect was calculated with compared to control based on the following equation and IC_{50} values were determined. EDTA-Na_2 was used as the reference standard.

Chelating activity (%) = [(Abs. control – Abs. sample)/ Abs. control] × 100.

Oxygen radical absorbance capacity (ORAC)

The oxygen radical absorbance capacity (ORAC) assay was conducted using a kinetic method [25] with modifications. Plant extracts were assayed in the assay concentration range of 1–100 μg/mL. Extracts (10 μL) were pre-incubated with phosphate buffer (40 μL) and fluorescein solution (4.8 μM, 100 μL) at 37 °C for 10 min and freshly prepared AAPH solution (40 μg/mL, 50 μL) was added. The decay of fluorescein was monitored at 1 min intervals for 35 min at the wavelengths of 494 nm (excitation) and λ = 535 nm (emission). Trolox was used as the reference standard. The net area under the curve of decay of fluorescein was determined using the calibration curve of trolox ($y = 0.035x + 0.08$, $R^2 = 0.999$) and expressed as mg trolox equivalents (TE)/g of extract.

Determination of Total polyphenolic content

The total polyphenolic content (TPC) of plant extracts was quantified by the modified Folin-Ciocalteu method [26]. Extracts were assayed within the assay concentration range of 50–500 μg/mL. Plant extracts (110 μL) were incubated with folin-ciocalteu reagent and sodium carbonate solution (10% *w*/*v*, 70 μL) for 30 min at room temperature (25 ± 2 °C). Absorbance was recorded at 765 nm. TPC was calculated using the calibration curve of Gallic acid standard curve ($y = 0.053x + 0.105$, $R^2 = 0.993$) and expressed as mg gallic acid equivalents (GAE)/g of extract.

Determination of Total flavonoid content

The total flavonoid content (TFC) of plant extracts was quantified by the aluminium chloride method [27]. Extracts were tested within the assay concentration range of 50–500 μg/mL. Extracts (100 μL) were incubated with $AlCl_3$-methanol solution (2%, 100 μL) for 10 min at room temperature (25 ± 2 °C) and absorbance was recorded at 415 nm. TFC was calculated using a calibration curve of quercetin ($y = 0.033x - 0.002$, $R^2 = 0.999$) and expressed in terms of mg quercetin equivalents (QE)/g of extract.

Gas chromatography - mass spectroscopy (GC-MS) analysis

The total ethanol extract of bark of *F. indica* was analysed by GC-MS using Thermoscientific Trace 1300 GC system, coupled with ISQ QD mass detector (EI mode, mass range of m/z 40–450). The GC system is equipped with a programmable temperature vaporization (PTV) inlet and a Supelcowax capillary column (30 m × 0.25 mm × 0.25 μm), fused with silica and polyethylene glycol as the stationary phase.

Sample was dissolved in ethanol (0.60 g/mL) and 500 μL of head space gas was introduced to the PTV inlet. The injector temperature was set at 250 °C with an initial oven temperature of 60 °C, which was set to increase at a rate of 5 °C min^{-1} to reach up to 220 °C. Helium was used as the carrier gas (Flow rate: 1 mL min^{-1}). The compounds in the extract were matched and identified using mass spectral database of NIST 11, USA.

Analysis of phenolic compounds using high Performanace liquid chromatography (HPLC)

The ethanol extract of *F. indica* was dissolved in methanol (5 mg/mL) and filtered through a membrane filter (0.25 μm) for HPLC analysis. The HPLC system was equipped with a Agilent 1260 Infinity II system, consisting of a quaternary pump (G7111A), vial sampler, coloumn heater and Diode array detector (WR G7115A). Separation was achieved on a reversed phase coloumn C 18 (250 mm × 4.6 mm × 5 μm). The eluates were detected at 254, 280 and 320 nm. Two solvent mixtures were used as the mobile phase in a gradient system. Water/formic acid (1000/0.005 *v*/v) was used as solvent A and methanol was used as solvent B. The total flow rate was 0.5 mL/min. The gradient profile of the mobile phase was from 10% B linearly to 70% B in 60 min followed by an isocratic flow for 10 min and back to 10% B at 90 min followed by isocratic flow for 10 min to re-equilibrate [28].

Statistical analysis

All analysis was carried out in triplicate and experimental results were expressed as mean ± standard error (SE), analysed with one-way ANOVA. Turkey's multiple range tests was applied for mean separation, when ANOVA was significant ($p < 0.05$). IC_{50} values were calculated using linear regression analysis. Pearson's correlation coefficient was used for the correlation analysis ($p < 0.05$) (IBM SPSS Statistics 22.0).

Results

Enzyme inhibitory activities of selected medicinal plants

Arachidonate 5-lipoxygenase inhibitory activity

Based on the percent inhibition in the screening, the results revealed that, the ethanol bark extract of *F. indica* had the highest A5-LOX inhibitory activity followed by the extracts of *S. cochinchinesis* and *C. innophyllum*, while the extract of *T. cordifolia* had the lowest activity (Table 2). Apart from the extracts of *A. pedunculata, L. zeylanica* and *B. nodiflorus*, the other extracts showed high to moderate A5-LOX inhibitory activities. Based on the IC_{50} values, the extract of *F. indica* (Fig. 1) showed the highest A5-LOX inhibitory activity followed by *S. cochinchinesis* and *C. innophyllum* in a dose dependent manner confirming the results of the initial screening (Table 2). The activities of the extracts were found to be significantly different from the positive control baicalein, which showed a strong dose dependent activity against A5-LOX enzyme activity.

Table 2 Anti-A5-LOX activity of ethanol extracts of medicinal plants

Plant name	A5-LOX Inhibiton (%)*	Anti-A5-LOX activity IC_{50} (μg mL^{-1})
Sphaeranthus indicus	32.45 ± 0.45^a	136.69 ± 1.79^a
Acronychiapedunculata	17.45 ± 0.94^b	294.68 ± 2.23^b
Calophyllum innophyllum	67.14 ± 0.51^c	74.82 ± 1.35^c
Symplocos cochinchinesis	70.12 ± 0.36^c	39.01 ± 0.91^d
Tinospora cordifolia	12.71 ± 0.71^b	393.63 ± 1.74^e
Flacourtia indica	89.35 ± 1.24^d	22.75 ± 1.94^f
Leucus zeylanica	19.37 ± 0.11^b	258.03 ± 1.91^g
Barathranthus nodiflorus	9.38 ± 0.32^e	213.27 ± 1.55^h
Diospyros ebenum	34.91 ± 0.84^a	143.76 ± 1.03^a
Argyreia populifolia	32.89 ± 0.17^a	152.41 ± 1.00^i
Baicalein	97.64 ± 0.65^f	1.76 ± 0.15^j

Data represented as mean ± SE ($N = 3$). *A5-LOX Inhibition at 100 μg/mL. Mean within each column followed by the same letter are not significantly different at $p < 0.05$

Hyaluronidase inhibitory activity

The hyaluronidase inhibitory activities ranged from 16.27 ± 1.00 to 42.31 ± 2.00% for the tested plant extracts. The ethanol bark extracts of *B. nodiflorus* and *D. ebenum* showed the highest activities followed by the extracts of *A. pedunculata* and *F. indica* (Table 3). The extracts of *S. indicus, C. innophyllum* and *T. cordifolia* showed no inhibitory activities against hyaluronidase

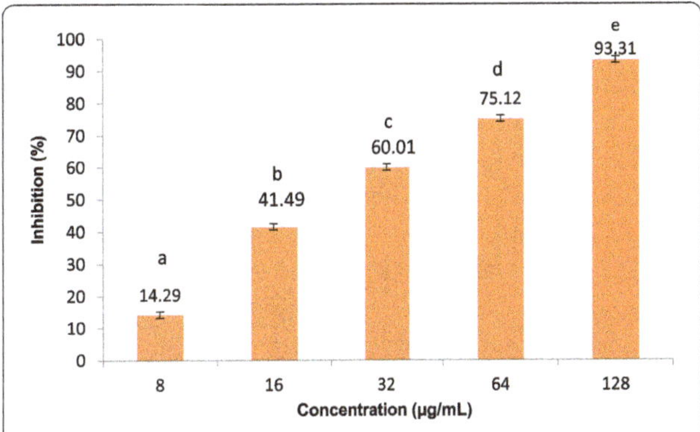

Fig. 1 A5-LOX inhibitory activities of ethanol extract of bark of *Flacourtia indica*. Results are presented as mean ± SE ($N = 3$). Means followed by the same letter are not significantly different at $p < 0.05$

Table 3 Xanthine oxidase and hyaluronidase enzyme inhibitory activities of total ethanol extracts of medicinal plants

Plant Name	Xanthine oxidase inhibition	Hyaluronidase inhibition
Sphaeranthus indicus	30.35 ± 0.32[a,f]	NI
Acronychia pedunculata	7.86 ± 0.14[b,d]	36.60 ± 1.02[a]
Calophyllum innophyllum	38.95 ± 1.28[c]	NI
Symplocos cochinchinesis	44.86 ± 1.43[c]	27.49 ± 1.09[b]
Tinospora cordifolia	17.92 ± 1.73[d]	NI
Flacourtia indica	70.46 ± 0.18[e]	36.67 ± 2.23[a]
Leucus zeylanica	13.26 ± 0.25[d]	24.38 ± 2.09[b]
Barathranthus nodiflorus	6.26 ± 0.93[b]	42.31 ± 2.00[d]
Diospyros ebenum	24.76 ± 2.16[a]	41.60 ± 1.18[d]
Argyreia populifolia	32.79 ± 2.16[f]	16.27 ± 1.00[e]
Allopurinol	99.26 ± 0.72[g]	NA
Tannic acid	NA	90.69 ± 0.50[f]

Inhibition (%) of xanthine oxidase and hyaluronidase is recorded at 250 and 500 µg/mL assay concentrations respectively
Data represented as mean ± SE ($N = 3$). Means followed by the same letter are not significantly different at $p < 0.05$, *NA* Not applicable

enzyme (Table 3). The extracts of *B. nodiflorus* and *D. ebenum* showed moderate activities (Table 3) compared to the reference standard tannic acid and good, comparable activities when compared with the reported activity of indomethacine (50%, 500 µg/mL) [28] a clinical drug in use against inflammation.

Xanthine oxidase inhibitory activity

All extracts showed some inhibitory activity against xanthine oxidase enzyme and activities ranged from 6.26 ± 0.93 to 70.74 ± 0.95%. The results revealed that, the ethanol bark extract of *F. indica* had the highest inhibitory activity followed by the extracts of *S. cochinchinesis* and *C. innophyllum* (Table 3). The extracts of *A. pedunculata* and *A. populifolia* showed significantly low inhibitory activities against xanthine oxidase enzyme with respect to the reference standard allopurinol (Table 3). The extract of *F. indica,* which showed the highest xanthine oxidase inhibitory activity showed significant ($p < 0.05$), dose dependent inhibitions within the concentration range of 31.25–500 µg/mL with a IC_{50} value of 176.62 ± 0.7 µg/mL (Fig. 2; Allopurinol: IC_{50}: 2.33 ± 0.51 µg/mL).

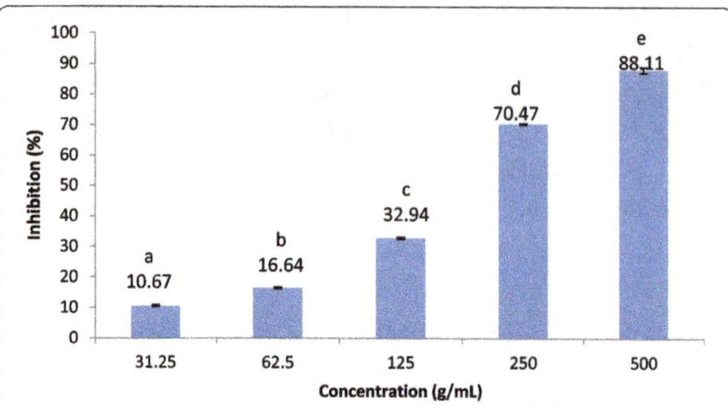

Fig. 2 Xanthine oxidase inhibitory activities of ethanol extract of bark of *Flacourtia indica.* Results are presented as mean ± SE ($N = 3$). Means followed by the same letter are not significantly different at $p < 0.05$

Nitric oxide production inhibitory activity and viability of LPS-activated RAW 264.7 macrophages

The inhibitory activities of extracts were moderate to low in comparison to the reference standard L-NMMA and ranged from 3.63 ± 0.69% to 38.07 ± 0.93%. Of the tested plant extracts, the extracts of *F. indica, S. cochinchinesis* and *C. innophyllum* showed significantly high activities, while that of *S. indicus, T. cordifolia, L. zeylanica* and *B. nodiflorus* showed significantly low activities (Table 4). The extracts showed no cytotoxicity (Cell viability: > 80%) at the tested concentration (Table 4).

Oxidative burst inhibition

The ethanol bark extract of *F indica,* which was identified as a highly anti-inflammatory extract was assessed for the effect on oxidative burst response on human whole blood and isolated PMNs. The extract showed a significant inhibition of ROS production on human whole blood (IC_{50}: 47.64 ± 2.32 µg/mL), which was found to be dose-dependent (12.5–200 µg/mL) (Fig. 3a). Interestingly, the extract showed promising, significant oxidative burst inhibitory effect when tested on isolated PMNs (IC_{50}:5.02 ± 0.38 µg/mL) (Fig. 3b), which is comparable with the reference drug Ibuprofen (IC_{50}: 5.12 ± 0.45 µg/mL).

Anti-oxidant activity

Anti-oxidant capacities of the extracts were evaluated using four different methods including the DPPH free radical scavenging, FIC, FRAP and ORAC assays. The extracts showed high to low DPPH free radical scavenging activities, having the IC_{50} values within the range of 6.99 ± 0.02–743.49 ± 1.94 µg/mL. The highest DPPH free radical scavenging activities were showed by the extracts of *C. innophyllum* and *S. cochinchinesis* followed by the extracts of *F. indica* and *S. indicus* in comparison to the reference standard trolox (Table 5).

In FIC assay, the extracts showed low chelating activities, indicating high IC_{50} values in comparison to the reference standard EDTA-Na_2. The extracts of *T. cordifolia, D. ebenum* and *A. populifolia* showed no chelating activity within the tested assay concentration range of 100–5000 µg/mL. Dose dependent activities were showed by the extracts of *A. pedunculata* and *S.*

Table 4 Inhibitory activities of ethanol extracts of medicinal plants on nitric oxide production and viability of LPS-activated RAW264.7 macrophages

Plant name	Nitric oxide production (μM)	% NO inhibition	% Cell viability
Sphaeranthus indicus	31.11 ± 0.17	9.46 ± 0.21[a,b]	87.21 ± 0.50
Acronychia pedunculata	30.39 ± 0.07	11.56 ± 0.21[b]	89.76 ± 0.35
Calophyllum innophyllum	23.67 ± 0.27	31.12 ± 0.78[c]	88.89 ± 0.82
Symplocos cochinchinesis	22.50 ± 0.28	34.52 ± 0.78[c]	82.15 ± 0.31
Tinospora cordifolia	32.89 ± 0.24	2.40 ± 0.69[a]	94.56 ± 2.57
Flacourtia indica	21.28 ± 0.32	38.07 ± 0.93[c]	87.31 ± 0.50
Leucus zeylanica	33.11 ± 0.24	3.63 ± 0.69[a]	93.02 ± 0.67
Barathranthus nodiflorus	31.22 ± 0.25	9.13 ± 0.72[a,b]	87.11 ± 1.16
Diospyros ebenum	29.08 ± 0.29	15.36 ± 0.85[d]	85.43 ± 1.22
Argyreia populifolia	27.64 ± 0.15	19.56 ± 0.43[d]	86.10 ± 0.61
L-NMMA	0.97 ± 0.12	97.10 ± 0.56[e]	97.54 ± 0.47

Data represented as mean ± SE ($N = 3$). Mean within each column followed by the same letter are not significantly different at $p < 0.05$. *Inhibition (%) at the assay concentration of 500 μg/mL

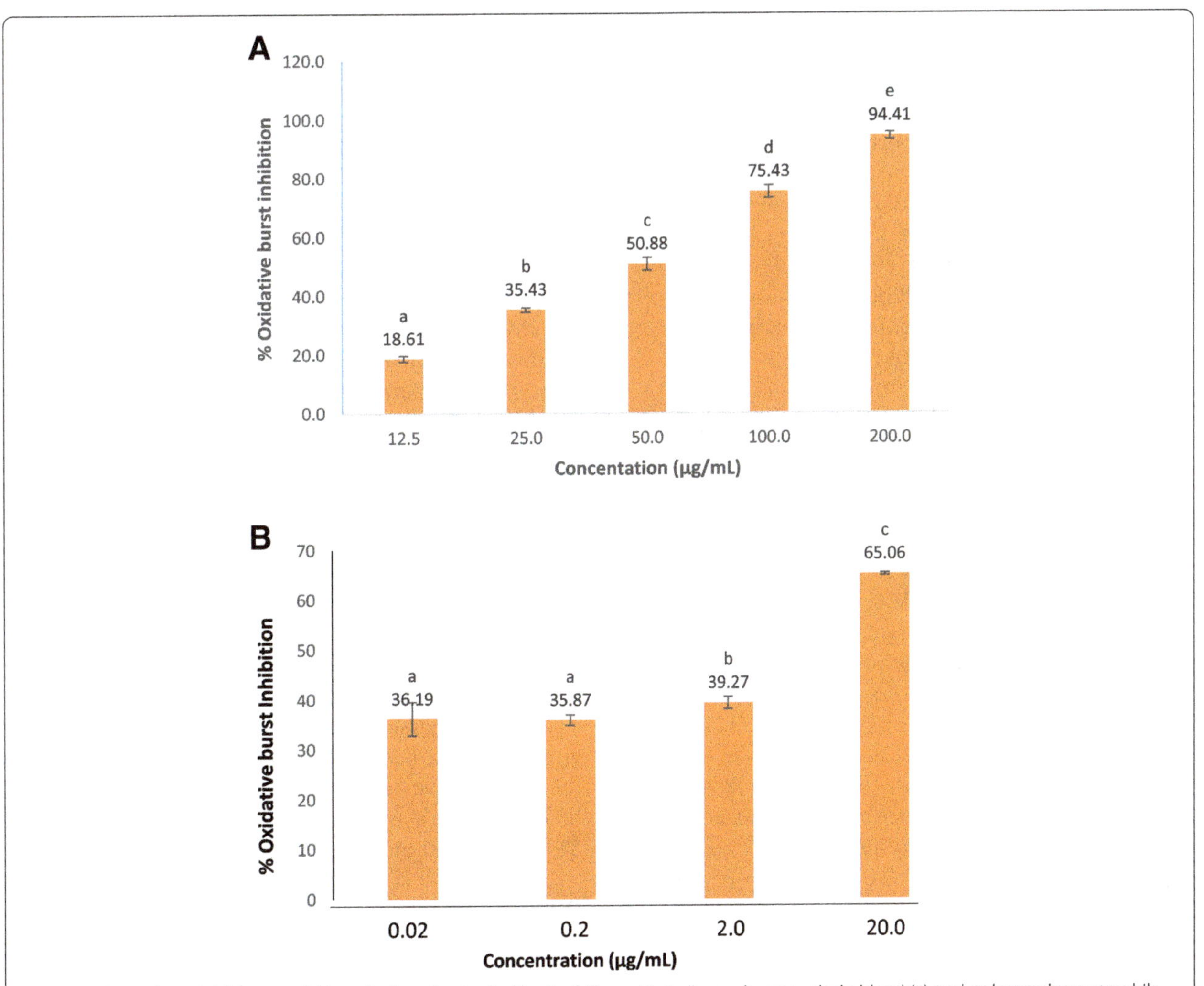

Fig. 3 Oxidative burst inhibitory activities of ethanol extract of bark of *Flacourtia indica* on human whole blood (**a**) and polymorphoneutrophils (**b**). Results are presented as mean ± SE(N = 3). Means followed by the same letter are not significantly different at $p < 0.05$

Table 5 Antioxidant activities of ethanol extracts of medicinal plants

Plant Name/Standard	IC_{50} (μgmL^{-1})/Inhibition (%)*		FRAP values (mg TE/g)	ORAC values (mg TE/g)
	DPPH	FIC		
Sphaeranthusindicus	109.33 ± 1.19[a]	19.21 ± 0.56*	326.15 ± 3.53[a]	1018.71 ± 9.96[a]
Acronychiapedunculata	743.49 ± 1.94[b]	974.56 ± 2.31[a]	741.64 ± 1.75[b]	322.67 ± 1.94[b]
Calophyllum nnophyllum	6.99 ± 0.02[c]	19.50 ± 0.71*	2613.00 ± 7.23[c]	2111.0 ± 6.35[c]
Symplocos cochinchinesis	9.85 ± 0.28[c]	1093.53 ± 4.04[b]	2181.61 ± 2.16[d]	2910.7 ± 12.9[d]
Tinospora cordifolia	389.20 ± 0.75[d]	NI	586.66 ± 3.29[e]	121.29 ± 2.12[e]
Flacourtia indica	26.37 ± 0.49[e]	8.29 ± 0.26*	375.20 ± 2.79[f]	1480.20 ± 11.5 [f]
Leucus zeylanica	352.65 ± 2.12[f]	33.46 ± 0.66*	157.69 ± 1.85[g]	63.69 ± 1.16[g]
Barathranthus nodiflorus	282.22 ± 1.78[g]	33.37 ± 0.40 *	427.29 ± 2.07[h]	18.07 ± 0.42[h]
Diospyros ebenum	177.32 ± 1.03[h]	NI	369.18 ± 0.61[f]	95.24 ± 0.00[e,g]
Argyreia populifolia	288.81 ± 1.45[g]	NI	268.01 ± 1.53[i]	479.55 ± 1.80 [i]
Trolox	5.29 ± 0.09[c]	NA	NA	NA
EDTA-Na_2	NA	13.07 ± 0.64 [c]	NA	NA
GreenTea	NA	NA	NA	1662.82 ± 0.22[j]

Data represented as mean ± SE ($N = 3$). Mean within each column followed by the same letter are not significantly different at $p < 0.05$. *Inhibition (%) at the assay concentration of 1000 μg/mL, *NA* Not applicable

cochinchinesis. For the remaining extracts, which showed chelating activity, dose response studies were not carried out due to the interference of turbidity of the reaction mixture at higher concentrations (> 1000 μg/mL) (Table 5).

In FRAP assay, the extracts showed low to high reducing power within the range of 157.69 ± 1.85–2613.00 ± 7.23 mg TE/g. The extract of *C. innophyllum* showed the highest FRAP value followed by the extracts of *S. cochinchinesis* and *A. pedunculata*. The extract of *L. zeylanica* showed the lowest FRAP (Table 5).

The ORAC of extracts ranged from 18.07 ± 0.42–2910.7 ± 12.9 mg TE/g. The extract of *S. cochinchinesis* showed the highest among the extracts and even significantly higher ORAC in comparison to the standard green tea extract. The extracts of *C. innophyllum, F. indica* and *S. indicus* also showed high ORAC values and that of *L. zeylanica* showed the lowest ORAC, compared to other extracts (Table 5).

Total polyphenol and flavonoid contents

The total polyphenol contents of the extracts ranged from 10.63 ± 0.22–661.42 ± 2.67 mg GAE/g. The extract of *S. cochinchinesis* showed the significantly highest polyphenol content followed by that of *C. innoplyllum* and *A. pedunculata*. The extracts of *L. zeylanicus* and *D. ebenum* showed the lowest polyphenolic contents (Fig. 4).

The flavonoid contents of the extracts ranged from 3.69 ± 0.15–72.74 ± 0.76 mg QE/g. The extract of *S. cochinchinesis* showed the highest flavonoid content and that of *S. indicus* and *F. indica* showed the lowest flavonoid contents. The extracts of *B. nodiflorus* (32.94 ± 0.88 mg QE/g) and *D. ebenum* (30.68 ± 0.30 mg QE/g) also showed significant flavonoid contents (Fig. 4).

Correlation between assays

The correlation analysis is important to get an understanding of statistical relationships between different assays. The *p* values resulted from the correlation analysis among ten assays are given in Table 6.

Gas chromatography - mass spectroscopy (GC-MS) analysis of ethanol extract of bark of Flacoutia indica

The GC-MS analysis of ethanol extract of bark of *F. indica* revealed the presence of six phytoconstituents including acid esters and fatty acid derrivatives (Table 7). Propan-2-yl tetradecanoate, [1,1'-Bicyclopropyl]-2-octanoic acid, 2′-hexyl-, methyl ester, Linoleic acid ethyl ester, Hexadecanoic acid, ethyl ester and Benzoic acid, ethyl ester were identified as major compounds (> 2% peak area) (Fig. 5).

Analysis of phenolic compounds using high performance liquid chromatography (HPLC)

The HPLC analysis produced a well resolved chromatogram representing peaks corresponding to retention time of phenolic compounds. The HPLC chromatogram of ethanol bark extract of *F. indica* at 254, 280 and 320 nm is given in Fig. 6.

Discussion

Enzyme inhibitory activities of selected medicinal plants

Arachidonate 5-lipoxygenase inhibitory activity

In this assay, all the extracts showed significant ($p < 0.05$) A5-LOX inhibitory activities at the tested concentrations.

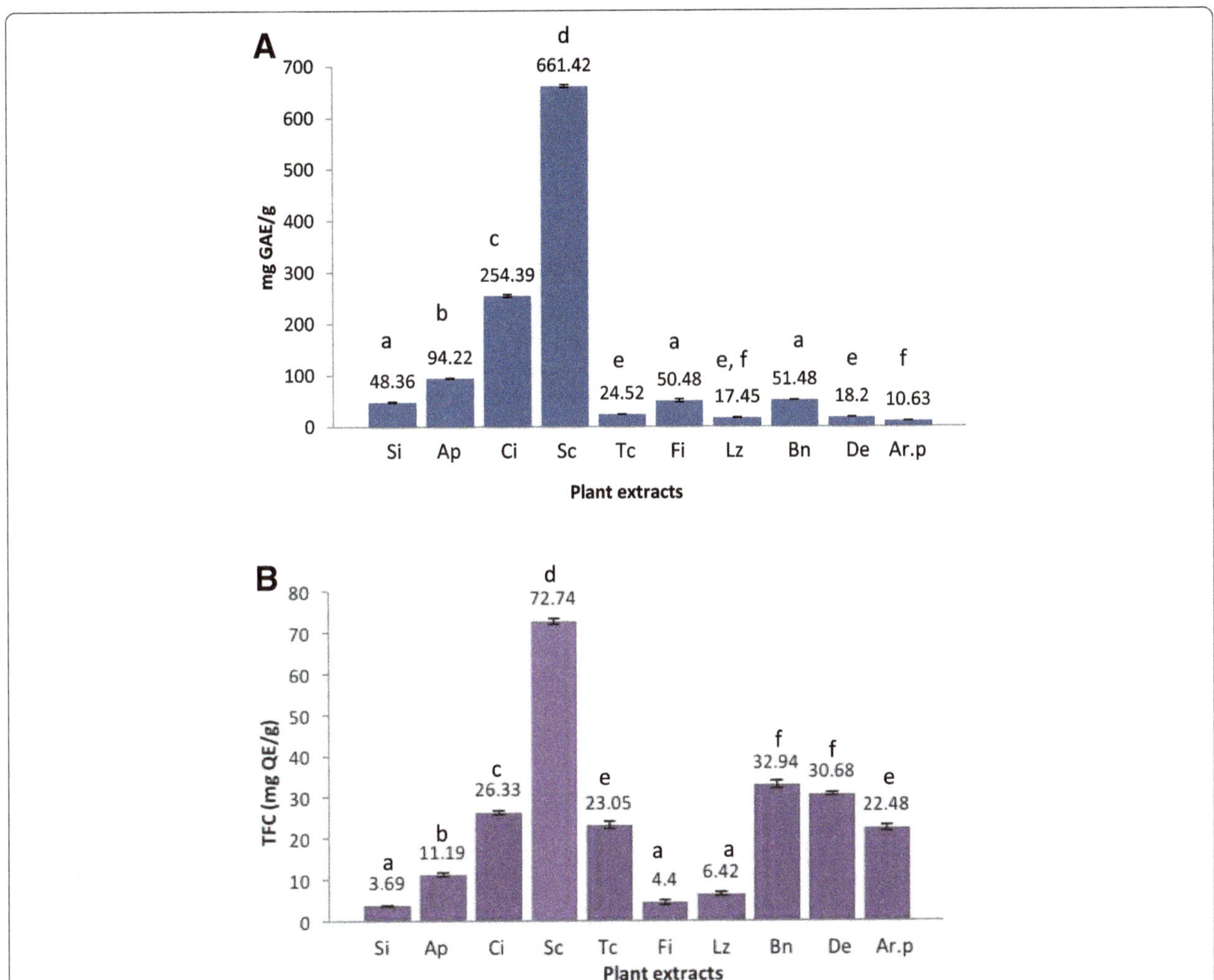

Fig. 4 Total polyphenolic contents (**a**) and total flavonoid Contents (**b**) of plant extracts. Results are presented as mean ± SE ($N = 3$). Means followed by the same letter are not significantly different at $p < 0.05$. Si:*Sphaeranthus indicus*, Ap:*Acronychia pedunculata*, Ci: *Calophyllum innophyllum*, Sc: *Symplocos cochinchinesis*, Tc:*Tinospora cordifolia*, Fi: *Flacourtia indica*, Lz: *Leucus zeylanica*, Bn:*Barathranthus nodiflorus*, De: *Diospyros ebenum*, Ar.p: *Argyria populiflia*.

Table 6 Pearson's correlation coefficients of in-vitro anti-inflammatory activities, antioxidant activities, total phenolic and total flavonoids content of extracts

	LOX	HYL	XO	NO	DPPH	FRAP	FIC	ORAC	TPC	TFC
A5-LOX	1	0.327^{ns}	0.930^{**}	0.950^{**}	-0.736^{**}	$.545^{**}$	$.150^{ns}$	$.844^{**}$	$.540^{**}$	0.228^{ns}
HYL		1	0.326^{ns}	0.371^{*}	-0.022^{ns}	$-.297^{ns}$	$.115^{ns}$	$-.043^{ns}$	$-.081^{ns}$	-0.059^{ns}
XO			1	0.864^{**}	$-.728^{**}$	$.287^{ns}$	$-.041^{ns}$	$.696^{**}$	$.326^{ns}$	0.069^{ns}
NO				1	$-.656^{**}$	$.592^{**}$	$.243^{ns}$	$.829^{**}$	$.587^{**}$	0.368^{*}
DPPH					1	$-.417^{*}$	$.270^{ns}$	$-.675^{**}$	$-.416^{*}$	-0.324^{ns}
FRAP						1	$.429^{*}$	$.811^{**}$	$.810^{**}$	0.607^{**}
FIC							1	$.436^{*}$	$.707^{**}$	0.520^{**}
ORAC								1	$.857^{**}$	0.523^{**}
TPC									1	0.821^{**}
TFC										1

The statistical significance is represented with $^{**}p < 0.01$ and $^{*}p < 0.05$. *ns* non-significant

Table 7 GC-MS data of ethanol bark extract of *Flacutia indica*

Retention time	Name of the compound	Molecular formula	Peak area %
16. 39	Benzoic acid, ethyl ester	$C_9H_{10}O_2$	2.42
24. 07	Propan-2-yl tetradecanoate	$C_{17}H_{34}O_2$	16.27
27. 87	Estra-1,3,5(10)-trien-17á-ol	$C_{18}H_{24}O$	0.94
28. 14	Hexadecanoic acid, ethyl ester	$C_{18}H_{36}O_2$	8.29
32. 83	Linoleic acid ethyl ester	$C_{20}H_{36}O_2$	7.72
38. 17	[1,1'-Bicyclopropyl]-2-octanoic acid, 2'-hexyl-, methyl ester	$C_{21}H_{38}O_2$	12.56

The ethanol bark extract of *F. indica* showed the highest A5-LOX inhibitory activity followed by that of *S. cochinchinesis* over the other extracts. When compared with the reported A5-LOX inhibitory activity of Caffeic acid, (IC_{50}: 57.0 μg/mL), [29] which is a known lipoxygenase inhibitor, the IC_{50} values of bark extracts of *F. indica* and *S. cochinchinesis* are about 2.5 fold and 1.5 fold lower than that of caffeic acid, respectively so that could be considered as even more potent than caffeic acid as A5-LOX inhibitors. To best of our knowledge, no previous studies have been conducted on A5-LOX inhibitory potential of extracts of *F. indica* and *S. cochinchinesis.*

Hyaluronidase inhibitory activity

In the hyaluronidase inhibitory assay, the extracts showed moderate to low anti-hyaluronidase activities at the tested concentration in comparison to the reference standard tannic acid. The extracts of *B. nodiflorus* and *D. ebenum* exhibited the highest anti-hyaluronidase activities compared to the other extracts. *B. nodiflorus* and *D. ebenum* are two medicinal plants endemic to Sri Lanka, that have been less exploited in the field of scientific research. The hyaluronidase inhibitory properties of these two plant extracts are recorded for the first time to upgrade the medicinal value of the species.

Xanthine oxidase inhibitory activity

All the extracts studied showed significant xanthine oxidase inhibitory activity ($p < 0.05$). The extract of *F. indica* showed the highest, xanthine oxidase inhibitory activity compared to the other extracts tested. This promising anti-xanthine oxidase potential of the extract of *F. indica* may be further supported by the traditional use of extracts of *F. indica* in the treatment of gouty arthritis. Specifically bark extracts have been used in the treatment of gout in the Unani system of medicine, where xanthine oxidase enzyme plays a major role in pathogenesis by imparting inflammation and catalyzing the formation of uric acid crystals leading to arthritic conditions [30].

Nitric oxide production inhibitory activity and viability of LPS-activated RAW 264.7 macrophages

Of the studied extracts, *F. indica* bark showed the highest NO production inhibitory activity. The NO production inhibitory activity could be either because of the direct inhibition of iNOs enzyme catalytic activity or expression of nitric oxide synthase. The high cell viability observed in the MTT cytotoxicity assay is evident for the non-toxic nature of the tested extracts confirming, that the observed NO production inhibitions are not due to any cytotoxic effect of extracts.

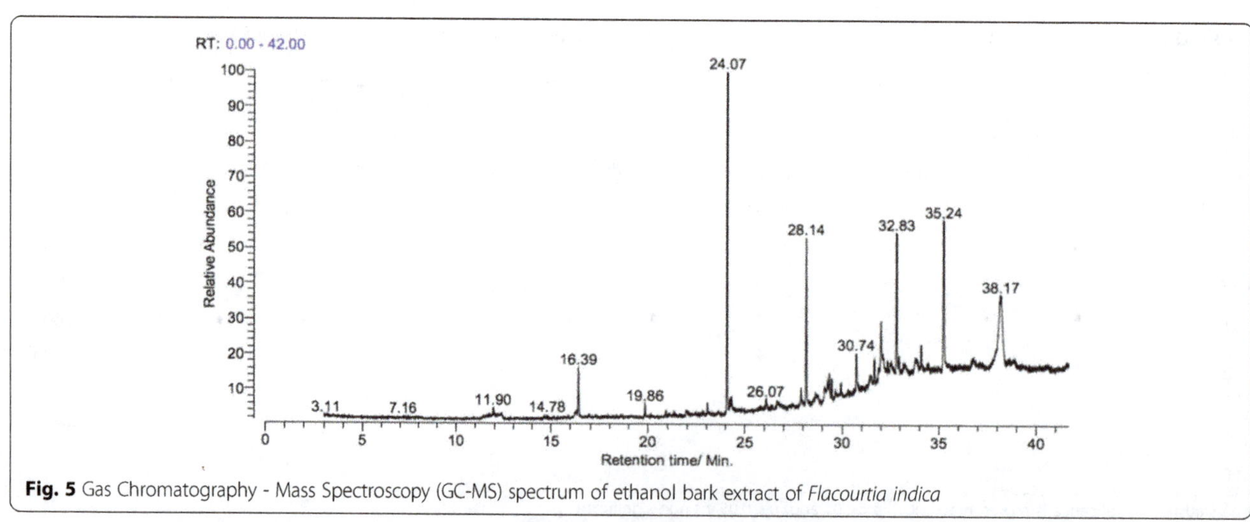

Fig. 5 Gas Chromatography - Mass Spectroscopy (GC-MS) spectrum of ethanol bark extract of *Flacourtia indica*

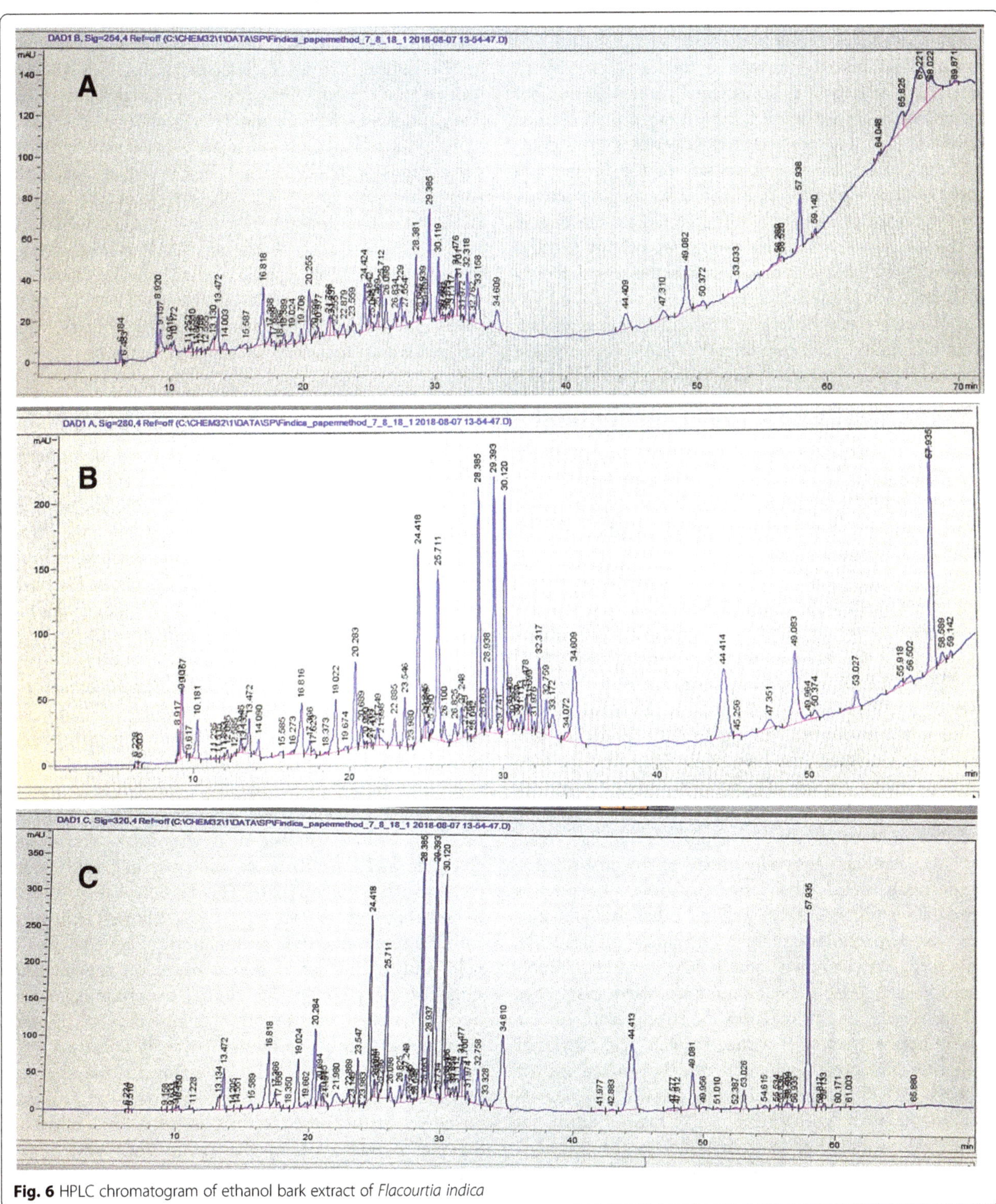

Fig. 6 HPLC chromatogram of ethanol bark extract of *Flacourtia indica*

Oxidative burst inhibitory activity

The bark extract of *F. indicia,* showed a pronounced oxidative burst inhibition in comparison to ibuprofen, when tested on PMNs. This observed activity may be due to the inhibition of NADPH oxidize enzyme, which catalyzes the generation of ROS or the direct scavenging of ROS upon the stimulation of opsonized zymosan [31].

Anti-oxidant activity

The bark extract of *C. innophyllum* showed the highest DPPH free radical scavenging activity and FRAP over other extracts, which may be attributed to the presence of major chemical compounds such as xanthones and coumarins abundantly present in the extracts [23]. *C. innophyllum* is known as a medicinal plant with number of curative properties and it has been extensively studied worldwide [23]. The present study ascertains the significant free radical scavenging activity of the Sri Lankan variety of *C. innophyllum* free radical scavenging activity with the means of marked DPPH free radical scavenging and FRAP. Lower chelating properties of the extracts may be due to the low contents of effective metal chelating compounds in the extracts.

ORAC evaluates a hydrogen atom transfer mechanism of anti-oxidants [25]. Significant ORAC of extracts indicates the peroxyl radical absorbance capacities of the extracts at different degrees. The extract of *S. cochinchinesis* showed the highest ORAC over the other extracts as well as the standard green tea extract. The presence of triterpenoids and flavonoid glycosides may be attributed to the anti oxidant potential of the extracts of *S. cochinchinesis.* It has been extensively studied for its anti-diabetic properties [32].

Total polyphenol and flavonoid contents

The moderate to weak and non-significant correlations of antioxidant and enzyme inhibitory activities with TPC and TFC (Table 6), respectively suggested that the polyphenolic and flavonoid compounds of the extracts may not be solely responsible for the enzyme inhibitory and antioxidant activities. It is further confirmed by the fact, that the ethanol extract of bark of *F. indica* has exhibited the highest bio-activities irrespective of possessing moderate to low contents of polyphenols and flavonoids (Fig. 4) Among the identified phytoconstitutents, hexadeconoic acid, ethyl ester is known to possess anti-oxidant properties as well as other bio-activities such as hypocholesterolemic, nematicide, pesticide, anti-androgenic, hemolytic and 5-alpha reductase inhibitory properties. Also the compound has flavor properties [33] which may be attributed to the strong aroma of the ethanol bark extract of *F. indica*. Linoleic acid ethylester is another bio-active compound detected in the extract of bark of *F. indica* which is known to possess anti-inflammatory properties and many more of bio-activities including anti-arthritic, anti-histaminic, anti-eczemic and anti-acne properties [33].

Correlation between assays

The A5-LOX, XO and NO inhibitory activities of plant extracts showed high, negative and significant correlations with DPPH free radical scavenging activity (IC_{50} values) ($r = -0.736$, -0.728 and -0.656 respectively at $p < 0.01$) and high, positive and significant correlations with ORAC assay ($r = 0.844$, 0.796 and 0.696 respectively at $p < 0.01$). This observation may be indicative of the dual function of bio-actives of plant extracts as free radical, peroxyl radical scavenging and A5-LOX, XO and NO production inhibitory compounds. Moreover, the A5-LOX, XO and NO inhibitory activities of plant extracts have showed high, positive and significant correlations with each other supporting the fact, that some common group of bio-actives of the extracts could be attributed for the enzyme inhibitory activities of the extracts (Table 6). FRAP of the extracts has showed a high, positive and significant correlation with TPC ($r = 0.810$, $p < 0.01$) so that the FRAP of the extracts may be due to the presence of polyphenols, which are well known to participate in redox reactions.

Gas chromatography - mass spectroscopy (GC-MS) analysis of ethanol extract of bark of Flacoutia indica

In previous studies the GC-MS analysis of methanol extract of root of *F. indica* has showed the presence of 4-Benzyol-3-methoxyisocoumarin as the major compound [34], which was not detected in the bark extract in this study. No other GC-MS analysis has been previously carried out on any species of the genus *Flacourtia* except for root of *F. indica* and this is the first report of the GC-MS analysis of Bark of *F. indica*.

Analysis of phenolic compounds using high performance liquid chromatography (HPLC)

According to a reported study, liquid chromatography-mass spectroscopy (LC-MS^n) analysis of aqueous methanolic fruit extract of *F. indica* has enabled identification of 35 phenolic compounds including rutin, feruloylquinic acid, esculin, gentisic acid glycoside, salicylic acid glycoside and derivatives of caffeolyquinic acids, quercetin and kaempferol [28]. The HPLC peak pattern of the ethanol bark extract of *F. indica* showed similarities with the reported HPLC peak pattern of aqueous methanolic fruit extract of *F. indica* based on the retention times of the peaks under similar experimental conditions. Therefore, the reported compounds of the fruit extract may also be present in the bark extract of *F. indica.* Further, the HPLC chromatogram may be used for standardization of ethanol bark extract of *F. indica.* However, further chemical Characterisation is needed for the identification of the compounds and activity guided fractionation is in progress.

In addition, presence of several other bio-active phytoconstituents including phenolic glycosides [35] coumarins (scoparon) [36, 37] and different types of polyphenolic compounds having radical scavenging properties such as coumaroylglucopyranose, tannins and butyrolactones [38] in the extracts of *F. indica* have been reported. Phenolic glycosides and coumarins have long been recognized as potent A5-LOX and xanthine oxidase inhibitors as well as antioxidants [39]. The bark of *F. indica* has been traditionally used to treat rhumatoid arthritis, [40] which is meadiated by inflammation. According to previous studies, The extracts of *F. indica* are known to possess a broad range of pharmacological activities including anti-inflammatory properties [34–36, 41] yet the pharmacological profile needs to be further investigated using more in vivo, in vitro and clinical studies [40]. This is the first report investigating the bio-activities of extract from bark of *F. indica* except for one study in which, the methanol extract of bark of *F. indica* has shown good DPPH free radical scavenging activity (IC_{50}: 17.5 ± 1.0 μg/ml) [38].

Conclusion

The extracts showed significant anti-inflammatory activities in vitro in terms of A5-LOX, xanthine oxidase, hyaluronidase and nitric oxide inhibitory activities along with promising anti-oxidant activities. Among the ten extracts, the ethanol extract of bark of *F. indica* showed the highest anti-inflammatory activity with good radical scavenging activities. Therefore, the ethanol extract of bark of *F. indica* is identified as a source of anti-inflammatory agents, which will be further studied to isolate and characterize bio-active constituents.

To the best of our knowledge, through this study, the pro-inflammatory enzyme inhibitory and anti-oxidant potential of ethanol bark extract of *F. indica* was identified and analysed by GC-MS and HPLC for the first time and selected for further bio-logical and chemical characterization.

Compounds studied

Benzoic acid, ethyl ester, Propan-2-yl tetradecanoate, Estra-1,3,5(10)-trien-17á-ol, Hexadecanoic acid, ethyl ester, Linoleic acid ethyl ester, [1,1'-Bicyclopropyl]-2-octanoic acid, 2′-hexyl-,methyl ester.

Abbreviations

A5-LOX : Arachidonate-5-lipoxygenase; AAPH: Potassium persulphate,2,2-azobis (2-amidinopropane) dihydrochloride; DMEM: Dulbecco's modified Eagle's medium; DMSO : Dimethyl sulfoxide; DPPH: 2,2-diphenyl-2-picryl-hydrazyl; EDTA-Na_2: Ethylenediamine tetra acetic acid disodium salt; FCS: Fetal calf serum; FIC: Ferrous ion chelating; FRAP: Ferric reducing antioxidant power; GC-MS: Gas chromatography-Mass spectrometry; HBSS: Hanks Balanced Salt Solution; HPLC: High performance liquid chromatography; LPS: Bacterial lipopolysaccharide,L-NMMA:NG-Monomethyl-L-argininep-dimethylamino benzaldehyde; MTT: 3-(4,5-dimethylthiazol-2-yl)-2,5-diphenyltetrazoliumbromide; NO: Nitric oxide; ORAC: Oxygen radical absorbance capacity; PDMAB: p-Dimethylaminobenzaldehyde; SOZ: Serum opsonized zymosan; XO: Xanthine oxidase

Acknowledgements

The technical staff at Dr. Panjwani Center for Molecular Medicine and Drug Research, International Center for Chemical and Biological Sciences, University of Karachi is highly acknowledged for their support.

Funding

The National Research Council of Sri Lanka (Grant No: 12–100).

Authors' contributions

Conception and design of in vitro experiments: HDSMP, JKRRS, SMH, AJ, OVDSJW, MIC. Conducted in vitro experiments: HDSMP. Conception and design of chemical characterisation: HDSMP, JKRRS, HDW. Conducted chemical characterisation: HDSMP, HDW. Data analysis and interpretation: HDSMP, JKRRS, SMH, OVDSJW, AJ. Manuscript drafting: HDSMP. Final approval and critical revision: JKRRS, SMH, OVDSJW, AJ, MIC. All authors read and approved the final manuscript.

Competing interest

The authors declare that they have no competing interest.

Author details

[1]Industrial Technology Institute (ITI), 363, Bauddhaloka Mawatha, Colombo 07, Sri Lanka. [2]Institute of Biochemistry, Molecular Biology and Biotechnology, University of Colombo, 90, Cumaratunga Munidasa Mawatha, Colombo 03, Sri Lanka. [3]Dr. Panjwani Center for Molecular Medicine and Drug Research, International Center for Chemical and Biological Sciences, University of Karachi, Karachi 75270, Pakistan. [4]H. E. J. Research Institute of Chemistry, International Center for Chemical and Biological Sciences, University of Karachi, Karachi 75270, Pakistan.

References

1. Sen S, Chakraborty R, Sridhar C, Pradesh A. Free radicals, antioxidants, diseases and phytomedicines: current status and future prospect. Int J Pharm Sci Rev Res. 2010;03:091-100.
2. Pala FS, Gürkan H. The role of free radicals in ethnopathogenesis of disease. Advances in Molecular Biology. 2008;1:1–9.
3. Dobrian AD, Lieb DC, Cole BK, Taylor-Fishwick DA, Chakrabarti SK, Nadler JL. Functional and pathological roles of the12- and15-lipoxygenases. Progress in Lipids Research. 2011;50:115–31.
4. Schneider I, Bucar F. Lipoxygenase inhibitors from natural plant sources. Part 1: medicinal plants with inhibitory activity on Arachidonate 5-lipoxygenase and 5-lipoxygenase/cyclooxygenase. Phytother Res. 2005;19:81–102.
5. González-Peña D, Colina-Coca C, Char CD, Cano MP, Ancos B, Sánchez-Moreno C. Hyaluronidase inhibiting activity and radical scavenging potential of Flavonols in processed onion. J Agric Food Chem. 2013;61:4862–72.
6. Cheenpracha S, et al. Inhibition of nitric oxide (NO) production in lipopolysaccharide (LPS)-activated murine macrophage RAW 264.7 cells by the norsesterterpene peroxide, epimuqubilin a. Mar Drugs. 2010;8(3):429–37.
7. Yumitha A, Suganda AG, Sukandar EY. Xanthine oxidase inhibitory activity of some Indonesian medicinal plants and active fraction of selected plants. Int J Pharmacy Pharm Sci. 2013;5:293–6.
8. Boukemara, H, Hurtado-Nedelec, M, Marzaioli, V., Bendjeddou, D, El Benna, J, & Marie, JC, *Anvillea garcinii* extract inhibits the oxidative burst of primary human neutrophils. BMC Complement Altern Med, 2016;16(1):433.
9. Rates SMK. Plants as source of drugs. Toxicon. 2001;39:603–13.
10. Arambewela LSR, Wimalasena S, Gunawardene N. Herbal medicine, phytopharmaceuticals and other natural products: trends and advances. 1st ed. Colombo: NAM S&T Centre, New Delhi and Institute of Chemistry Ceylon; 2006.
11. Perera HDSM, Samarasekara R, Handunnetti S, Weerasena OVDS. In vitro anti-inflammatory and anti-oxidant activities of ten medicinal plants traditionally used to treat inflammatory diseases in Sri Lanka. Ind Crop Prod. 2016;94:610–20.
12. Samaradivakara SP, Samarasekera R, Handunnetti SM, Weerasena OVDSJ. Cholinesterase, protease inhibitory and antioxidant capacities of Sri Lankan medicinal plants. Ind Crop Prod. 2016;83:227–34.
13. Wu MJ, Wang L, Weng CY, Yen JH. Antioxidant activity of methanol extract of the *N. nucifera* leaf (*Nelumbo nucifera* gertn.). Chin. Med J. 2003;31(5):987–98.
14. Tappel AL. Methods in enzymology. Academic press, New York. USA. 1962: 539.

15. Sahasrabudhe A, Dedhar M. Anti-hyaluronidase, anti-elastase activity of Garciniaindica. Int J Bot. 2010;6(3):299–303.
16. Lee SK, Mbwambo ZH, Chung H, Luyengi L, Gamez EJ, Mehta RG, Pezzuto JM. Evaluation of the antioxidant potential of natural products. Comb Chem High Throughput Screen. 1998;1(1):35–46.
17. Min HY, Kim MS, Jang DS, Park EJ, Seo EK, Lee SK. Suppression of lipopolysaccharide-stimulated inducible nitric oxide synthase (iNOS) expression by a novel humulene derivative in macrophage cells. Int Immunopharmacol. 2009;9(7):844–9.
18. Yang EJ, Yim EY, Song G, Kim GO, Hyun CG. Inhibition of nitric oxide production in lipopolysaccharide-activated RAW 264.7 macrophages by Jeju plant extracts. InterdiscipToxicol. 2009;2(4):245–9.
19. Hansen MB, Nielsen SE, Berg K. Re-examination and further development of a precise and rapid dye method for measuring cell growth/cell kill. J Immunol Methods. 1989;119(2):203–10.
20. Mesaik MA, Ul-Haq Z, Murad S, Ismail Z, Abdullah NR, Gill HK, et al. Biological and molecular docking studies on coagulin-H: human IL-2 novel natural inhibitor. MolImmunol. 2006;43:1855–163.
21. Helfand S, Werkmeister J, Roader J. Chemiluminescence response of human natural killer cells. I. the relationship between target cell binding, chemiluminescence and cytolysis. J Exp Med. 1982;156:492–505.
22. Blois MS. Antioxidant determination by use of stable free radical. Nature. 1958;181:1199–200.
23. Benzie IFF, Szeto YT. Total antioxidant capacity of teas by the ferric reducing antioxidant power assay. J Agric Food Chem. 1991;47:633–6.
24. Kim MY. Free radical scavenging and ferrous ion chelating activities of citrus fruits derived from induced mutations with gamma irradiation. Life Sci. 2013;10:401–3.
25. Ou B, Hampsch-Woodill M, Prior RL. Development and validation of an improved oxygen radical absorbance capacity assay using fluorescein as the fluorescent. J Agric Food Chem. 2001;49:4619–26.
26. Singleton VL, Orthofer R, Lamuela-Raventos RM. Analysis of total phenols and other oxidation substrates and antioxidants by means of Folin-Ciocaltue reagent. Meth Enzymol. 1999;299:152–78.
27. Siddhuraju P, Becker K. Antioxidant properties of various solvent extracts of total phenolic constituents from three different agro climatic origins of drumstick tree (*Moringaoleifera* lam.) leaves. J Agric Food Chem. 2003;51:2144–55.
28. Alakolanga AGAW, Siriwardene AMDA, SavitriKumar N, Jayasinghe L, Jaiswal R, Kuhnert N. LC-MS^n identification and characterization of the phenolic compounds from the fruits of *Flacourtia indica* (Burm. F.) Merr. And *Flacourtia inermis* Roxb. Food Res Int. 2014;62:388–96.
29. Torres-Carro R, Isla MI, Thomas-Valdes S, Jiménez-Aspee F, Schmeda-Hirschmann G, Alberto MR. Inhibition of pro-inflammatory enzymes by medicinal plants from the Argentinean highlands (Puna). J Ethnopharmacol. 2017;205:57–68.
30. Akram M, Usmanghani K, Ahmed I, Azhar I, Hamid A, Pak J. Comprehensive review on therapeutic strategies of gouty arthritis. Pharm Sci. 2014;27:1575–82.
31. Mahomoodally F, et al. In vitro modulation of oxidative burst via release of reactive oxygen species from immune cells by extracts of selected tropical medicinal herbs and food plants. Asian Pac J Trop Med. 2012;5:440–7.
32. Rashed KN. Antioxidant activity from *Diospyros Ebenum* stems extracts and phytochemical profile. JAIS. 2013;1:70–2.
33. Duke's Phytochemical and Ethnobotanical Databases U.S. Department of Agriculture, Agricultural Research Service 992–1996. [Online]. Available: http://phytochem.nal.usda.gov [Accessed 12 July 2017].
34. Eramma N, Devaraja G. Antibacterial potential and phytochemical analysis of *Flacourtia indica* (Burm.F.) Merr. Root extract against human pathogens. Indo Am J Pharm Res. 2013;3:3832–46.
35. Kamatou GPP, Viljoen AM, Steenkamp P. Antioxidant, anti-inflammatory activities and HPLC analysis of south African Salvia species. Food Chem. 2010;119:684–8.
36. Nazneen N, Mazid MA, Kundu JK, et al. Protective effects of *Flacourtia indica* aerial parts extract against paracetamol-induced hepatotoxicity in rats. J Taibah Univ Sci. 2009;2:1–6.
37. Jang SI, Kim YJ, Lee WY, et al. Scoparone from *Artemisia capillaris* inhibits the release of inflammatory mediators in RAW 264.7 cells upon stimulation cells by interferon-gamma plus LPS. Arch Pharm Res. 2005;28:203–8.
38. Swati M, Nath SG, Yatendra K, Kanchan K, Mohan SR, Prakash O. Phytochemical analysis and free-radical scavenging activity of Flacourtia indica (Burm. F.) Merr. J Pharm Res. 2009;8:81–4.
39. Werz O. Inhibition of 5-lipoxygenase product synthesis by natural compounds of plant origin. Planta Med. 2007;73:1331–57.
40. Ancy P, Padmaja V, Radha K, Jomy J, Hisham A. Diuretic activity of the roots of *Flacourtia indica*. Hygeia J D Med. 2013;5:79–83.
41. Kundu J, Roy M, Bachar SC, Chun KS, Kundu JK. Analgesic, anti-inflammatory, and diuretic activity of methanol extract of *Flacourtia indica*. Arch Basic Appl Med. 2013;1:39–44.
42. Jayaweera DMA, Senaratna LK. Medicinal plants (indigenous and exotic) used in Ceylon. Part II. National Sci Found. 2006;69.
43. Su CR, Kuo PC, Wang ML, Liou MJ, Damu AG, Wu TS. Acetophenone derivatives from *Acronychia pedunculata*. J Nat Prod. 2003;66:990–3.
44. Prabakaran K, Britto J. Biology, agroforesty and medicinal value of *Calophyllum inophyllum* L. (Clusiaceae): a review. J Asian Nat Prod Res. 2012;1:24–33.
45. Vadivu R, Lakshmi KS. In vitro and in vivo anti-inflammatory activity of leaves of *Symplocos cochinchinensis* (Lour) Moore ssp Laurina. Bangladesh J Pharmacol. 2008;3:121–4.
46. Jayaweera DMA, plants M. (indigenous and exotic) used in Ceylon. Part IV. National Sci Counc Sri Lanka. 1982:81.
47. Patro SK, Behera PC, Kumar PM, Sasmal D. Pharmacological review of *Flacourtia sepiaria*. SAJP. 2013;2:89–93.
48. Jain D, Baheti AM, Jain SR, Khandelwal KR. Use of medicinal plants among tribes in Satpursa region of Dhule and Jalgaon district of Maharastra- an ethnobotanical survey. Indian J Tradit Know. 2010;9:152–7.
49. Samaranayake GVP, Pushpakumara AAJ. A literary review on traditional medical systems for bone fractures in Sri Lanka. IJTRD. 2016;3:534–6.
50. Jayaweera DMA, Senaratna LK. Medicinal plants (indigenous and exotic) used in Ceylon. Part II. National Sci Found. 2006;89.

3

Complementary medicine products used in pregnancy and lactation and an examination of the information sources accessed pertaining to maternal health literacy

Larisa Ariadne Justine Barnes[1,2*], Lesley Barclay[2,3], Kirsten McCaffery[4] and Parisa Aslani[5]

Abstract

Background: The prevalence of complementary medicine use in pregnancy and lactation has been increasingly noted internationally. This systematic review aimed to determine the complementary medicine products (CMPs) used in pregnancy and/or lactation for the benefit of the mother, the pregnancy, child and/or the breastfeeding process. Additionally, it aimed to explore the resources women used, and to examine the role of maternal health literacy in this process.

Methods: Seven databases were comprehensively searched to identify studies published in peer-reviewed journals (1995–2017). Relevant data were extracted and thematic analysis undertaken to identify key themes related to the review objectives.

Results: A total of 4574 articles were identified; 28 qualitative studies met the inclusion criteria. Quantitative studies were removed for a separate, concurrent review. Herbal medicines were the main CMPs identified ($n = 21$ papers) in the qualitative studies, with a smaller number examining vitamin and mineral supplements together with herbal medicines ($n = 3$), and micronutrient supplements ($n = 3$). Shared cultural knowledge and traditions, followed by women elders and health care professionals were the information sources most accessed by women when choosing to use CMPs. Women used CMPs for perceived physical, mental-emotional, spiritual and cultural benefits for their pregnancies, their own health, the health of their unborn or breastfeeding babies, and/or the breastfeeding process. Two over-arching motives were identified: 1) to protect themselves or their babies from adverse events; 2) to facilitate the normal physiological processes of pregnancy, birth and lactation. Decisions to use CMPs were made within the context of their own cultures, reflected in the locus of control regarding decision-making in pregnancy and lactation, and in the health literacy environment. Medical pluralism was very common and women navigated through and between different health care services and systems throughout their pregnancies and breastfeeding journeys.

(Continued on next page)

* Correspondence: larisa.barnes@sydney.edu.au
[1]Faculty of Pharmacy, The University of Sydney, Camperdown, NSW 2006, Australia
[2]University Centre for Rural Health, The University of Sydney, PO Box 3074, Lismore, NSW 2480, Australia
Full list of author information is available at the end of the article

(Continued from previous page)
Conclusions: Pregnant and breastfeeding women use herbal medicines and micronutrient supplements for a variety of perceived benefits to their babies' and their own holistic health. Women access a range of CMP-related information sources with shared cultural knowledge and women elders the most frequently accessed sources, followed by HCPs. Culture influences maternal health literacy and thus women's health care choices including CMP use.

Keywords: Pregnancy, Lactation, Breastfeeding, Complementary medicine products, Health literacy, Culture, Medical pluralism, Health care choices,

Background

Medical pluralism, or the co-existence of different medical or therapeutic systems and traditions in one local setting has been recognised in most societies around the world [1]. Studies in both low and high income countries show that women routinely seek pre and postnatal health care from both traditional and allopathic providers, even when access to care from biomedically trained midwives and doctors is available [2–6]. In some places this is due to different cultural understandings of health and illness regarding specific needs for care during the reproductive phases of a woman's life [7, 8], but can also be to receive specific services from the different forms of care sought, or for specific pregnancy or breastfeeding related concerns [9–11]. Internationally and across economic strata, the desire for holistic care has also been associated with women's choices to use traditional or complementary medicines in pregnancy, birth and lactation [12–16]. Holism can be seen simply as the recognition and care for both the physical body and the mind and emotions [17], or be a more multifaceted concept that incorporates the health of body, mind and spirit [18]. First Nations' concepts of holism also encompass social and cultural connections to Land, Elders, and Nation, and views political, cultural and social determinants of health as interconnected [19–21].

The prevalence of complementary medicine use in pregnancy and lactation has been increasingly noted globally. One multinational study found that of 23 countries, rates of herbal medicine use in pregnancy were the highest in Russia (69.0%), Australia (43.8%) and Poland (49.8%) [22]. A cross-sectional survey of Hispanic women in Indianapolis USA found that 14.2 and 13.0% of women surveyed began using herbal remedies in pregnancy and breastfeeding, respectively [23]. A UK study investigating various forms of complementary and alternative medicine (CAM) used in pregnancy found that 5.1% of women surveyed used dietary supplements, 34.9% used vitamins and 5.4% used herbal medicines, and that 35% of women who used CAM also visited a trained CAM practitioner [24]. Complementary medicine use in lower income countries has also been documented. For example 12% of Kenyan women living in Nairobi, and 52.4% of Malaysian women in the Tumpat district used herbal medicine in their recent pregnancies [25, 26]. Concerns with complementary medicine use in pregnancy and lactation are frequently raised for the health of the mothers, in pregnancy due to unknown effects of complementary medicine products (CMPs) on the baby in utero. Lactation is also a concern as little is known about risks associated with CMP exposure through breastmilk [27–29].

Health literacy refers to an individual's ability to search for, understand, and apply health information when making decisions about their health [30], and influences the health care decisions women make during pregnancy and lactation. Maternal health literacy can be defined as "the cognitive and social skills that determine the motivation and ability of women to gain access to, understand and use information in ways that promote and maintain their health and that of their children" ([31], p381). In short, the knowledge, skills and confidence a woman has will influence the health care choices she makes whilst pregnant and breastfeeding. The World Health Organisation identifies four overarching factors in health literacy: (i) the health care team and system, (ii) the condition or illness, (iii) therapy (medications, lifestyle modifications, exercise prescriptions, etc.), and (iv) patient-related factors such as prior knowledge of health and health care, literacy, numeracy and communication skills and cultural background [32]. Access to appropriate information sources, as well as the ability to appraise the information obtained in order to make safe and pertinent decisions, are also key components of health literacy [33, 34].

The objectives of this systematic review were to determine what sources of information on complementary and alternative medicine products (CMPs) have been described in the literature from a range of countries, and are used in pregnancy and lactation for the benefit of the mother, the pregnancy, child and/or the breastfeeding process. The role of maternal health literacy in these practices was also examined. This paper focuses on the results from the qualitative studies included in this systematic review. It complements a concurrent synthesis of the quantitative papers looking at the same question.

Methods

Protocol and registration number

Details of the protocol for this systematic review were registered on PROSPERO and can be accessed at: https://www.crd.york.ac.uk/PROSPERO/display_record.asp?ID=CRD42016052283.

Literature search strategy and criteria

An electronic search of seven databases was undertaken: AMED Allied and Complementary Medicine (via Ovid SP), CINAHL (via Ebsco), Cochrane Database of Systematic Reviews (via Ovid SP), EMBASE (via Ovid SP), Maternity and Infant Care (via Ovid SP), Medline (via Ovid SP), and PubMed. The date range was set between 1995 and 2015 to reflect developments in the field of health literacy over this time, as well as increases in the documentation of complementary medicine use in pregnancy world-wide and in complementary medicine research [35]. A second search of the seven databases was also performed to check for subsequent publications published from 2015-Jun 2017 before completing this review. A variety of terms were used to cover the four central themes of the review: pregnancy, lactation, complementary and alternative medicine products (CMPs) and health literacy. CMPs were operationally defined as ingested herbal medicines given for specific therapeutic purposes in foods, tea, decoction, tablet, capsule or ethanolic extract forms, topical herbal preparations such as herbal washes, creams or ointments, and aromatherapy oils for inhalation, as well as dietary vitamin and mineral supplements and pre and probiotic supplements. Terms within each concept (pregnancy, lactation, complementary medicine and health literacy) were combined with OR, and results from each concept combined with AND (Additional file 1). Reference lists from relevant studies and review papers were also hand searched. An initial systematic literature search was conducted and papers' titles were screened for inclusion or exclusion based on set criteria (Table 1). This was followed by a screening of all remaining papers' abstracts and then full text versions of papers against the same criteria. The lead author (LAJB) screened all papers by title, abstract and full text. PA participated in the screening of titles and full text papers. Differences regarding study selection were resolved by discussion between LAJB and PA. Although the transition from non-pregnant woman through conception, pregnancy, labour, birth, and the postpartum period is a continuum experienced by each childbearing woman, these different stages are described differently within the literature. For the purposes of this systematic review, the use of complementary therapies across the childbearing continuum of pregnancy, labour and birth, and breastfeeding in the postpartum period (defined as up to 24 months) [36] have been examined.

Table 1 Inclusion and exclusion criteria

Inclusion criteria
1. Use of qualitative methods for data collection including focus group discussions or in-depth interviews
2. Focus on the use of complementary medicine products as defined operationally above
3. Described CMP use in pregnancy and/or lactation
4. CMPs were used by the woman for the benefit of her own health in pregnancy, the pregnancy itself, the baby and/or the breastfeeding process
5. Information sources the woman accessed with regards to the CMPs used are reported
6. Health literacy, or related concepts, were discussed
Exclusion criteria
• Pre-conceptual folic acid supplementation only
• Trials of CMPs in pregnancy or lactation (trial would have been the information source on the CMP studied)
• Information sources not clearly identifiable
• Potential information sources identified by the authors, but not clearly identified by participants
• Data not collected from pregnant and breastfeeding women themselves
• Data only collected from health care practitioners
• Study protocols or social marketing campaigns
• Overview or commentary papers on CAM modalities, philosophies or practices regarding women's health
• Overview or commentary papers on biomedical maternity care philosophies
• Commentary papers on CMP use or the lack of uptake of recommended nutritional supplements in pregnancy, including iron, folic acid and iodine.
• Studies where CMPs were given directly to infants, and not the breastfeeding mothers
• Studies focussing on CAM use to treat infertility

Critical appraisal of reporting quality

Each paper was assessed according to the 32 item checklist *Consolidated Criteria for Reporting Qualitative Research (COREQ)* [37]. The COREQ checklist aims to assess how comprehensively and explicitly qualitative studies are reported and covers three main domains: 1) research team and reflexivity, 2) study design and 3) analysis and findings [37]. Use of the COREQ checklist guided the assessment of the rigour and methodological coherence of the included papers and contributed to the synthesis required as part of the systematic review process.

Data extraction

All papers included were analysed comprehensively in order to extract applicable data including: author and year, country study was performed in, number of participants, data collection and analysis methods, major factors explored, CMP type discussed, childbearing stage of relevance to the CMP use, and CMP-related information sources accessed. Following this, major and minor themes were identified and data from each study was summarised within these themes with illustrating participant quotes, where relevant.

Thematic analysis

Findings across the studies were aggregated following the methods set out by Thomas and Harden [38] and Braun and Clarke [39]. Firstly descriptive themes were developed to describe the use of CMPs by pregnant and breastfeeding women for the benefit of their own health whilst pregnant, the pregnancy, baby or breastfeeding process, and to describe the information sources women accessed when choosing to use CMPs in pregnancy and lactation. Following this, analytical themes were developed in order to delve deeper into the concept of CMP use in pregnancy and lactation and women's access to information sources – the reasons for CMP use, the perceived and actual benefits of CMP use and what influences women to use CMPs in pregnancy and lactation.

During the coding process, it was necessary to delineate between perceived benefits of taking CMPs for the mother, the pregnancy, the growing baby, and the breastfeeding process. For clarity these perceived benefits are divided into these different themes, but it should also be recognised that there is overlap. For example, it is of benefit to the mother's health to avoid miscarriage, but also obviously of benefit to the pregnancy. Papers were also analysed for specific results on health literacy.

Results

Study selection

The search strategy generated 4574 citations after duplicates were eliminated (Fig. 1). After reviewing titles and abstracts 683 papers were examined by full text. After studies focussing only on folic acid supplementation were removed, 22 qualitative studies were identified for inclusion. The reference lists of these 22 qualitative studies were examined by title, abstract and full text, and a further two studies were found that fulfilled the inclusion criteria. The second search of the seven databases yielded an additional 506 citations. After screening, a further four papers were identified, making a total of 28 papers covering 26 studies for inclusion in this qualitative synthesis. The three publications by Westfall [10, 40, 41] report on different aspects of one large study. Therefore, although the 28 included publications present the findings of 26 investigations, for clarity, the total number of studies will be referred to as 28 hereafter.

COREQ appraisal results

The studies included varied in how comprehensively they fulfilled the criteria for each domain of the COREQ checklist (Additional file 2). Critical appraisal of the papers identified a number of gaps in the reporting of the papers overall.

For the first domain *Research team and reflexivity*, overall the papers reported well on who conducted the interviews and focus groups (19/28), researchers' credentials (19/28), but less than half (13/28) reported on gender of the researchers. Interviewer characteristics, occupation, experience and whether a relationship was established between researchers and participants prior to the start of a study, and whether participants knew the researchers' goals and reasons for doing the research were not well reported.

For domain two *Study design*, only 20/28 papers identified the methodological orientation of the research reported. Sampling method was reported clearly in 25/28 papers as was the number of participants (26/28), and to a lesser extent, place of data collection (21/28) and description of the sample (23/28). However, gaps across the studies can be seen in reporting the method of approaching participants (13/28 reported this), non-participation rates (9/28) and whether any other people were present during data collection besides researchers and participants (6/28). Data saturation was only discussed in 7/28 papers and transcripts were returned for participant comment in only 7/28 papers.

For Domain 3 *Analysis and findings*, the coding tree was only provided in 7/28 papers and in 10/28 studies participants provided feedback on the findings. Additionally, 11/28 papers reported on the number of coders. The presentation of the analysis and findings were clearly reported across most of the papers with major themes being clearly presented in the results sections of all 28 papers, and 24/28 papers also included descriptions of diverse cases or minor themes.

Pertinent features of included studies

Table 2 describes significant features of the studies included in this synthesis.

Geographical and economic classifications

Countries from all World Bank economic classifications [42] are represented in the sample, although the majority of studies come from countries with Low-Income Economies (LICs) or Lower-Middle-Income Economies (LMICs) classifications, and two of the studies from High-Income Economies (HICs) included actually focus on the experiences of women from poorer countries: immigrants to Canada from India, a LMIC [43]; and Hmong refugees from Thailand, an Upper-Middle-Income Economy (UPIC) living in Australia (HIC) with very low education and income levels [44]. Additionally, three of the included studies from Canada (HIC) [10, 40, 41] were from the same study, so the number of women involved from HIC backgrounds in the overall synthesis is only 143 out of more than 1075 total participants across all studies (for Waiswa et al. [45] exact numbers in the 10 FGDs were not given). Thirteen studies were from African nations: 12 from the Sub-Saharan region and one from North Africa and eight studies focussed on East or South Asian women's experiences.

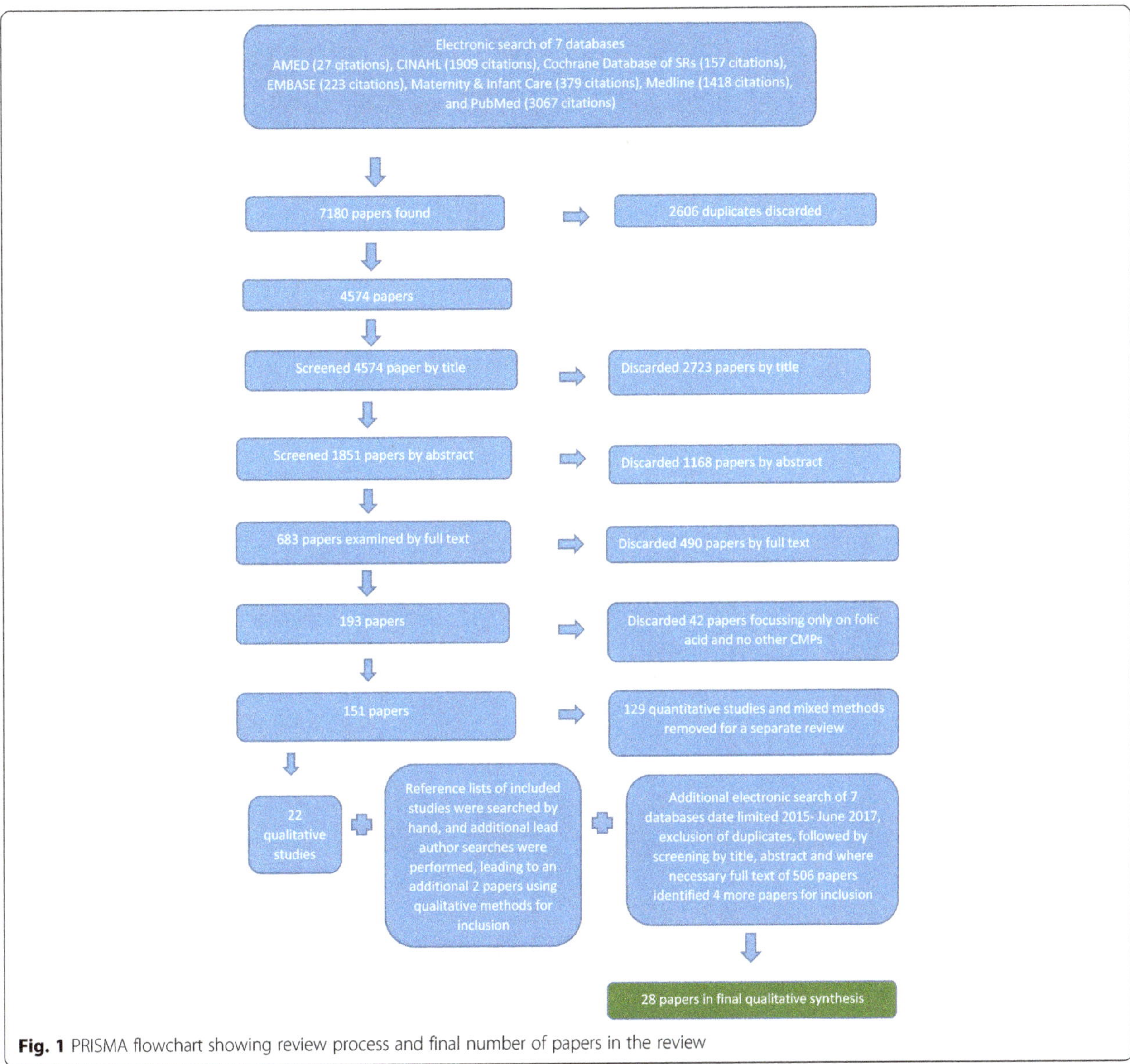

Fig. 1 PRISMA flowchart showing review process and final number of papers in the review

Theoretical frameworks for the data analysis methods

The theoretical frameworks for the studies varied: seven used an ethnographical basis [7, 44, 46–50], one combined ethnography with content analysis [51], four others used some form of content analysis [45, 52–54], and four reported using thematic analysis [10, 40, 41, 55]. Ethnobotanical research [56], narrative analysis [57], and naturalistic qualitative descriptive processes [43] provided the theoretical framework for one paper each. Phenomenology was used in two papers [4, 58]. The final five papers did not state the theoretical framework used [8, 59–62].

Data collection methods

Eleven studies utilised in-depth interviews only [4, 10, 40, 41, 43, 49, 53, 55, 57, 61, 63] and two studies used focus group discussions only [8, 52] to collect data. Five studies combined focus group discussions and in-depth interviews [45, 51, 54, 60, 62], four studies combined in-depth interviews with participant observation [44, 46, 48, 58], and one study combined informal conversations, in-depth interviews, focus group discussions and participant observation [50]. Data was collected using open-ended interviews and participatory observation [7], group interviews and individual interviews [56], unstructured one-on-one interviews [64], semi-structured interviews [59] and unstructured interviews [47] in the final five studies.

Number of participants across and within studies

The total number of participants that can be counted across all studies was 1075 but would actually be higher as exact numbers of participants were not reported in one study [45] and additional quotes from HCPs are given in

Table 2 Pertinent features of included studies

Author (date)	Country (economic classification [a])	Number of participants	Data collection method	Data analysis method	Study aims	CMPs reported on in the papers [b]	Stage in the continuum of childbearing reporting use of the CMP as interpreted by the author [c]	Information sources women access for CMPs
Aborigo et al. (2012) [60]	Ghana (LMIC)	253 (including 35 women with newborn infants; 8 traditional birth attendants and local healers; 16 community leaders; 4 Focus Group Discussions [FGDs] with 8–10 grandmothers each; and 12 compound heads)	In-depth interviews [IDIs] and Focus group discussions [FGDs]	Not stated	To explore breastfeeding initiation and supplementation; cultural practices around breastfeeding initiation; and implications for the improvement of infant health	Herbal medicines	Breastfeeding	Traditional Birth Attendants (TBAs); herbalists; other local healers; women's mothers-in-law and grandmothers; heads of households
Callister et al. (2011) [61]	Three countries: The People's Republic of China (UPIC), Taiwain (HIC) and USA (HIC)	34 Chinese women (10 living in Guangzhou, China, 12 living Taiwan, and 12 who had immigrated to western United States.)	In-depth interviews	Not stated	Comparison of childbirth experiences of Chinese women in their countries of origin with those who had immigrated to the USA before giving birth; provide insights on Chinese women's cultural practices and beliefs associated with giving birth for nurses and midwives in the USA.	Herbal medicines	Pregnancy and postnatal month	Shared cultural traditions; women's mothers and mothers-in-law
Dako-Gyeke et al. (2013) [62]	Ghana (LMIC)	55 (including 17 pregnant and 15 postnatal women; 10 nurse-midwives; 2 medical doctors; 3 community members; 3 spiritualists; 1 traditional birth attendant; 1 herbalist)	In-depth interviews and Focus group discussions	Not stated	Describe the beliefs, perspectives and knowledge of pregnancy and birth of peri-Urban Ghanaian women and how these influence the health care seeking behaviour these women.	Herbal medicines	Pregnancy, labour and birth	Herbalists, TBAs and some spiritualists
Damanik (2009) [51]	Indonesia (LMIC)	64 (including 24 current mothers; 36 grandmothers)	In-depth interviews and Focus group discussions	Content analysis and Ethnography	To gather information about cultural beliefs and practices around the use of the plant Torbangun (*Coleus amboinicus Lour*) as a galactagogue by Indonesian women postnatally.	Herbal medicines	Breastfeeding and the postpartum month	Shared cultural traditions; mothers, mothers-in-law, and husbands of the new mother
Ejidokun (2000) [54]	Nigeria (LMIC)	25 (23 pregnant women; 2 health care providers who were also local grandmothers and midwives)	Focus group discussions (23 pregnant women) and in depth interviews (2 health	Thematic content analysis	Assess the knowledge, attitudes and practices related to maternal anaemia among pregnant women, health workers land the community in	Iron and folic acid tablets	Pregnancy	Media: radio & printed advertisements on buses; health clinic workers; information given in places of worship like mosques.

Table 2 Pertinent features of included studies *(Continued)*

Author (date)	Country (economic classification [a])	Number of participants	Data collection method	Data analysis method	Study aims	CMPs reported on in the papers [b]	Stage in the continuum of childbearing reporting use of the CMP as interpreted by the author [c]	Information sources women access for CMPs
			professionals)		two Nigerian sites; to identify barriers and enablers to the use of folic acid and iron tablets by pregnant women; assess family members' and maternal health care providers' awareness of maternal anaemia, and how much importance they attach to it.			
Elter et al. (2016) [58]	Thailand (UPIC)	16 (all pregnant women)	In-depth interviews, participant observations, and a demographic record	Interpretive phenomenology	To explore first-time Thai mothers' experiences of postpartum family practices, particularly their experiences and understandings of spiritual healing.	Herbal medicines	Early postnatal period including breastfeeding	Shared cultural knowledge; family elders
Grewal et al. (2008) [43]	Canada (HIC)	15 (postnatal women with babies less than 3 months) [N.B. 5 health care professionals and community leaders also provided recommendations based on the study findings]	In-depth interviews	Naturalistic qualitative descriptive design	Describe knowledge and cultural traditions of newly immigrated Punjabi women's pregnancy, birth and postnatal experiences in Canada; the role of family and community in these experiences and how women incorporate these beliefs and practices into the Canadian health care system; and women's interactions with the Canadian health care system	Herbal medicines	Labour and birth, early postnatal period and breastfeeding	Shared cultural knowledge; elders especially female family members including mothers, mothers-in-law, and sisters-in-law and husbands (if no extended family around) prepared the herbs in foods and teas for the women
Holst et al. (2009) [52]	United Kingdom (HIC)	6 pregnant women (all women were recruited from an antenatal clinic and had used herbs in pregnancy)	One Focus Group Discussion	Content analysis	To increase understanding of women's reasons for using herbal products during pregnancy	Herbal medicines	Pregnancy	Family and friends; internet; CAM and biomedical HCPs
Juntunen et al. (2000) [7]	Tanzania (LIC)	49 (including 28 women; 21 men; informant also included a pastor; traditional healer; farmers; teachers; village health workers; traditional birth attendant; and trained hospital staff)	Open-ended interviews and participatory observation	Ethnography	To identify cultural care practices and beliefs around health protection the Bena people use throughout their lifetime	Herbal medicines	Pregnancy, labour and birth, early postnatal period	Local traditional African healers; older women in the community

Table 2 Pertinent features of included studies *(Continued)*

Author (date)	Country (economic classification [a])	Number of participants	Data collection method	Data analysis method	Study aims	CMPs reported on in the papers [b]	Stage in the continuum of childbearing reporting use of the CMP as interpreted by the author [c]	Information sources women access for CMPs
Lamxay et al. (2011) [56]	Lao People's Democratic Republic (LMIC)	30 (23 women; 7 men)	Group interviews and individual interviews	Ethnobotanical research	To study the activities and diet followed by the Kry ethnic group in Lao People's Democratic Republic during pregnancy, childbirth and postpartum confinement period, and identify medicinal plants used during these times.	Herbal medicines	Pregnancy, labour and birth, postpartum period and breastfeeding	Husbands and other relatives, other mothers who had given birth several times and acted as assistants to the birthing woman
Liamputtong et al. (2005) [4]	Thailand (UPIC)	30 (all women - most had recently given birth; a few were currently pregnant)	In-depth interviews	Phenomenology	To understand women's traditional beliefs and practices regarding pregnancy and childbirth among women in Northern Thailand, including the role of a traditional midwife.	Herbal medicines	Pregnancy, labour and birth	Mothers or women and men of older generations; *mor mon*, a magical healer or older man who has knowledge about magical cures and healing
Mogawane et al. (2015) [64]	South Africa (UPIC)	15 (all currently pregnant women)	Unstructured one-on-one interviews	Qualitative, explorative, descriptive, and contextual research design	Investigate the Indigenous [medical] practices of pregnant women attending the Dilokong hospital, Limpopo Province, South Africa	Herbal medicines	Pregnancy, labour and birth	Traditional African Healers, TBAs, also community elders and church leaders
Ngomane & Mulaudzi (2012) [57]	South Africa (UPIC)	12 (all currently pregnant women)	Unstructured in-depth interviews	Narrative analysis	To explore and describe the Indigenous beliefs and practices that influence late antenatal clinic attendance by pregnant women	Herbal medicines	Pregnancy, labour and birth	TBAs and family members
Obermeyer (2000) [46]	Morocco (LMIC)	151 (including 126 postnatal women; 20 modern (biomedical) health care providers; 5 traditional birth attendants)	Semi-structured in-depth interviews and observation in homes and clinics	Ethnography	Model the ethnophysiology and symbolism of pregnancy and birth in Morocco and what this implies for women's maternal health; understand women's health care and decision-making actions regarding birth	Herbal medicines and vitamin supplements	Pregnancy, labour and birth	Traditional midwives and traditional healers
Okafor et al. (2014) [8]	Nigeria (LMIC)	25 (all women who had delivered a baby in the previous 2 years)	Focus group discussions	No theory stated except Framework Method used to analyse data	Discover rural women's preferred choice of health care provider for pregnancy and delivery services in Lagos, Nigeria; inform maternal health care services for rural Nigerian women	Herbal medicines	Pregnancy, labour and birth	TBAs
Rice (2000) [44]	Australia (HIC)	33 (including 27 women; three shamans; two medicine women; one magic healer)	In-depth interviews and participant observation	Ethnography	To examine cultural beliefs and practices related to the 30 day confinement period after birth in Hmong society for Hmong women now residing in Australia. Also to discuss traditional and changing patterns of childbearing for	Herbal medicines	Breastfeeding and the postpartum month	Shared cultural knowledge; Medicine Women, Shamans, Traditional Hmong healers.

Table 2 Pertinent features of included studies *(Continued)*

Author (date)	Country (economic classification [a])	Number of participants	Data collection method	Data analysis method	Study aims	CMPs reported on in the papers [b]	Stage in the continuum of childbearing reporting use of the CMP as interpreted by the author [c]	Information sources women access for CMPs
					these women in their new social environment.			
Rutakumwa & Krogman (2007) [59]	Uganda (LIC)	63 (all rural women living in Uganda)	Semi-structured interviews	Not stated, except constant comparative method of analysis to develop descriptive categories	Identify rural Ugandan women's perspectives on their own health problems, their solutions and coping strategies, and their recommendations for improving services to suit their health needs.	Herbal medicines	Pregnancy	Shared cultural knowledge, older female family members, TBAs.
Sim et al. (2014) [55]	Australia (HIC)	20 (women all currently breastfeeding, or who had breastfed in previous 12 months; all had used herbal galactagogues)	In-depth, semi-structured interviews	Thematic analysis - transcripts were analysed using descriptive and qualitative approaches	Understand women's perspectives and attitudes towards using herbal galactagogues during breastfeeding; understand women's choices in using alternative medicine to promote breastfeeding; identify factors that influence their decision-making.	Herbal medicines	Breastfeeding	Internet and social-media based mothers' groups, family and friends, trusted HCPS [biomedical HCPs, and CAM HCPs, and Lactation Consultants]
Thwala et al. (2011) [47]	Swaziland (LMIC)	15 (all women with at least 1 child, the youngest less than 2 years old)	Unstructured interviews	Ethnography	Describe the values, beliefs and childbirth practices of rural Swazi women in pregnancy, labour and the postpartum period.	Herbal medicines	Pregnancy	Shared cultural traditions, Traditional African Healers, mothers-in-law.
Waiswa et al. (2008) [45]	Uganda (LIC)	10 focus group discussions with mothers under 30 years of age, older mothers including grandmothers, fathers and childminders [but no exact number given for each FGD]; 6 key informant interviews with 6 health workers and 4 TBAs	Focus group discussions and in depth key informant interviews	Latent thematic content analysis	Assess the acceptability of Millennium Development Goals to reduce infant and maternal mortality in rural Ugandan communities; identify acceptable factors and barriers and to ante and postnatal care.	Herbal medicines	Pregnancy	Shared cultural traditions and practices; TBAs.
Warriner et al. (2014) [63]	United Kingdom (HIC)	10 (all currently pregnant women)	In-depth interviews	Not stated just thematic analysis used in analysis of transcripts	To investigate over the counter [OTC] use of complementary medicines and pharmaceutical medications in pregnancy, the role of others in influencing women's choice to use CMPs, and how issues of choice and control influence women's use of OTC CMPs and pharmaceuticals in pregnancy.	Vitamin and mineral supplements, homoeopathic remedies and herbal medicines available over the counter	Pregnancy	Homoeopaths, doctors and midwives, other pregnant women.

Table 2 Pertinent features of included studies *(Continued)*

Author (date)	Country (economic classification [a])	Number of participants	Data collection method	Data analysis method	Study aims	CMPs reported on in the papers [b]	Stage in the continuum of childbearing reporting use of the CMP as interpreted by the author [c]	Information sources women access for CMPs
Westfall (2003a) [40] *Herbal healing*	Canada (HIC)	33 (27 currently pregnant women, of whom 26 used herbal medicines in pregnancy; 6 mentors including herbalists, authors and midwives)	In-depth interviews	Thematic analysis	To give voice to women's self-prescription of herbal medicines in pregnancy; understand women's perceptions of the roles and safety of herbal medicine use in pregnancy, and the choice to use herbal medicine in pregnancy.	Herbal medicines	Pregnancy	Own knowledge, own intuition, and trusted sources including books, friends, family members, biomedical HCP maternity care providers, CAM HCPs (herbalists), herbal shops, and the internet. Six mentors were listed by participants – these were midwives and childbirth educators and herbalists
Westfall (2003b) [10] *Galactagogue herbs*	Canada (HIC)	23 (women, all currently breastfeeding; 14 had used herbal galactagogues)	In-depth interviews	Thematic analysis	To discuss the potential value of five galactagogue herbs used by breastfeeding women, including the women's own observations, historical use safety and efficacy; inform future research.	Herbal medicines	Breastfeeding	Midwives, friends, mothers, public health nurse, doula.
Westfall (2004) [41] *Anti-emetic herbs in pregnancy*	Canada (HIC)	27 (all currently pregnant; 20 had nausea and vomiting of pregnancy, and of these 10 had used herbal medicines to treat)	In-depth interviews	Thematic analysis	Discuss the details of the herbal medicines used by women to treat pregnancy-induced nausea and vomiting.	Herbal medicines	Pregnancy	Herbalists
Wilkinson & Callister (2010) [48]	Ghana (LMIC)	24 (all pregnant women; some HCP quotes also included)	In-depth interviews and participant observation	Ethnography with the Health Belief Model	Describe the perceptions of childbirth held by Ghanaian women; inform health policy makers and health care providers to insure women receive clinically safe and culturally sensitive care.	Herbal medicines and vitamins	Pregnancy	Herbalists, biomedical midwives
Wulandari & Whelan (2011) [53]	Indonesia (Bali) (LMIC)	18 (all currently pregnant women)	In-depth interviews	Content analysis	Explore the beliefs, attitudes and behaviours of pregnant women in Bali, Indonesia	Herbal medicines and iron tablets	Pregnancy	Shared cultural knowledge, family members
Yeo et al. (2000) [49]	USA (HIC)	22 (11 couples - 11 women and their 11 husbands in were interviewed in pregnancy and then postnatally)	In-depth interviews	Ethnography	Examine Japanese couple's perceptions and experiences of prenatal care and childbirth in Michigan, USA; explore implications for providing culturally competent care.	Pre and postnatal vitamins	Pregnancy and breastfeeding	Shared cultural knowledge, doctors, family and friends.
Young & Ali (2005) [50]	Tanzania (Zanzibar) (LIC)	52 (including 25 mothers; 27 health care workers including	Informal conversations,	Ethnography	Using ethnography as the basis, to describe traditional	Traditional iron remedies and iron	Pregnancy and the postpartum month	Iron tablets – hospital and nurses; Traditional

Table 2 Pertinent features of included studies *(Continued)*

Author (date)	Country (economic classification [a])	Number of participants	Data collection method	Data analysis method	Study aims	CMPs reported on in the papers [b]	Stage in the continuum of childbearing reporting use of the CMP as interpreted by the author [c]	Information sources women access for CMPs
		4 government health officials; 3 biomedical doctors; 2 maternity ward nurses; 4 health aides; 2 pharmacists; 3 three TBAs; 1 diviner/healer; 3 traditional medicine makers; 5 employees at private pharmacies)	in-depth interviews, focus group discussions and participant observation		(non-biomedical) treatments for maternal iron deficiency anaemia in Zanzibar; describe women's choices in choosing treatments; inform health planners of these choices so that and culturally appropriate care can be provided, with the aim to reduce maternal anaemia.	tablets		remedies – traditional healers

TBAs Traditional Birth Assistants or Attendants, *Biomedical HCPs* biomedically trained health care practitioners - nurses, midwives, doctors and obstetricians; *CAM HCPs* Western complementary medicine health care practitioners including naturopaths and herbalists trained in Western Herbal Medicine

[a] *LIC* low income economy, *LMIC* lower middle income economy, *UPIC* upper middle income economy, *HIC* high income economy according to The World Bank Classifications [33], based on 2015 gross national income per capita

[b] Complementary medicine type discussed in the paper, as identified by the first author (LAJB)

[c] For the purposes of this review and analysis of the identified studies, the first author (LAJB) conceptualised the continuum of childbearing from pregnancy, birth, the early postpartum period, longer postpartum period and breastfeeding as separate but related stages

another [48] without information on how many HCPs participated. Additionally, some studies [7, 45, 56, 59] included discussions with pregnant or lactating women as well as other community members, family members and health care practitioners without reporting numbers of each type of participant. Hence the total number of pregnant and/or breastfeeding women across all studies that can actually be counted is 566, but will have been larger. For those studies where the number of pregnant and lactating women is clearly stated, sample sizes ranged between six and one hundred and twenty-six, and averaged 31. Overall, there was a wide variety in the number of participants, with the smallest being a UK study with just one focus group of six women [52] and the largest including 126 semi-structured interviews with women who had recently given birth in Morocco [46]. Most studies had between 15 and 35 participants.

Types of CMP discussed

Herbal medicine use was the main CMP discussed, with 21/28 focussing on herbal medicines exclusively, 3/28 discussing herbal medicines and vitamin supplements [46, 48, 53], and 3/25 discussing iron and folic acid [54], pre and postnatal vitamins [49], and traditional iron remedies and iron supplements [50] respectively. In addition to vitamin and mineral supplements and herbal medicines, homoeopathic remedies were also included in one paper [63].

Focus on pregnancy and/or breastfeeding

Although the continuum of childbearing can be conceptualised from pre-conception through pregnancy, birth, the postpartum period and breastfeeding, there was great variety in the foci of the papers included (Fig. 2). Only nine papers discussed CMP use during breastfeeding [10, 43, 44, 49, 51, 55, 56, 58, 60]. The remaining 19 papers discussed CMP use in pregnancy and other childbearing stages without reference to breastfeeding.

Information sources accessed by women around the world

The information sources accessed by women when choosing to use CMPs in pregnancy and lactation are illustrated in Fig. 3 (and by country groups, see Additional file 3). Shared cultural knowledge and traditions (14 papers) followed by women elders (women's own mothers, mothers-in-law and grandmothers, other older experienced female family members) (11 papers) were information sources identified most commonly. Following this, women accessed their health care providers for information – for women from LMIC and LIC countries and backgrounds this included Traditional Birth Assistants, traditional (non-Western) herbalists or healers, medicine women, magical healers or shamans [4, 7, 8, 44–47, 59, 60, 62, 64] but also included biomedical health care practitioners in some studies [48, 50, 54]. Similarly, women from HIC backgrounds often sought information from biomedical health care providers as well as Western herbalists or naturopathic practitioners [40, 52, 55, 63]. One significant difference between women in high income countries and low to middle income countries, was that women in HICs reported accessing CMP information via the Internet, whereas women from low and low-middle income countries did not. The studies involving immigrant women from lower income countries into HICs (Punjabi women to

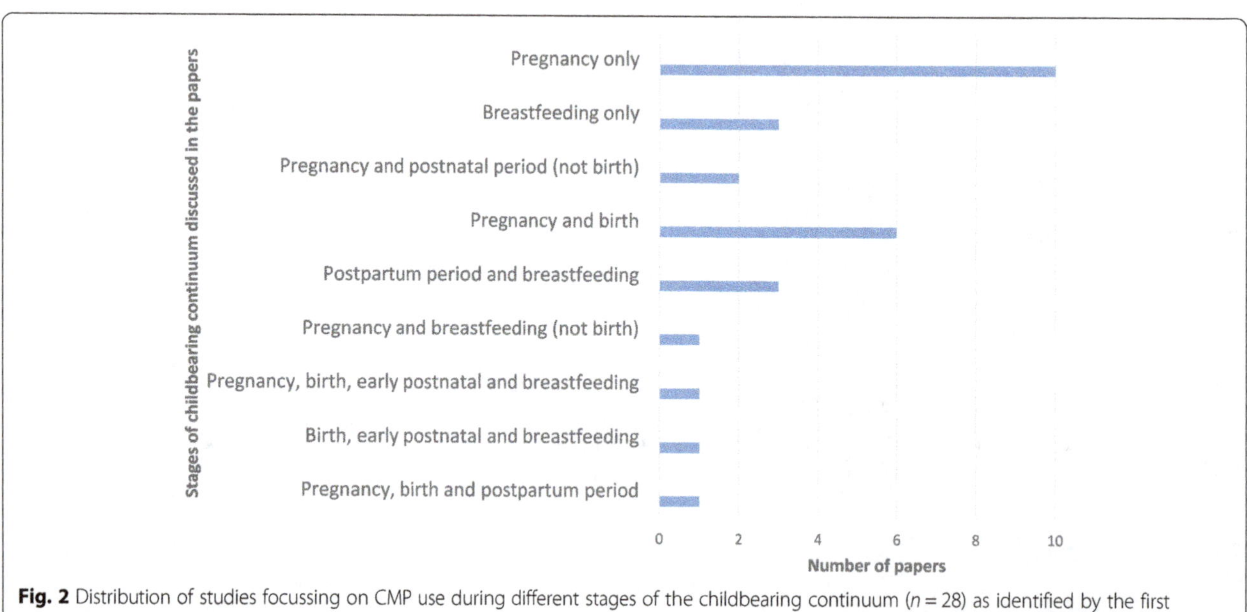

Fig. 2 Distribution of studies focussing on CMP use during different stages of the childbearing continuum ($n = 28$) as identified by the first author (LAJB)

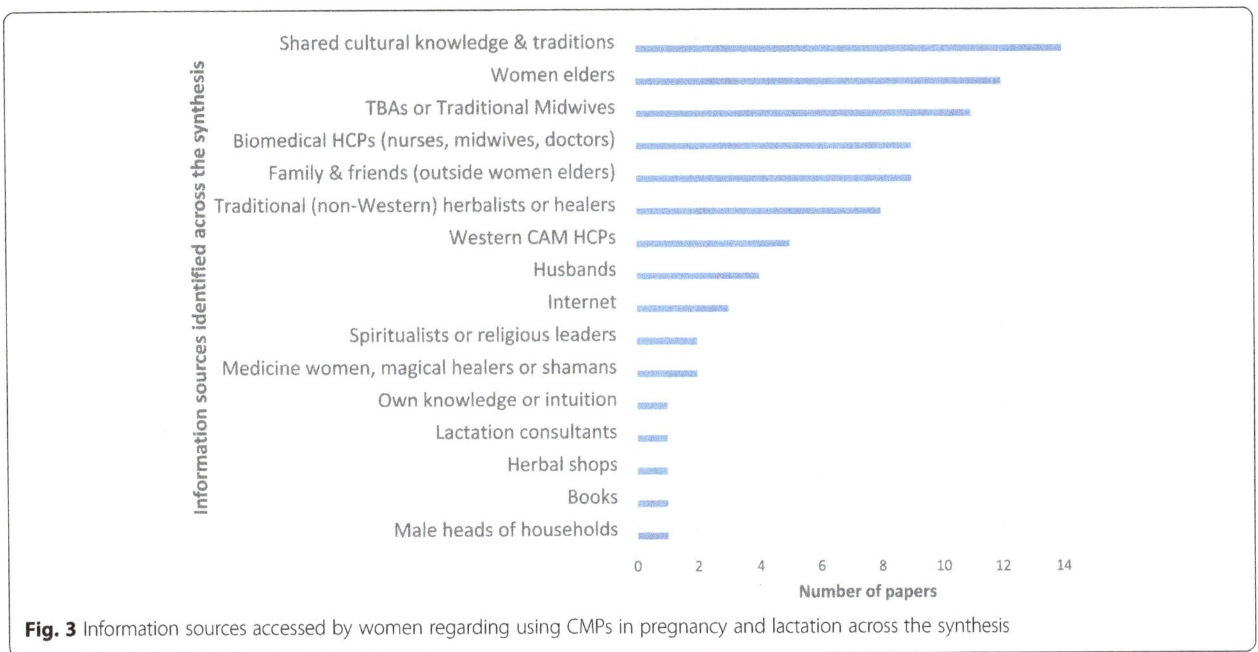

Fig. 3 Information sources accessed by women regarding using CMPs in pregnancy and lactation across the synthesis

Canada, Hmong women to Australia) showed that the women brought their cultural traditions and knowledge with them to their new countries and that traditional knowledge and practices remained important. Similarly, Yeo, Fetters [49] found that the strong cultural beliefs held by Japanese women living in the USA influenced their willingness to take prenatal vitamin supplements. The near-universality of family and friends being reported as information sources is evident when combining the group reporting women elders and other female family members, husbands and family and friends together.

Discussion of health literacy in the papers

For the included studies, the role of health literacy in women's use of CMPs during pregnancy and lactation was complex. The reasons why mothers make decisions about their own and their children's health care are influenced by women's individual skills and abilities to access and evaluate health information, as well as individual skills and knowledge [65, 66]. None of the included studies directly measured the health literacy levels of participants and nor did any discuss findings explicitly in relation to health literacy as an over-arching concept. However, participants' knowledge, attitudes and practices, all of which are concepts related to health literacy, were discussed.

Knowledge, attitudes and practices

All studies discussed participants' knowledge, attitudes and practices. 'Health beliefs and practices' was the most commonly discussed aspect of health (18/28 papers) followed by 'health knowledge, attitudes and practices' (12/28), 'health care seeking behaviours' (12/28) and 'health behaviours' (11/28). Health beliefs and practices were the greatest influence on women's use of CMPs across the papers – women took CMPs because of perceived health benefits to themselves and/or their babies (discussed further below). The cultural importance regarding use of CMPs was also evident, especially for women from LICs and LMICs [45–47, 50, 51, 53, 54, 59, 60], but also for women in UPICs and HICs who described the importance of specific cultural practices during pregnancy, childbirth and the postpartum period [4, 43, 44, 49, 58, 61]. For many, the information regarding the cultural importance of CMP use during the childbearing continuum was passed on to them through women elders in their communities [7, 43, 44, 47, 51, 53, 57–61, 64] (also see Fig. 3).

Women's health beliefs, practices, and health behaviours were influenced by their health knowledge and attitudes. For women in developing countries, knowledge of the biomedical model of pregnancy and birthing care was often poor. Women did not understand how regular antenatal care could help reduce their own and their babies' risks of morbidity and mortality [45, 57, 62]. Women's cultural knowledge regarding needs for traditional medical care along with their needs for psychosocial support led them to seek traditional care, and their albeit limited understanding of the biomedical model motivated them to access biomedical care [8, 45–48, 59, 62, 64]. In more wealthy economies, women's engagement in medical pluralism was also discussed in relation to health beliefs and practices. Women's perceptions of CMPs as being safer than pharmaceutical medications was explored [10, 40, 41, 52, 55, 63], as was their use of CMPs as part of efforts to increase autonomy, and self-responsibility for their own and their infants' health [40, 55, 63]. Knowledge regarding the safety profiles of herbal medicine especially was also considered low in several of the studies across income streams [52, 53, 63], although this was usually discussed from the perspective of a biomedical outsider, with requisite concerns regarding lack of scientific testing of the CMPs being the basis of authors' concerns.

The focus of almost half the discussions (13/28) was on how to improve patient outcomes through culturally competent care [4, 43–45, 47, 49, 50, 53, 54, 56, 57, 61, 64]. Women's health knowledge, attitudes, beliefs, and practices were all discussed in relation to their health care seeking behaviours and especially in the poorer countries where maternal morbidity and mortality are high, in relation to their health outcomes. For these poorer communities, whole of community approaches to improving the health literacy through education and information dissemination were commonly proposed [45, 50, 53, 54, 57, 60], as often pregnant or breastfeeding women experienced significant barriers to accessing biomedical health care. These barriers included geographical isolation and/or gender inequities [47, 59, 60], as well as cultural norms that advocated family decision-making over individual decision-making and where family based care during pregnancy and the postpartum period was the norm [45, 47, 53, 58, 60]. For women in wealthier economies where culturally competent care was also discussed, the focus was more on what biomedical HCPs could do to improve provider-patient communication and understand the culturally based needs of pregnant and breastfeeding women [43, 44, 49, 61].

Women's use of CMPs in pregnancy and lactation and their perceived benefits

Thematic analysis revealed that women's use of CMPs in pregnancy and lactation could be separated into several themes with associated subthemes. Additionally, women's use of CMPs in pregnancy and lactation can be separated into two main over-arching motives, 'Protective or preventative actions' or 'Facilitation of a normal process' (Table 3). These themes and subthemes are further elaborated in Additional file 4.

Discussion

All mothers want what is best for themselves and their unborn and breastfeeding babies and this review has identified that mothers from a range of economically advantaged countries use CMPs to help facilitate this. Underpinning this desire and the decision-making associated with it are several factors: a woman's individual health literacy, the health literacy environments she moves in, her own culture and the cultures at play in the health literacy environment, considerations of safety and where the locus of control regarding decision making in pregnancy and lactation sits.

Culture, health literacy and holistic health

This review's identification of shared cultural knowledge as a major information source for women choosing to use CMPs in pregnancy and lactation warrants further discussion of culture, health literacy and holistic health.

The United Nations Educational, Scientific and Cultural Organization defines culture as "the set of distinctive spiritual, material, intellectual and emotional features of society or a social group, and that it encompasses, in addition to art and literature, lifestyles, ways of living together, value systems, traditions and beliefs" [67]. This definition has been accepted by the World Health Organisation's expert group on the cultural contexts of health and wellbeing [68]. Culture is a way of life, and can include religious, social or ethnic characteristics, but is also dynamic as values and practices can change over time. It is also important to acknowledge that all kinds of knowledge are cultural, including the practices of traditional health care systems, Western complementary health care systems, and scientific and biomedical practices [68]. A mother's own culture influences both her individual health literacy skills and abilities, and how she accesses, evaluates and uses health care information and services in her health literacy environment when making decisions about her own and her children's health. Additionally she may also encounter different cultural knowledge bases within both the health system infrastructure and in the people and relationships within the health literacy environment including other care-givers, the health care team and systems accessed, each with their own personal and medical cultural knowledge bases [31, 32, 65]. Thus it can be argued that women make the decisions to use CMPs in pregnancy and lactation both within the context of their own cultures and the cultures of the health literacy environment. This is illustrated in Fig. 4 which builds on Parker's [66] model, used by the Australian Commission on Safety and Quality in Health Care in their working definition of health literacy [65]. The cultural components of health literacy and the ways they impact on individual health literacy and the health literacy environments are depicted in the orange boxes added to the original model (in green and white). In this way, the original model is expanded to include both (i) an individual mother's culture, and how her culture influences the ways she uses her skills and abilities to access and interpret health information; and (ii) the different cultural knowledge bases extant in the health literacy environment in which she moves.

'Protection and prevention' and 'Facilitation of normal physiological processes'.

Table 3 Thematic analysis: women's use of CMPs in pregnancy and lactation and perceived benefits

Use of CMPs during pregnancy			
Major themes	*Subthemes*	*Over-arching motive 'Protective or preventative action' OR 'Facilitation of a normal process'*	*Selected examples (full thematic analysis can be seen in* Additional file 3*)* *(in italics – participant direct quotes; in* Roman (non-italicised) - text quotes (the papers did not always include quotes)
Women's use of CMPs – perceived physical benefits			
For the benefit of the pregnancy	• Prevention of vaginal bleeding and miscarriage in early pregnancy • Protect against vaginal leaking and bleeding in both early and late pregnancy	Protective or preventative action	*"At the initial stages of my pregnancy I was bleeding and I came to the hospital for drugs but it was persistent. So I went for herbal medicine and it helped me" (Focus group participant, ANC client, Madina)"* (Dako-Gyeke et al. 2013, p211) [62]
	• Ensure a safe pregnancy	Facilitation of a normal process	*"I have been advised to drink boiled herbs (Mbita) for the preservation and protection of my unborn baby, so that I may have a safe pregnancy and labour."* (Ngomane & Mulaudzi, 2012, p34) [57]
For the benefit of the baby	• Promotion of the developing baby's physical health - assist the baby's intrauterine growth and support their well-being, health and vitality • Monitor the baby's health and growth	Facilitation of a normal process	*"I think both [iron pills and herbal medicine] are important, aren't they? I take the herbals regularly and I feel that my baby is healthy that was also what I did in my first pregnancy. I regularly took the herbals and nothing's wrong with my baby. In fact, he was very vigorous. (Woman 6)"* (Wulandari & Whelan, 2011, p868–9) [53]
	• No perceived benefit for the use of CMPs in pregnancy – taking vitamins was incompatible with Japanese cultural beliefs around taking medications in pregnancy	Neither	*"I have been eating Japanese food in the United States just like I did in Japan when I had my first child. I never took a vitamin with my first child. .. and it did not have any bad effects on my child. .. then American doctors told me that it's better to take vitamins. .. I don't mind taking it, but I don't know why I need to take it, as nothing bad happened with my first child in Japan." (Yeo* et al.*, 2000, p194)* [49]
For the benefit of the mother	• Prevention or treatment of common illnesses associated with pregnancy like thrush and urinary tract infections • Prevention or treatment of non-pregnancy related illnesses • First line treatment of maternal danger signs in pregnancy • Protection against the development of pregnancy complications	Protective or preventative action	"The participants identified *'aseje'*, (a special concoction, mainly herbs) as one of the attractions of seeking care from TBAs. It is believed that the *'aseje'* prevents development of any complications during pregnancy and labour and keeps pregnant women healthy" (Okafor et al. 2014, p46) [8]
	• Safe support for mother's own physical health • Treatment of maternal anaemia; provision of nourishment • Safe form of treatment for nausea and vomiting of pregnancy • Treatment of abdominal pain in pregnancy	Facilitation of a normal process	"Tonic herbs can be thought of as lying somewhere in between food and drugs; they are used therapeutically, to treat sub-clinical conditions or to prevent health degeneration. They are used to strengthen, nourish and support the body, to prevent rather than cure disease [...] The most popular herb was raspberry leaf *(Rubus idaeus)* - a uterine tonic - used by 22 women." (Westfall 2003 – herbal healing, pp26–27) [40].
For the benefit of the labour and birthing processes	• Prevention of vaginal tearing during birth and reducing risk of caesarean section • Prevention of foetal distress	Protective or preventative action	"A typical example is what is locally known as *amalagala*, a product of crushed sweet-potato leaves mixed with water. This mixture is administered to pregnant women, who bathe in it or sit on it to lessen the risk of requiring a Caesarean section or of vaginal tearing during delivery. The women did not discuss trial and error for this concoction but unanimously reported confidence in its efficacy"

Table 3 Thematic analysis: women's use of CMPs in pregnancy and lactation and perceived benefits *(Continued)*

			(Rutakumwa & Krogman, 2007) [59]
	• Use of herbal tonics to tone the uterus and strengthen it in preparation for labour • Prepare for an easy birth • Enhance or induce labour • Relieve labour pains • Induce expulsion of retained placenta • Relieve afterbirth pains	Facilitation of a normal process	"Consumption of traditional herbal medicine was also mentioned as a way of preparing for an easy birth. The traditional herbal medicine was referred to as *ya tom*. A woman must consume *ya tom* three times per day for three consecutive days. Women can purchase dried herbal medicine and boil it until it reduces to small cup quantity and drink it as tea. This is believed to make the baby strong, hence facilitating an easy birth." (Liamputtong et al. 2005, p146) [4]
Women's use of CMPs in pregnancy to protect against spiritual threats to themselves and their unborn babies – perceived benefits involving spiritual protection			
For the benefit of both mother and baby	• Protect the baby from spiritual threats that could cause physical harm including death of the foetus or preterm labour	Protective or preventative action	"All the women in this study stated that both the mother and baby might fall ill because of *kuhabula*. To prevent illness therefore, the women expressed belief in the power of traditional doctors and medicine, or divine prayer if the women or family was religious". .. *[traditional medicines are taken] to make sure that the baby is protected on all fronts; protected from kuhabula [acquisition of illnesses from bad spirits in the environment] through the use of traditional medicine"* (Thwala et al., 2011, p95) [47]
II. Use of CMPs during breastfeeding			
Women's use of CMPs – perceived physical benefits			
For the benefit of the breastfeeding process	• Increased breastmilk production – perceived and diagnosed milk insufficiency • Use of galactagogues 'just in case' breastmilk supply needs support • Use of galactagogues to build supply as part of a cultural tradition (note, no mention of perceived insufficiency)	Facilitation of a normal process	*"I think it's [fenugreek] worth trying. And as for me, I certainly find that useful and reassuring that I have found something effective to increase my milk supply. As a new mum, you just never know, you never know what is coming, what problems you will encounter and I certainly did not anticipate that milk supply will be an issue. I have always thought that breastfeeding is easy and will come naturally because everyone else does it, and I wasn't told about it being an issue". (BW 12).* (Sim et al., 2014, p216) [55]
For the benefit of the breastfeeding process and the mother's physical health	• Use of galactagogues supports post-birth recovery and also builds breastmilk supply	Facilitation of a normal process Protective or preventative action	"During the early postpartum period as women recovered, family members again provided certain foods that were believed to have 'hot effects' and bring the body into balance. These types of food are seen as essential for healing and recovery from the birthing process (arising from Ayurveda traditions), including relieving back pain, promoting menstrual flow to cleanse the body, building the mother's milk supply, and preventing weakness and illness in later life. 'Hot foods' included … chai (fennel seed tea with ginger) … and other special foods … made from 'heat-producing' ingredients such as ginger powder, fennel seeds … and special herbs." (Grewal, 2008, p294) [43]
For the benefit of the mother's physical health	• Expulsion of lochia through 'uterine cleansing' and control of postpartum bleeding • Assists in recovery after childbirth • Restoration of physical balance through heat	Facilitation of a normal process	*"You eat them [chicken herbal medicine] so that your body will settle back to normal quicker and if you don't use them then it will take you a long time to get back to normal. The bleeding will go on for a long time and that will make you very thin. That is not good.. . If you bleed too long the body won't get back to normal again and this can make you pale and skinny. If you have the chicken herbs to eat then your*

Table 3 Thematic analysis: women's use of CMPs in pregnancy and lactation and perceived benefits *(Continued)*

			blood will be good and you will feel strong quickly.. . You eat them to give you strength and also to wash out your blood quickly too" (Rice, 2000, p29) [44]
	• Treatment of a prolapsed uterus • Protection of the mother's future health	Protective or preventative action	"Considered the most important Chinese cultural practice is 'doing (or sitting) the month' (*zuoyuezi*). … 'Doing the month' includes activity restrictions, avoiding 'wind chill' ... and eating raw ginger soup with Chinese herbs to 'rid the body of cold' … If such practices as described are not followed, the new mother is at risk for 'the month disease,' which is thought to have deleterious effects on their health for the rest of their lives (Callister et al., 2011, pp390–1) [61]
For the benefit of the breastfeeding baby	• Protection of the breastfeeding baby through the mother's use of CMPs • Purification of mother's breasts in preparation for breastfeeding and to ensure breastmilk is sweet	Protective or 2preventative action	"The ingestion of local herbs is used as a means of warding off any harmful effects to the baby […] To protect the baby from health problems … the newly delivered mother, her mother, and her mother-in-law - should take local drugs [herbal medicines] before the grandmother sees the baby for the first time" (Juntunen et al., 2011, p177) [7]
	• Promotion of the baby's health through enabling the mother to continue to breastfeed	Facilitation of a normal process	"All participants seemed to have adopted the 'breast is best' philosophy. These women acknowledged and appreciated the health, physical and psychological benefits of breastfeeding to both mothers and infants. […] Recognition of the importance and significance of breastfeeding was identified as the main facilitator to develop perseverance and a determined attitude to breastfeed: *"I mean honestly, if drinking snake oil would make me have more breast milk I would have done it, anything that helps!"* (Sim et al., 2014, p216) [55]
Women's use of CMPs during breastfeeding – perceived mental-emotional benefits			
For the benefit of the mother	• Increased self-confidence, self-empowerment and reassurance • Increases my ability for self-care	Facilitation of a normal process	"Many participants also mentioned the feeling of reassurance through the use of herbal supplements during breastfeeding, which was especially important for first-time mothers. Hence, the use of herbal galactagogue was described as a method of reassurance in the context of their own perceptions. The positive emotional impact contributed to the success of breastfeeding practices amongst the participants." (Sim et al., 2014, p216) [55]
	• Restoration of mind-body balance	Protective or preventative action	"The herbs in hot bath, such as leaves of *Nat*, release aromatic oils, which are believed to relieve mind–heart, emotional, and psychological stress. LD said *'the water for a hot bath is boiled with leaves of an herb named Nat. The leaves will prevent her from feeling dizzy or being intoxicated.'* Leaves of *Nat* … can be used for treating fatigue, exhaustion, psychological and emotional imbalances, and postpartum depression [and also] to ward off a malevolent spirit and to make holy water. The women in this study used both the medicinal and supernatural properties of Nat leaves to treat the mind–heart essence" (Elter et al., 2016, p253) [58].
Women's use of CMPs during breastfeeding – perceived benefits involving spiritual protection			
For the benefit of the mother	• Spiritual protection in the postpartum period	Protective or preventative action	In Thailand, *Nat* leaves are also used to ward off a malevolent spirit and to make holy water.

Table 3 Thematic analysis: women's use of CMPs in pregnancy and lactation and perceived benefits *(Continued)*

			The women in this study used both the medicinal and supernatural properties of Nat leaves to treat the mind–heart essence" (Elter et al., 2016, p253) [58]
Women's use of CMPs during breastfeeding – perceived cultural benefits			
For the benefit of the mother	• Cultural cleansing rituals after childbirth	Facilitation of a normal process	"Also first-time mothers are expected to go through a cultural cleansing known as *sooru* in Kasem and *kosoto* in Nankani, regardless of the bitterness of their breastmilk. The process involves the pouring of warm herbal water over the mother for a period of 3 days if the child is a male and for 4 days if the child is female" (Aborigo et al. 2012, p76) [60]
III. Additional themes relating to perceived benefits of women's use of CMPs throughout the childbearing continuum			
Perceptions of safety regarding CMP use in pregnancy and lactation	• Complementary medicines are safer than pharmaceutical medications • Receiving reassurance that herbal medicines are safe during pregnancy and breastfeeding	Protective or preventative action	*'I am certainly not opposed to the idea of using herbs during breastfeeding, as long as I know and have checked with my child health nurses and doctors or even ringing up a pharmacist' (BW 12)"* (Sim et al., 2014, p216) [55]
Using both CMPs and concurrently accessing biomedical care promotes best care for both mother and baby	• Better management of maternity complications in pregnancy and birth • Protection of the baby from diseases understood to arise from spiritual causes as well as from diseases treatable with biomedical medicines	Protective or preventative action	*"I use traditional medicines during the pregnancy … I also go to the hospital every month to have check-ups. They give me pills which I take home to drink together with the traditional medicines [...I use both traditional medicines and hospital medicines] to make sure that the baby is protected on all fronts; protected from kuhabula [acquisition of illnesses from bad spirits in the environment] through the use of traditional medicine as well as protected from the hospital diseases by using their modern medicine."* (Thwala et al., 2012, p95) [69]

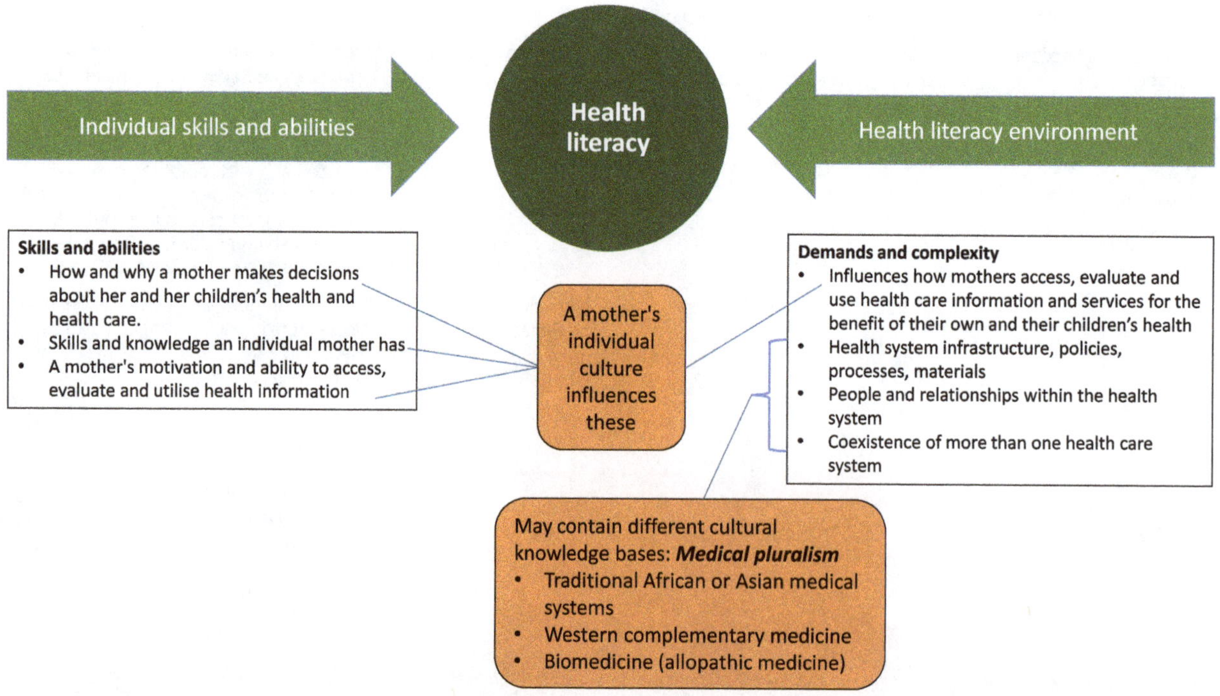

Individual skills and abilities

Health literacy

Health literacy environment

Skills and abilities
- How and why a mother makes decisions about her and her children's health and health care.
- Skills and knowledge an individual mother has
- A mother's motivation and ability to access, evaluate and utilise health information

A mother's individual culture influences these

Demands and complexity
- Influences how mothers access, evaluate and use health care information and services for the benefit of their own and their children's health
- Health system infrastructure, policies, processes, materials
- People and relationships within the health system
- Coexistence of more than one health care system

May contain different cultural knowledge bases: ***Medical pluralism***
- Traditional African or Asian medical systems
- Western complementary medicine
- Biomedicine (allopathic medicine)

Fig. 4 Impact of culture on health literacy, modified from Parker [66] and the Australian Commission on Safety and Quality in Health Care's working definition of health literacy [65]

Pregnant and lactating women in the countries sampled choose to use complementary medicine products based on two over-arching themes identified in this synthesis, *'Protective or preventative action' and/or 'Facilitation of a normal process'*. Women's motivation to use CMPs is based on the desire to both protect themselves and their babies from adverse events, and to facilitate the normal physiological processes of pregnancy, birth and breastfeeding. Women attempted to prevent adverse outcomes in pregnancy including miscarriage or malformation of the baby, ill health of the mother during pregnancy, and to prevent foetal distress and vaginal tearing in labour and birth. Additionally, CMPs were used to prevent future health problems for both mother and baby through the restoration of the mother's health in the postnatal period and the establishment of breastfeeding. Whilst this synthesis predominantly identified perceived physical benefits relating to CMP use in pregnancy and lactation, perceived mental-emotional, cultural and spiritual benefits were also found. Again, the impact of culture cannot be underestimated when examining women's health care choices in pregnancy and lactation. Whilst pregnancy, labour, birth and breastfeeding are physiologically comparable for all women, there is great variety in the social and cultural contexts within which these events occur, as well as in the individual customs, beliefs, morals and values women will bring to their individual experiences [7, 47, 69]. A woman's cultural heritage and her cultural environment will influence her health care decisions in pregnancy and lactation [61, 70]. Finlayson & Downe's [71] systematic review found that cultural beliefs regarding the need to protect a pregnancy from supernatural threats, combined with women's preferences for traditional medicines, contributed to the low use of biomedical antenatal services in LICs and LMICs. Also contributing to this low utilisation was the commonly held cultural view of pregnancy as a normal physiological state, as opposed to a biomedical perception of pregnancy as a risky situation [71]. These results support the current review's identification of the two overarching motivating themes 'protection and prevention' and 'facilitation of normal physiological processes' as strong motivators for women's use of CMPs during pregnancy and breastfeeding for women in developing economies. Studies from LIC and LMIC countries included in the present review also identified that traditional and cultural beliefs contribute to CMP use in pregnancy and lactation, and that women view herbal and traditional medicines as being safer, more effective, affordable and more easily accessed than pharmaceutical medications, [47, 57, 62, 72]. Regarding women in HICs, motivations for their CMP use during pregnancy have been examined in four systematic reviews. Pallivalappila et al. [73] were unable to make definitive conclusions regarding pregnant women's motivations regarding use of complementary medicine, or their perceptions of the effectiveness and safety of CMPs, due to substantial flaws in study design and reporting. However, three other reviews of CMP use by pregnant women in HICs [12–14] did find links between CMP use and women's preferences for holistic approaches to health, along with women's perceptions that use of complementary medicine facilitated better health, wellbeing and quality of life in pregnancy, and could help them prepare for a normal labour and birth. In line with the theme 'facilitation of normal physiological processes', women's desire for autonomy and control over individual pregnancy health were also identified as motivating factors for women's use of CMPs [12–14]. Consistent with the theme 'protection and prevention' Adams et al.'s [12] review also identified that women perceived their CMPs to be safer than pharmaceutical prescriptions when using CMPs to relieve pregnancy-related complaints.

Locus of control, culture and CMP use in pregnancy and lactation

Studies examining the health locus of control aim to describe what health beliefs influence people's health behaviours [74]. For pregnancy this could include measuring perceived responsibility pregnant women hold (internal locus of control) and the extent external forces like chance and health professionals (termed 'powerful others') will affect the health outcomes of their babies [75, 76]. For pregnant and breastfeeding women from LIC, LMIC and UPIC countries, powerful others also included their mothers and mothers-in-law and other extended family members who often provided both antenatal and postpartum care within a context of culturally prescribed practices. In contrast, for women from HICs, the use of CMPs was associated with increasing autonomy and taking self-responsibility for their own, and their babies' health [10, 55, 63]. This finding has also been documented in other qualitative and quantitative CAM research [77–79]. Locus of control can be seen as part of the wider cultural context and differs between cultures and for women living in countries of low versus high economic backgrounds.

Figure 5 illustrates how the two over-arching motivators for CMP use, *'Protective or preventative action' or 'Facilitation of a normal process',* and considerations of locus of control sit within the context of culture and its influence on health literacy. Pregnant and lactating women use CMPs for their perceived benefits for the mother, the pregnancy, the child and/or the breastfeeding process. Overlaying but also integral to this is the interactive model of health literacy [65, 66] which illustrates how each individual woman is influenced by her

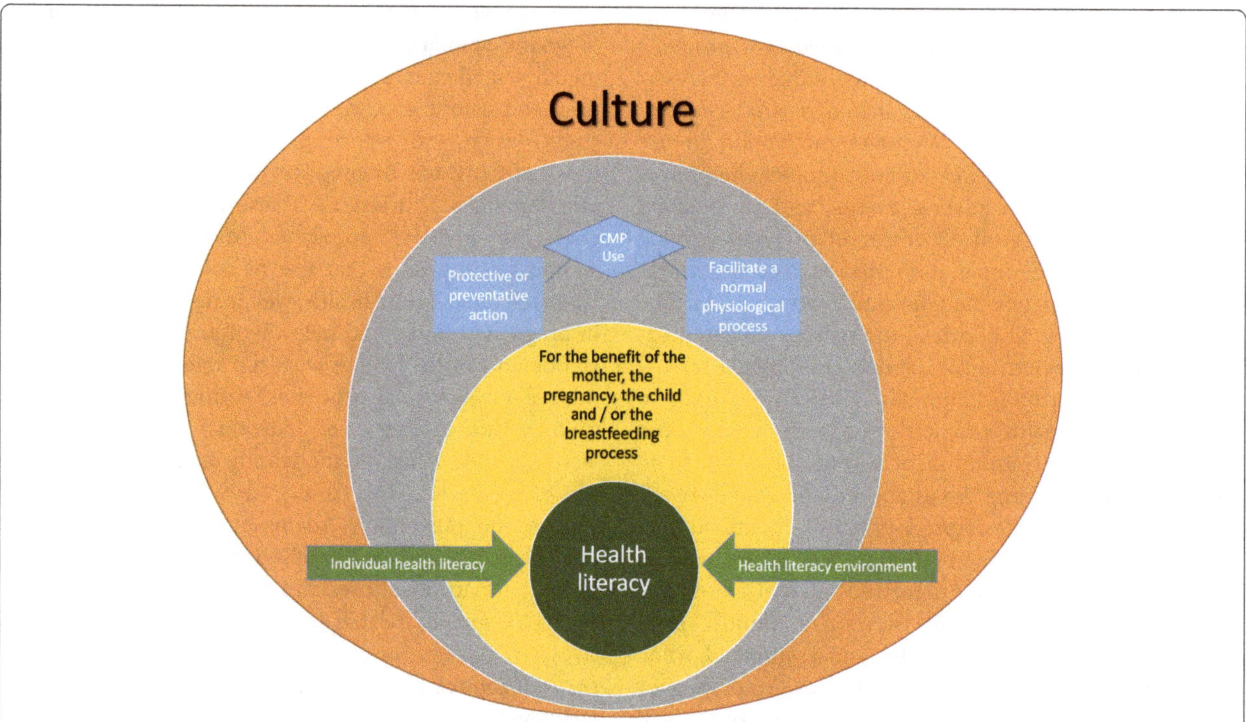

Fig. 5 Health literacy and women's decisions to use CMPs in pregnancy and lactation, within the overarching influence of culture, modified from Parker [66] and the Australian Commission on Safety and Quality in Health Care's working definition of health literacy [65]

individual health literacy and her health literacy environment. Culture is integral to both these components: it influences a woman's individual health literacy, and different cultural influences come into play at different levels of the model, including within different elements of the health literacy environment.

Medical pluralism and considerations of cultural influences on health care decision-making in pregnancy and lactation

The concurrent use of CAM and biomedicine has been well documented in many cultures [17, 80] and in pregnancy and lactation around the world [45, 47, 81–83]. This synthesis also highlights that many women used CMPs within a context of *medical pluralism,* defined as the co-occurrence of different medical or therapeutic systems and traditions in one local setting [1, 11]. Medical pluralism can also be seen as a patient centred model where individual consumers chose the level of integration between co-occurring health systems, which in turn facilitates a recognition of paradigm differences between biomedicine and complementary or traditional medical systems [84]. Both the autonomy of the individual woman, and the integrity of the different treatment systems she moves through are maintained [84]. Similarly to this current review, medical pluralism was identified as a contributor to women's choices in Nagata et al.'s [80] systematic review investigating social determinants of iron supplementation in women of reproductive age. Herbal medicines and home remedies were identified as being popular, and often utilised more readily in areas where medical pluralism allowed women to choose between these and biomedical or public health measures. The success of iron supplementation often depended on collaboration or mutual respect between biomedical and traditional medical or complementary medicine systems of healing [80]. Yixi & Rancine's [85] integrative review of the healthcare experiences of Chinese women immigrants in English-speaking countries also found that women embraced medical pluralism and utilised both Traditional Chinese and the Western biomedical healthcare approaches in a pragmatic way that allowed them to expand their healthcare choices and gave them more comprehensive ways of understanding and managing their health concerns. The current review also showed that women's engagement with medical pluralism increased their healthcare choices in pregnancy and lactation. Additionally, it was found that women's health literacy environments also reflect medical pluralism as the important information sources many accessed included biomedical HCPs as well as traditional healers and Western complementary medicine practitioners. As a result, for most of the studies, women navigated through and between different heath care services and systems, seeking and receiving care from both biomedical practitioners and CAM or traditional medical practitioners. However, this does not mean that women asked all their biomedical, traditional or CAM

HCPs for information on CMPs. In studies involving women from East or South Asia (Indonesia, Thailand, China, Lao and India), HCPs were not identified as information sources on CMPs, rather shared cultural knowledge, women elders or other family members were the important information sources on herbal medicines [4, 43, 44, 51, 53, 56, 58, 61]. However, except for the study on Kry women from Lao [56], the women in all these studies did engage in medical pluralism as it is evident from the papers that they accessed biomedical care whilst pregnant or breastfeeding. Additionally, their exclusion of HCPs as information sources for CMPs may reflect more the questions asked to investigate the aims of each study, as other studies included in this synthesis showed that biomedical and traditional health care practitioners were important sources of information on CMPs for pregnant and lactating women originating from East Asia (Lao and Japan) [44, 49].

Medical pluralism and the concept of holism

It is useful to examine the reasons behind women's engagement in medical pluralism further. MacArtney and Wahlberg [17] argue that some opponents of complementary medicine frame CAM users as ignorant of scientific methods of research, deceived by false advertising or claims, or irrational believers with a distrust of science itself, and view CAM practitioners or advocates as immoral in offering placebo or inferior treatments in place of biomedical options. This judgemental approach is unhelpful as it prevents any understanding of the evidence for why people choose to use CAM or CMPs, and polarises the debate into automatically generated positive or negative responses [17]. It also discounts the evidence showing that engagement in medical pluralism is common, and disregards wider issues that may be at play including individual health literacy and the health literacy environment, factors that play important roles in the wellbeing of women and their babies. As discussed above, engagement with plural medical systems can be seen to expand a woman's healthcare choices [80, 85] and to determine the information sources she accesses as part of her health literacy environment when seeking to support her own and her children's health. Conversely, there are also risks women may miss out on important health-promoting care if co-occurring medical systems are perceived to be dichotomous or in conflict [54, 80] Women's engagement with holistic health is also a factor that plays an important role in the wellbeing of women and their babies.

There are diverse interpretations regarding the concept of holism. The simplest concept of holism, common in both CAM and biomedical texts, recognises both the physical body and the mind and emotions, originally separated in Descartes' philosophy [17]. Some CAM texts build on this to include connections between the body, mind and spirit and/or discussions of wider social and political contexts of health [18]. First Nations' concepts of holistic health encompass an individual's physical, mental-emotional, spiritual, social and cultural connections to health (including connections to Land, Elders, and Nation), and see political, cultural and social determinants of health as interconnected [19–21]. The importance of information from women elders, from family and friends, and other lay people can be put into the context of the broad definitions of holistic health such as defined by First Nations' concepts. The concept of locus of control may play a factor in women's health care decisions, the accessing of a variety of information sources, including interpersonal, non-health care professional relations and cultural information, can likewise be viewed within these broader concepts of holism whilst also considering medical pluralism. A mother may seek help for a health care concern from several sources depending on which recommendations she feels will be safe and effective, what sources she can access, and which sources support her worldview and understandings of health and illness. If seeking support from a clinician, rapport and trust may also play a role [86]. Empowerment may also play a role, especially for women from HICs [10, 55, 77, 86].

Safety considerations in women's choices to use CMPs in pregnancy and lactation

This synthesis revealed that for women from HICs, the use of CMPs throughout the childbearing continuum was associated with the perceptions that CMPs were safer than pharmaceutical medications, and that these women sought reassurance that the herbal medicines they used were safe for pregnancy and breastfeeding. This perception of safety has been found previously in systematic reviews on the use of CAM generally in HIC populations [87, 88] but may not have been explored adequately in developing countries. Although the perception of safety was not a large theme explaining women's use of CMPs in developing countries, this synthesis did reveal that for women from some LMICs and UPICs, safety for mother and baby was believed to be facilitated by the concurrent use of biomedical care with CMPs, including the prevention of maternity complications in pregnancy and birth, and protection from diseases arising from spiritual forces not treatable with biomedical drugs.

Perceptions of safety may not always be correct. Cultural influences on health care choices cannot always be considered the safest or best outcome options. Some traditional practices may endanger the lives of both mothers and their unborn babies, especially for women in some of the studies from developing nations. As an example, for some countries, one of the perceived benefits of herbal medicine use post-birth was to expel lochia and induce 'uterine cleansing' [43, 44, 51]. However, inducing bleeding post-birth can be very dangerous for post-partum women, and the possibility of dying during childbirth is a reality for many of the women in the LICs and LMICs in this review [45, 48].

Implications for policy and practice

For the large proportion of studies from economically disadvantaged countries included in this review, policy and practice implications mainly centre on reducing high maternal and infant morbidity and mortality rates. Specific national policies [46, 57], the United Nations Millennium Development Goals [89], or the World Health Organisation's policies aimed at increasing maternal and neonatal health through education, health checks and micronutrient supplements as part of regular antenatal care [45, 50, 53, 54, 57, 62, 64] or the initiation of exclusive breastfeeding immediately post-birth [60] are discussed. Several factors are implicated in implementing policies in developing countries, including the need to identify and reduce cultural, social, geographical, economic and gender barriers to adequate biomedical antenatal, birthing and postnatal care [45–47, 59, 71, 90]. Additionally, intervention strategies aimed at promoting heath seeking behaviours to support reductions in child and maternal mortality must consider pregnant and breastfeeding women's use of CMPs, within the context of their perceptions of health risks, the safe promotion of health and where to go for support with these [90]. This is true for women in developing nations, as well as for women in HICs. Whilst the women participants and their babies in the included studies from USA, Canada, and the UK (all HICs) were at far less risk of pregnancy and birth-related morbidity and mortality than the participants from LIC, LMIC and UPIC countries, the contexts within which these HIC women chose to use CMPs include their own cultural perceptions of how to best support their pregnancies, postnatal health and the health of their babies.

Central to discussions on policy with regard to medical pluralism is an awareness that cultural awareness, including the provision of culturally appropriate care, and consultation and involvement of the whole community is necessary if any policy changes aimed at reducing maternal and infant mortality and increasing maternal and infant survival and health are to succeed [8, 45, 48, 60, 64, 71]. Community-wide consultation is essential to successfully remove barriers to maternal and infant care [45, 57, 62, 64, 71], to identify possible solutions, and educate women's family-members, including husbands and/or mothers-in-law, who often hold the power to make decisions regarding the health care a woman is able to seek for herself or her baby [45, 59, 60]. Policies that encourage collaboration between biomedical HCPs and TBAs, traditional herbalists and other traditional healers may help improve maternal and child health outcomes [47, 57, 59, 60]. These include policies to enable further training of Traditional Birth Attendants [8, 57, 64] in recognition that TBAs are usually the providers of culturally sensitive, affordable care, are identified as being active participants in helping promote maternal and infant health, and are ideally placed to refer and accompany women at risk to biomedical care in a timely manner when necessary [8, 47, 57, 60]. Additionally, for rural women, TBAs may often be the only HCPs they regularly see [15, 47, 48, 59]. Training of TBAs in minor surgical procedures like suturing, especially in areas where birthing often takes place outside biomedical health care institutions [59] is recommended, but policy changes to encourage more broader collaboration with TBAs and traditional healers and community health workers in education around the importance of antenatal and postnatal care, micronutrient supplementation and other important measures to improve maternal and infant health outcomes is also necessary [47, 54, 57, 59, 60].

For more economically advantaged nations, policy discussions centre on educational needs of biomedical HCPs regarding complementary medicine and CMPs due to policy and practice shifts that emphasise consumers' rights, choices, and active involvement in health care, and providers' responsibilities when pregnant or breastfeeding women autonomously choose to incorporate CMPs as part of their health care practices [12, 63]. In HICs policy implications call for biomedical HCPs to be better educated about CMPs, in order to be more able and willing to discuss their use openly and non-judgementally with pregnant or breastfeeding women [3, 23, 24, 52, 55, 63, 91, 92] and to realise the importance of holism to mothers as well as women's desire for autonomy and control [55, 93, 94]. Regarding breastfeeding specifically, policy implications need to ensure HCPs receive sufficient education in lactation and in helping women to breastfeed successfully in order to be able identify and provide help with breastfeeding difficulties and improve services for breastfeeding women [55, 95–97].

An important practice implication for biomedical HCPs across all economic strata centres on balancing the provision of evidence-based biomedical care that aims to ensure the safety and health of both mother and baby, and the need to accommodate culturally different health care practices and women's choices regarding maternal health care. The recognition of the need for culturally appropriate services is linked to the perception that provision of culturally sensitive care has the potential to enhance women's wellbeing, and in turn the health of their babies and whole communities, provided that other social determinants of health like gender, age, income and personal and ethnic history are also taken into consideration [98–100]. Cultural understandings shape how women and their caregivers receive information and how they make health care choices [70]. The provision of culturally sensitive care facilitates communication between biomedical and other HCPs, the women they provide care for, and within the whole community. By considering and respecting women's values and beliefs around pregnancy and childbirth, women's use of CMPs can be discussed openly. Studies across all economic strata have shown that if a woman perceives her biomedical HCP to have negative or uninterested views on CMPs, she will not candidly discuss her use of them with her HCP [24, 48, 52, 53, 63]. For developing economies, recommendations to provide training of biomedical nurses and midwives in culturally appropriate care aim at reducing cultural barriers to biomedical care and strengthening relationships between biomedical HCPs and the whole community, including traditional practitioners [7, 47, 57]. As mutual respect and communication are facilitated through the provision of culturally appropriate care, it can also help find ways to intervene appropriately if unsafe practices are identified in pregnancy or the postnatal period [47, 58, 60].

Discussions on culturally appropriate care in HICs and UPICs again centre around promoting maternal and infant health, although the focus is less on reducing morbidity and mortality, and more on increasing biomedical HCPs' understanding and respect for cultural differences when working with women from diverse backgrounds who engage in traditional practices that may not be taught in biomedical education [43, 44, 58, 61]. The need for cultural safety to be taught in universities and health services so that HCPs can develop a critical understanding of social determinants on both their own and others' health is crucial if culturally sensitive care is to be provided effectively [98, 100]. Recommendations for practice include recognition of the involvement of extended family as influential care-givers in providing pregnancy and postpartum care for many women [43, 58, 61] and recognition of beliefs, experiences and practices that women engage in to promote their holistic health and recovery from childbirth, and prevent future ill-health, especially in the postnatal period [44, 51, 58, 61]. HCPs can help facilitate positive health behaviours through hands-on educational activities, by identifying and working with medical and other influential leaders in the community and women's partners [49]. Recognising language differences as a potential barrier is also an important aspect of providing culturally competent, good quality maternity care [43, 49, 61]. The use of clear pictorial-based information when communicating with pregnant or breastfeeding women is recommended regardless of a woman's literacy or education levels, as is the provision of health information in a woman's own language and the use of translation services [43, 49, 61].

Future research on the inter-professional relationships between biomedical, traditional and/or CAM HCPs providing care to pregnant and breastfeeding women, as well as power dynamics between women and their non-HCP information providers, would be useful in pointing out how to make women's reproductive journeys whilst engaging in medical pluralism safe and supportive. Additionally, future research needs to encompass explicit measurements of health literacy, and investigation of how different literacy levels impact on women's understandings and use of CMPs in pregnancy and lactation.

Limitations

The exclusion of articles in languages other than English is a limiting factor, as important studies from all over the world discussing CMP use in pregnancy and lactation may be missing from this review. Additionally, the proportion of studies from LIC and LMIC countries was substantially larger than those from UPIC and HIC countries. This may have increased the importance of cultural knowledge and women elders as information sources identified in this synthesis.

The hand searches identified additional papers which were not identified in the original search, possibly because of the use of different keywords encompassing the terms 'ethnobotanical' or 'ethnopharmacology'. The heterogeneity in research design and methodology of the included papers in this review may also restrict the ability to make larger conclusions about CMP use in pregnancy and lactation. However, this review does provide the first qualitative synthesis regarding CMP use in pregnancy and lactation, the perceived benefits of these, and the information sources women access regarding the use of CMPs in pregnancy and lactation. This provides important information for health care planners and practitioners across the world, and emphasises the importance of culture and health literacy when working with pregnant and lactating women.

Conclusions

This review shows that women use CMPs in pregnancy and lactation in order to optimise their own holistic health, and the health of their babies, according to the benefits they perceive to be associated with the CMPs. Herbal medicines were the most commonly reported type of CMP used, followed by vitamin and mineral supplements. Women utilise a range of information sources, with shared cultural knowledge and traditions, and women elders being the most commonly identified information sources, followed by health care practitioners. This review found that culture plays a pivotal role in women's decisions to use CMPs. The role of maternal health literacy in explaining women's choices to use CMPs in pregnancy and lactation is explored using an interactive health literacy framework. Women choosing to use CMPs as well as accessing biomedical care can be seen to be either supplementing biomedical care, or choosing to complement it with their CMP use for the benefit of themselves and their babies, with the aim to prevent or protect themselves and their babies from adverse events, or to facilitate the normal physiological processes of pregnancy and lactation. The influence of culture on maternal health literacy and health care choices shows that women act on beliefs and practices important to their own cultural understandings of health and illness. Biomedical maternity care providers and complementary medicine health care professionals can use this information to inform their best practice and care when working with pregnant and breastfeeding women, and to understand how and why women may make decisions to use CMPs during pregnancy and lactation.

Abbreviations

Biomedical HCPs: Biomedical health care practitioners. (Biomedically trained health care practitioners - nurses, midwives, doctors and obstetricians); CAM HCPs: Complementary medicine health care practitioners. (Western complementary medicine health care practitioners including naturopaths and herbalists trained in Western Herbal Medicine); CAM: Complementary and alternative medicine; CMP: Complementary medicine product; CMPs: Complementary medicine products; COREQ: Consolidated Criteria for Reporting Qualitative Research; FGDs: Focus group discussions; HCPs: Health Care Professionals; HIC : High Income Economy*; HICs: High Income Economies*; IDIs: In-depth interviews; LIC: Low Income Economy*; LICs: Low Income Economies*; LMIC: Lower Middle Income Economy*; LMICs: Lower Middle Income Economies*; Non-HCP information providers: Non-health care professional information providers (including women elders, family and friends); TBAs: Traditional Birth Assistants or Attendants; UK: United Kingdom; UPIC: Upper Middle Income Economy*; UPICs: Upper Middle Income Economies*; USA: United States of America; : * According to The World Bank Classifications [42], based on 2015 gross national income per capita

Acknowledgements

The authors would like to acknowledge librarian Loraine Evison for her assistance with drafting the search strategies and training in searching electronic databases, and Dr. Claire O'Reilly for her expertise and help with specific terms used in the search strategies.

Funding

Philanthropical funding from Blackmores Ltd. funds Larisa Barnes' PhD scholarship at The University of Sydney. Blackmores have no input into the design, execution or the dissemination of her research.

Availability of data and materials

Additional files are included with this submission, ensuring readers will have access to the following:

1. Example search strategy (Additional file 1)
2. Full COREQ analysis of the included papers as per Tong et al. [37] (Additional file 2)
3. Information sources accessed by women by country groupings (Additional file 3)
4. The full thematic analysis regarding perceived benefits of complementary medicine product (CMP) use in different stages of the childbearing continuum (Additional file 4)

As this paper is a Systematic Review, and uses previously published results, there is no further data to share.

Authors' contributions

LAJB drafted the search strategies, performed the searches, screened all papers by title, abstract and full text, did the thematic analysis, and drafted the manuscript. PA provided feedback on the search strategies, screened papers by title, provided feedback on the thematic analysis and interpretation of data, and critically revised the manuscript. LB provided feedback on the qualitative synthesis and critically revised the manuscript. KM provided feedback on the search strategies, and critically revised the manuscript. All authors have read and approved the manuscript.

Authors' information

Ms. Larisa Barnes, BA, BNat (Hons), is a PhD candidate with the Faculty of Pharmacy, The University of Sydney. Larisa also works in the allied health education team at the University Centre for Rural Health, Lismore Campus, The University of Sydney.

Professor Parisa Aslani, PhD, BPharm (Hons), MSc, G Cert Ed Stud (Higher Ed), is the Professor in Medicines Use Optimisation at the Faculty of Pharmacy, The University of Sydney.

Emeritus Professor Lesley Barclay, AO, PhD, is an Emeritus Professor with the Sydney School of Public Health, The University of Sydney, and formerly Professor and Director of the University Centre for Rural Health, Lismore Campus, The University of Sydney.

Professor Kirsten McCaffery, BSc (Hons), PhD, is the Sub-Dean of Research and NHMRC Career Research Fellow at Sydney School of Public Health, The University of Sydney.

Consent for publication

Not applicable.

Regarding Figs. 4 and 5: these figures build on a model designed by Ruth Parker [66] and used by the Australian Commission on Safety and Quality in Health Care as their working definition of health literacy [65]. As Figs. 4 and 5 build on the original model, and we have added more than 50% to the original model, Ruth Parker and the Australian Commission on Safety and Quality in Health Care have been cited in the text appropriately. Consent to use the original model in this paper was sought and received from Ruth Parker and forwarded to the Editor.

Competing interests

The authors declare that they have no competing interests.

Author details

[1]Faculty of Pharmacy, The University of Sydney, Camperdown, NSW 2006, Australia. [2]University Centre for Rural Health, The University of Sydney, PO Box 3074, Lismore, NSW 2480, Australia. [3]Sydney School of Public Health, The University of Sydney, Edward Ford Building (A27), Camperdown, NSW 2006, Australia. [4]Sydney School of Public Health, Sydney Medical School, The University of Sydney, Rm 128B, Edward Ford Building A27, Camperdown, NSW 2006, Australia. [5]Faculty of Pharmacy, The University of Sydney, Rm N502, Pharmacy & Bank Building (A15), Science Rd, Camperdown, NSW 2006, Australia.

References

1. Krause K, Alex G, Parkin D. Medical knowledge, therapeutic practice and processes of diversification. MMG working paper; 2012. p. 12. http://pubman.mpdl.mpg.de/pubman/item/escidoc:1615151:4/component/escidoc:1615150/WP_12-11_Concept-Paper_MEDDIV.pdf
2. Hill E, Hess R, Aborigo R, Adongo P, Hodgson A, Engmann C, et al. "I don't know anything about their culture": the disconnect between allopathic and traditional maternity care providers in rural northern Ghana. Afr J Reprod Health. 2014;18:36–45.
3. Frawley J, Adams J, Sibbritt D, Steel A, Broom A, Gallois C. Prevalence and determinants of complementary and alternative medicine use during pregnancy: results from a nationally representative sample of Australian pregnant women. Aust N Z J Obstet Gynaecol. 2013;53:347–52. https://doi.org/10.1111/ajo.12056.
4. Liamputtong P, Yimyam S, Parisunyakul S, Baosoung C, Sansiriphun N. Traditional beliefs about pregnancy and child birth among women from Chiang Mai, Northern Thailand. Midwifery. 2005;21:139–53.
5. Holst L, Wright D, Haavik S, Nordeng H. The use and the user of herbal remedies during pregnancy. J Altern Complement Med. 2009;15:787–92. https://doi.org/10.1089/acm.2008.0467.

6. Frawley JE. Women's use of complementary and alternative medicine products and services during pregnancy: insights for safe, informed maternity care. Sydney: University of Technology Sydney; 2015.
7. Juntunen A, Nikkonen M, Janhonen S. Utilising the concept of protection in health maintenance among the Bena in Tanzania. J Transcult Nurs. 2000;11:174–81.
8. Okafor IP, Sekoni AO, Ezeiru SS, Ugboaja JO, Inem V. Orthodox versus unorthodox care: a qualitative study on where rural women seek healthcare during pregnancy and childbirth in Southwest, Nigeria. Malawi Med J. 2014;26:45–9. http://www.ncbi.nlm.nih.gov/pmc/articles/PMC4141242/pdf/MMJ2602-0045.pdf
9. Steel A, Adams J, Sibbritt D, Broom A, Gallois C, Frawley J. Utilisation of complementary and alternative medicine (CAM) practitioners within maternity care provision: results from a nationally representative cohort study of 1,835 pregnant women. BMC Pregnancy Childbirth. 2012;12 https://doi.org/10.1186/1471-2393-12-146.
10. Westfall RE. Galactagogue herbs: a qualitative study and review. Can J Midwifery Res Pract. 2003;2:22–7.
11. Main I. Biomedical practices from a patient perspective. Experiences of polish female migrants in Barcelona, Berlin and London. Anthropol Med. 2016;23:188–204.
12. Adams J, Lui CW, Sibbritt D, Broom A, Wardle J, Homer C. Women's use of complementary and alternative medicine during pregnancy: a critical review of the literature. Birth. 2009;36 https://doi.org/10.1111/j.1523-536X.2009.00328.x.
13. Hall HG, Griffiths DL, McKenna LG. The use of complementary and alternative medicine by pregnant women: a literature review. Midwifery. 2011;27:817–24.
14. Rayner J-A, Willis K, Burgess R. Women's use of complementary and alternative medicine for fertility enhancement: a review of the literature. J Altern Complement Med. 2011;17:685–90. https://doi.org/10.1089/acm.2010.0435.
15. Ebuehi OM, Akintujoye I. Perception and utilization of traditional birth attendants by pregnant women attending primary health care clinics in a rural local government area in Ogun State, Nigeria. Int J Womens Health. 2012;4:25–34.
16. O'Driscoll T, Payne L, Kelly L, Cromarty H, St Pierre-Hansen N, Terry C. Traditional first nations birthing practices: interviews with elders in Northwestern Ontario. J Obstet Gynaecol Can. 2011;33:24–9. https://doi.org/10.1016/S1701-2163(16)34768-5.
17. MacArtney JI, Wahlberg A. The problem of complementary and alternative medicine use today: eyes half closed? Qual Health Res. 2014;24:114–23.
18. Evans S. Response to baer and colleagues: the politics of holism. Med Anthropol Q. 2012;26:271–4. https://doi.org/10.1111/j.1548-1387.2012.01205.x.
19. Raven M, Katz I, Kinnane S, Gorring B, Griffiths A. Renewed framework for the social and emotional wellbeing of aboriginal and Torres Strait Islander peoples report to the department of health and ageing. Sydney: Social Policy Research Centre, University of New South Wales; 2013.
20. Bartlett JG. Health and well-being for Métis women in Manitoba. Can J Public Health. 2005;96:S22–7.
21. McIvor O, Napoleon A. Language and culture as protective factors for at-risk communities. J Aborig Health. 2009;5:6–25.
22. Kennedy DA, Lupattelli A, Koren G, Nordeng H. Herbal medicine use in pregnancy: results of a multinational study. BMC Complement Altern Med. 2013;13:355. http://www.biomedcentral.com/1472-6882/13/355
23. Kochhar K, Saywell RM Jr, Zollinger TW, Mandzuk CA, Haas DM, Howell LK, et al. Herbal remedy use among Hispanic women during pregnancy and while breastfeeding: are physicians informed? Hispanic Health Care Int. 2010;8:93–106. https://doi.org/10.1891/1540-4153.8.2.93.
24. Hall HR, Jolly K. Women's use of complementary and alternative medicines during pregnancy: a cross-sectional study. Midwifery. 2014;30:499–505. https://doi.org/10.1016/j.midw.2013.06.001.
25. Rahman AA, Daud WNW, Sulaiman SA, Ahmad Z, Hamid AM. The impact of knowledge and sociodemographic factors on the dangerous use of herbal medicines during pregnancy in Tumpat district. Intern Med J. 2008;15:209–12.
26. Mothupi MC. Use of herbal medicine during pregnancy among women with access to public healthcare in Nairobi, Kenya: a cross-sectional survey. BMC Complement Altern Med. 2014;14:432. https://doi.org/10.1186/1472-6882-14-432
27. Mills E, Dugoua J-J, Perri D, Koren G. Herbal medicines in pregnancy and lactation: an evidence-based approach. London and New York: Taylor & Francis; 2006.
28. Dugoua J-J. Herbal medicines and pregnancy. J Popul Ther Clin Pharmacol. 2010;17:e370–e8.
29. Amer MR, Cipriano GC, Venci JV, Gandhi MA. Safety of popular herbal supplements in lactating women. J Hum Lact. 2015;31:348–53.
30. Jordan JE, Buchbinder R, Briggs AM, Elsworth GR, Busija L, Batterham R, et al. The Health Literacy Management Scale (HeLMS): a measure of an individual's capacity to seek, understand and use health information within the healthcare setting. Patient Educ Couns. 2013;91:228–35.
31. Renkert S, Nutbeam D. Opportunities to improve maternal health literacy through antenatal education: an exploratory study. Health Promot Int. 2001;16:381–8.
32. Ostini R, Kairuz T. Investigating the association between health literacy and non-adherence. Int J Clin Pharm. 2014;36:36–44.
33. Chinn D. Critical health literacy: a review and critical analysis. Soc Sci Med. 2011;73:60–7. https://doi.org/10.1016/j.socscimed.2011.04.004.
34. Nutbeam D. The evolving concept of health literacy. Soc Sci Med. 2008;67:2072–8. https://doi.org/10.1016/j.socscimed.2008.09.050.
35. Berkman ND, Davis TC, McCormack L. Health literacy: what is it? J Health Commun. 2010;15:9–19. https://doi.org/10.1080/10810730.2010.499985.
36. Rallis S, Skouteris H, McCabe M, Milgrom J. The transition to motherhood: towards a broader understanding of perinatal distress. Women Birth. 2014;27:68–71. https://doi.org/10.1016/j.wombi.2013.12.004.
37. Tong A, Sainsbury P, Craig J. Consolidated criteria for reporting qualitative research (COREQ): a 32-item checklist for interviews and focus groups. Int J Qual Health Care. 2007;19:349–57. https://doi.org/10.1093/intqhc/mzm042.
38. Thomas J, Harden A. Methods for the thematic synthesis of qualitative research in systematic reviews. BMC Med Res Methodol. 2008;8:45.
39. Braun V, Clarke V. Using thematic analysis in psychology. Qual Res Psychol. 2006;3:77–101. https://doi.org/10.1191/1478088706qp063oa.
40. Westfall RE. Herbal healing in pregnancy: women's experiences. J Herb Pharmacother. 2003;3:17–39.
41. Westfall RE. Use of anti-emetic herbs in pregnancy: women's choices, and the question of safety and efficacy. Complement Ther Nurs Midwifery. 2004;10:30–6.
42. The World Bank. World bank country and lending groups: The World Bank group; 2017. Available from: https://datahelpdesk.worldbank.org/knowledgebase/articles/906519-world-bank-country-and-lending-groups. Cited 3 Mar 2017.
43. Grewal SK, Bhagat R, Balneaves LG. Perinatal beliefs and practices of immigrant Punjabi women living in Canada. J Obstet Gynecol Neonatal Nurs. 2008;37:290–300. https://doi.org/10.1111/j.1552-6909.2008.00234.x.
44. Rice PL. Nyo dua hli -- 30 days confinement: traditions and changed childbearing beliefs and practices among Hmong women in Australia. Midwifery. 2000;16:22–34.
45. Waiswa P, Kemigisa M, Kiguli J, Naikoba S, Pariyo GW, Peterson S. Acceptability of evidence-based neonatal care practices in rural Uganda - implications for programming. BMC Pregnancy Childbirth. 2008;8:21. https://doi.org/10.1186/1471-2393-8-21.
46. Obermeyer CM. Pluralism and pragmatism: knowledge and practice of birth in Morocco. Med Anthropol Q. 2000;14:180–201.
47. Thwala SB, Jones LK, Holroyd E. Swaziland rural maternal care: ethnography of the interface of custom and biomedicine. Int J Nurs Pract. 2011;17:93–101. https://doi.org/10.1111/j.1440-172X.2010.01911.x.
48. Wilkinson SE, Callister LC. Giving birth: the voices of Ghanaian women. Health Care Women Int. 2010;31:201–20. https://doi.org/10.1080/07399330903343858.
49. Yeo S, Fetters M, Maeda Y. Japanese couples' childbirth experiences in Michigan: implications for care. Birth. 2000;27:191–8.
50. Young SL, Ali SM. Linking traditional treatments of maternal anaemia to iron supplement use: an ethnographic case study from Pemba Island, Zanzibar. Matern Child Nutr. 2005;1:51–8. https://doi.org/10.1111/j.1740-8709.2004.00002.x.
51. Damanik R. Torbangun (Coleus amboinicus Lour): a Bataknese traditional cuisine perceived as lactagogue by Bataknese lactating women in Simalungun, North Sumatera, Indonesia. J Hum Lact. 2009;25:64–72. https://doi.org/10.1177/0890334408326086.
52. Holst L, Wright D, Nordeng H, Haavik S. Use of herbal preparations during pregnancy: focus group discussion among expectant mothers attending a hospital antenatal clinic in Norwich, UK. Complement Ther Clin Pract. 2009;15:225–9.
53. Wulandari LPL, Whelan AK. Beliefs, attitudes and behaviours of pregnant women in Bali. Midwifery. 2011;27:867–71. https://doi.org/10.1016/j.midw.2010.09.005.
54. Ejidokun OO. Community attitudes to pregnancy, anaemia, iron and folate supplementation in urban and rural Lagos, South-Western Nigeria. Midwifery. 2000;16:89–95. https://doi.org/10.1054/midw.1999.0196.

55. Sim TF, Hattingh HL, Sherriff J, Tee LB. Perspectives and attitudes of breastfeeding women using herbal galactagogues during breastfeeding: a qualitative study. BMC Complement Altern Med. 2014;14:216. https://doi.org/10.1186/1472-6882-14-216.
56. Lamxay V, de Boer HJ, Björk L. Traditions and plant use during pregnancy, childbirth and postpartum recovery by the Kry ethnic group in Lao PDR. J Ethnobiol Ethnomed. 2011;7:14. https://doi.org/10.1186/1746-4269-7-14.
57. Ngomane S, Mulaudzi FM. Indigenous beliefs and practices that influence the delayed attendance of antenatal clinics by women in the Bohlabelo district in Limpopo, South Africa. Midwifery. 2012;28:30–8. https://doi.org/10.1016/j.midw.2010.11.002.
58. Elter PT, Kennedy HP, Chesla CA, Yimyam S. Spiritual healing practices among rural postpartum Thai women. J Transcult Nurs. 2016;27:249–55.
59. Rutakumwa W, Krogman N. Women's health in rural Uganda: problems, coping strategies, and recommendations for change. Can J Nurs Res. 2007; 39:105–25.
60. Aborigo RA, Moyer CA, Rominski S, Adongo P, Williams J, Logonia G, et al. Infant nutrition in the first seven days of life in rural northern Ghana. BMC Pregnancy Childbirth. 2012;12:76. https://doi.org/10.1186/1471-2393-12-76.
61. Callister LC, Eads MN, Diehl JPSY. Perceptions of giving birth adherence to cultural practices in Chinese women. MCN Am J Matern Child Nurs. 2011;36: 387–94. https://doi.org/10.1097/NMC.0b013e31822de397.
62. Dako-Gyeke P, Aikins M, Aryeetey R, McCough L, Adongo PB. The influence of socio-cultural interpretations of pregnancy threats on health-seeking behavior among pregnant women in urban Accra, Ghana. BMC Pregnancy Childbirth. 2013;13:211. https://doi.org/10.1186/1471-2393-13-211.
63. Warriner S, Bryan K, Brown AM. Women's attitude towards the use of complementary and alternative medicines (CAM) in pregnancy. Midwifery. 2014;30:138–43. doi: https://doi.org/10.1016/j.midw.2013.03.004
64. Mogawane MA, Mothiba TM, Malema RN. Indigenous practices of pregnant women at Dilokong hospital in Limpopo province, South Africa. Curationis. 2015;38:1–8.
65. Australian Commission on Safety and Quality in Health Care. Health literacy: taking action to improve safety and quality. Sydney: ACSQHC; 2014.
66. Parker R. Measuring health literacy: what? So what? Now what? In: Hernandez L, editor. Measures of health literacy: workshop summary; roundtable on health literacy. Washington, DC: National Academies Press (US); 2009.
67. United Nations Educational Scientific and Cultural Organization. UNESCO universal declaration on cultural diversity Paris 2001 [Wednesday, July 12th 2017]. Available from: http://portal.unesco.org/en/ev.php-URL_ID=13179&URL_DO=DO_TOPIC&URL_SECTION=201.html.
68. World Health Organisation. Beyond bias: exploring the cultural contexts of health and well-being measurement. Copenhagen Ø: World Health Organisation; 2015.
69. Thwala SB, Holroyd E, Jones LK. Health belief dualism in the postnatal practices of rural Swazi women: an ethnographic account. Women Birth. 2012;25:e68–74. https://doi.org/10.1016/j.wombi.2011.10.006.
70. Webb R. Culturally appropriate care. AJN Am J Nurs. 2008;108:30. https://doi.org/10.1097/01.NAJ.0000336409.30001.1d.
71. Finlayson K, Downe S. Why do women not use antenatal services in low- and middle-income countries? A meta-synthesis of qualitative studies. PLoS Med. 2013;10:e1001373.
72. Fakeye TO, Adisa R, Musa IE. Attitude and use of herbal medicines among pregnant women in Nigeria. BMC Complement Altern Med. 2009;9:53.
73. Pallivalappila AR, Stewart D, Shetty A, Pande B, McLay JS. Complementary and alternative medicines use during pregnancy: a systematic review of pregnant women and healthcare professional views and experiences. Evid Based Complement Alternat Med. 2013;2013:205639.
74. Wallston KA. The validity of the multidimensional health locus of control scales. J Health Psychol. 2005;10:623–31. https://doi.org/10.1177/1359105305055304.
75. Wulandari LPL, Craig P, Whelan AK. Foetal health locus of control and iron supplementation adherence among pregnant women in Bali. J Reprod Infant Psychol. 2013;31:94–101. https://doi.org/10.1080/02646838.2012.751585.
76. Labs SM, Wurtele SK. Fetal health locus of control scale: development and validation. J Consult Clin Psychol. 1986;54:814–9.
77. Frawley J, Sibbritt D, Broom A, Gallois C, Steel A, Adams J. Women's attitudes towards the use of complementary and alternative medicine products during pregnancy. J Obstet Gynaecol. 2016;36:462–7. https://doi.org/10.3109/01443615.2015.1072804.
78. Barrett B, Marchand L, Scheder J, Plane MB, Maberry R, Appelbaum D, et al. Themes of holism, empowerment, access, and legitimacy define complementary, alternative, and integrative medicine in relation to conventional biomedicine. J Altern Complement Med. 2003;9:937–47.
79. Fries CJ. Self-care and complementary and alternative medicine as care for the self: an embodied basis for distinction. Health Sociol Rev. 2013;22:37–51.
80. Nagata JM, Gatti LR, Barg FK. Social determinants of iron supplementation among women of reproductive age: a systematic review of qualitative data. Matern Child Nutr. 2012;8:1–18. https://doi.org/10.1111/j.1740-8709.2011.00338.x.
81. Kalder M, Knoblauch K, Hrgovic I, Munstedt K. Use of complementary and alternative medicine during pregnancy and delivery. Arch Gynecol Obstet. 2011;283:475–82. https://doi.org/10.1007/s00404-010-1388-2.
82. Sibbritt D, Adams J, Lui CW. Health service utilisation by pregnant women over a seven-year period. Midwifery. 2011;27:474–6. https://doi.org/10.1016/j.midw.2010.03.005.
83. Smith JA, Badell ML, Kunther A, Palmer JL, Dalrymple JL, Ramin SM. Use of complementary and alternative medications among patients in an obstetrics and gynecology clinic. J Reprod Med. 2012;57:390–6.
84. Wiese M, Oster C, Pincombe J. Understanding the emerging relationship between complementary medicine and mainstream health care: a review of the literature. Health (London). 2010;14:326–42. https://doi.org/10.1177/1363459309358594.
85. Lu Y, Racine L. Reviewing Chinese immigrant women's health experiences in English-speaking Western Countries: a postcolonial feminist analysis. Health Sociol Rev. 2015;24:15–28. https://doi.org/10.1080/14461242.2015.1006656.
86. Golden I, Stranieri A, Sahama T, Pilapitiya S, Siribaddana S, Vaughan S. Informatics to support patient choice between diverse medical systems. In: Proceedings of the 16th International Conference on E-health Networking, Application and Services (Healthcom); 2014 Oct 15-18; IEEE, Natal, Brazil, 2014. pp. 111-5.
87. Bishop FL, Yardley L, Lewith GT. A systematic review of beliefs involved in the use of complementary and alternative medicine. J Health Psychol. 2007; 12:851–67.
88. Reid R, Steel A, Wardle J, Trubody A, Adams J. Complementary medicine use by the Australian population: a critical mixed studies systematic review of utilisation, perceptions and factors associated with use. BMC Complement Altern Med. 2016;16:1–23. https://doi.org/10.1186/s12906-016-1143-8.
89. United Nations Economic Commission for Europe. Millennium development goals Geneva: United Nations economic Commission for Europe; 2000. Available from: http://www.unece.org/hk/sustainable-development/millennium-development-goals/millennium-development-goals.html. Cited 7 July 2017.
90. Winch PJ, Alam MA, Akther A, Afroz D, Ali NA, Ellis AA, et al. Local understandings of vulnerability and protection during the neonatal period in Sylhet District, Bangladesh: a qualitative study. Lancet. 2005;366:478–85. https://doi.org/10.1016/s0140-6736(05)66836-5.
91. Frawley J, Adams J, Steel A, Broom A, Gallois C, Sibbritt D. Women's use and self-prescription of herbal medicine during pregnancy: an examination of 1,835 pregnant women. Womens Health Issues. 2015;25:396–402. https://doi.org/10.1016/j.whi.2015.03.001.
92. Sim TF, Hattingh HL, Sherriff J, Tee LB. What do breastfeeding women taking herbal galactagogues perceive of community pharmacists' role in breastfeeding support? A qualitative study. Int J Environ Res Public Health. 2015;12:11132–45. https://doi.org/10.3390/ijerph120911132.
93. Warriner S. Over-the-counter culture: complementary therapy for pregnancy. Br J Midwifery. 2007;15:770–2.
94. Gaffney L, Smith C. The views of pregnant women towards the use of complementary therapies and medicines. Birth Issues. 2004;13:43–50.
95. Sim TF, Hattingh HL, Sherriff J, Tee LB. Towards the implementation of breastfeeding-related health services in community pharmacies: pharmacists' perspectives. Res Soc Adm Pharm. 2017;13:980. http://www.sciencedirect.com/science/article/pii/S1551741116303266
96. Wilson DR. Breastfeeding: a woman's health issue. Beginnings. 2010;30:6–9.
97. Watkins AL, Dodgson JE. Breastfeeding educational interventions for health professionals: a synthesis of intervention studies. J Spec Pediatr Nurs. 2010; 15:223–32.
98. Kruske S, Kildea S, Barclay L. Cultural safety and maternity care for Aboriginal and Torres Strait Islander Australians. Women Birth. 2006;19:73–7.
99. Williamson M, Harrison L. Providing culturally appropriate care: a literature review. Int J Nurs Stud. 2010;47:761–9.
100. Correa-Velez I, Ryan J. Developing a best practice model of refugee maternity care. Women Birth. 2012;25:13–22. https://doi.org/10.1016/j.wombi.2011.01.002.

4

Gender specific association between the use of complementary and alternative medicine (CAM) and alcohol consumption and injuries caused by drinking in the sixth Tromsø study

Kristina Sivertsen[1], Marko Lukic[2] and Agnete E. Kristoffersen[3*]

Abstract

Background: Alcohol is consumed almost worldwide and is the most widely used recreational drug in the world. Harmful use of alcohol is known to cause a large disease-, social- and economic burden on society. Only a few studies have examined the relationship between CAM use and alcohol consumption. To our knowledge there has been no such research in Norway. The aim of this study is to describe and compare alcohol consumption and injuries related to alcohol across gender and different CAM approaches.

Methods: The data used in this study is based on questionnaire data gathered from the sixth Tromsø Study conducted between 2007 and 2008. Information on CAM use and alcohol consumption was available for 6819 women and 5994 men, 64.8% of the invited individuals. Pearson chi-square tests and independent sample t-tests were used to describe the basic characteristics of the participants and to calculate the differences between men and women regarding these variables. Binary logistic regression analyses were used to investigate the associations between the different CAM approaches and alcohol consumptions and injuries caused by drinking.

Results: Women who drank alcohol more than once a month were more likely to have applied herbal or "natural" medicine and self-treatment techniques (meditation, yoga, qi gong or tai-chi), compared to those who never drank, and those who only drank monthly or less. For women, an association was also found between having experienced injuries caused by drinking and use of self-treatment techniques and visit to a CAM practitioner. No association was found between amount of alcohol consumed and use of CAM approaches. For men, an association was found between injuries caused by drinking and use of herbal or "natural" medicine.

Conclusion: The findings from this cross-sectional study suggests that women who drink frequently are more likely to use "natural" medicine and self-treatment techniques. Both men and women who had experienced injuries because of their drinking were more likely to have used CAM approaches.

Keywords: Complementary and alternative medicine, CAM, Herbal medicine, Self-treatment, Alternative medical practitioner, Alcohol consumption, Alcohol-related injuries, Cross-sectional study, The Tromsø study

* Correspondence: agnete.kristoffersen@uit.no
[3]National Research Center in Complementary and Alternative Medicine (NAFKAM), Department of Community Medicine, Faculty of Health Sciences, UiT The Arctic University of Norway, Tromsø, Norway
Full list of author information is available at the end of the article

Background

Alcohol is consumed almost worldwide and is the most widely used recreational drug in the world [1]. However, alcohol consumption varies across countries and cultures and there are wide variations within global estimates [1, 2]. The highest levels of alcohol consumption are found in Europe (10.9 l per inhabitant over the age of 15 (15+)), followed by the Americas (8.4 l) the Western Pacific Region (6.8 l) and Africa (6.0 l). The lowest level is found in South-East Asia, especially in the Eastern Mediterranean (0.7 l) [1]. In Norway, people drink on average six litres of pure alcohol a year [3]. When unrecorded consumption, such as border trade and tax-free commerce is included, the number is estimated to be about 7.7 l per inhabitant (15+) [1, 4]. In the Norwegian city Tromsø, the general alcohol consumption is found to be relatively low, reflecting the modest alcohol consumption in Norway [5].

Harmful use of alcohol is known to cause a large disease-, social- and economic burden on society [1, 6]. Despite varying estimates of alcohol use, most countries show substantial disease and death rates attributed to alcohol consumption [1, 2]. Harmful alcohol use is among the five leading risk factors for disease, disability and preventable death [1, 7, 8], and contributes to 7.4% of total diseases burden for men and 3% for women [1].

Complementary and alternative medicine (CAM) is used worldwide, but have often been an underestimated part of health care. More countries are now increasingly recognizing and accepting CAM's contribution to individual's health and well-being and its contribution to health care [9]. In the last 30 years there has been an increasing interest and use of CAM, particularly in Western societies [10–12].

The definition of CAM differ across countries and organizations. According to the World Health Organization (WHO), CAM is defined as a broad spectre of health services that are not incorporated in a countries traditional health care system and is not part of public health services [9]. In Norway, CAM providers offers treatment both as an alternative to, and complementary to conventional treatment. As such, the CAM providers offers therapies that are not usually a part of the public health care system and are paid by out of pockets payments [13].

CAM is often used by people suffering from chronic conditions or life-threatening and serious illness such as cancer [11, 13], chronic pain [14, 15], mental disorders [16] and/or in situations when conventional treatment options are limited [15]. However, motives for use also include a range of other reasons, including using CAM as preventive therapies, CAM being more congruent with their personal belief system, CAM's ability to provide hope, the notion that CAM offers a more holistic view of health care, the therapeutic value of CAM, more emphasis on patient control, and a perception that CAM practitioners offers a more supportive role compared to conventional health care personal [10].

CAM use is believed to be closely associated with sociodemographic variables such as female gender, young to middle age, middle to high income, high level of education and poorer self-perceived health [10, 17–19]. According to a Norwegian survey, close to half of the female participants reported to have used some kind of CAM, while one out of four male participants reported the same [20]. Gender differences in use of CAM has also been found in other Norwegian [20, 21] and international studies [10, 22].

Although there has been focus on a range of sociodemographic characteristics associated with use of CAM, only a few studies have examined the relationship between CAM use and alcohol consumption. They indicated that use of CAM is associated with different level of alcohol use [23–26]. Having consumed alcohol in one's life but not being a heavy drinker [27] as well as less frequent alcohol consumption [28] was associated with CAM use. The findings have, however, been ambiguous. Another study found an inverse relationship between alcohol consumption and CAM use [29], while several other studies failed to find any significant association between the two [30–32].

To our knowledge, there has been no research comparing alcohol consumption between users and non-users of CAM in Norway. Since both alcohol patterns and use of CAM is strongly associated with gender, the aim of this study is to describe and compare gender specific alcohol consumption and injuries related to alcohol across gender and use of different CAM approaches.

Methods

The study population

The Tromsø Study is a population-based, prospective study of a range of health related issues and is considered a great resource for surveillance of risk factors and disease in the population [33]. This study is based on the sixth Tromsø Study conducted between October 2007 and December 2008. The invited population came from four groups: people who participated in the second visit in the fourth Tromsø study conducted in 1994/1995, a 10 % random sample of people aged 30–39, all individuals aged 40–42 and 60–87 and a 40% random sample of people aged 43–59 years, all residing in the municipality of Tromsø [34].

An invitation containing information and a four-page questionnaire (Q1) was sent by mail to the participants within 2 wks of a suggested appointment for a physical examination [35]. A total of 19,762 people between 30 and 87 years were invited [36], with a participation rate of 65.7% (12,981 participants).

Q1 was filled out at home and brought to the examination. Q1 included questions on various health issues, symptoms and diseases, use of medication and healthcare services, disability, employment, income, lifestyle, and reproduction. The second questionnaire (Q2), of 28 pages, was handed out during the examination, and the participants could either fill it out at the spot or return it later in prepaid postage envelopes. Q2-data was available for 95.8% of the participants who filled out Q1, and contained follow-up questions of topics covered in Q1 [36].

As shown in Fig. 1, we excluded participants who refrained from answering any of the three included CAM questions and/or any of the three included alcohol questions ($n = 168$). A total of 12,813 participants (64.8% of the invited individuals), 6819 women and 5994 men were included in the analyses.

Assessment of CAM use and alcohol consumption

Use of alcohol is based on self-reported consumption of alcohol gathered from Q1 [37] and Q2 [38]. From Q1, the two following questions were used: Firstly: *"How often do you drink alcohol?"* with the response options: *"Never"*, *"Monthly or more infrequently"*, *"2-4 times a month"*, *"2-3 times a week"*, *"More than 3 times a week"*. The first category *"Never"* was used as the reference category for all analyses including alcohol frequency. Secondly, *"How many units of alcohol (a beer, a glass of wine or a drink) do you usually drink when you drink alcohol?"*, with five possible answers: *"1–2"*, *"3–4"*, *"5–6"*, *"7–9"*, *"10 or more"*. The categories with highest level of consumption had few respondents and were collapsed into the category *"5 or more"* as five or more drinks in one occasion is defined as heavy episodic drinking and have been associated with increased risk of harm [1, 39, 40]. The first option, *"1–2"* units, was set as the reference category. From Q2, the following question was included in the analyses: *"Have you or someone else been injured because of your drinking?"*, with *"Never"*, *"Yes, but not in the last year"* and *"Yes, during the last year"* as the response options. Due to few respondents in the two last categories, these were merged into one *"Yes"*-category. *"Never"* was set as the reference category.

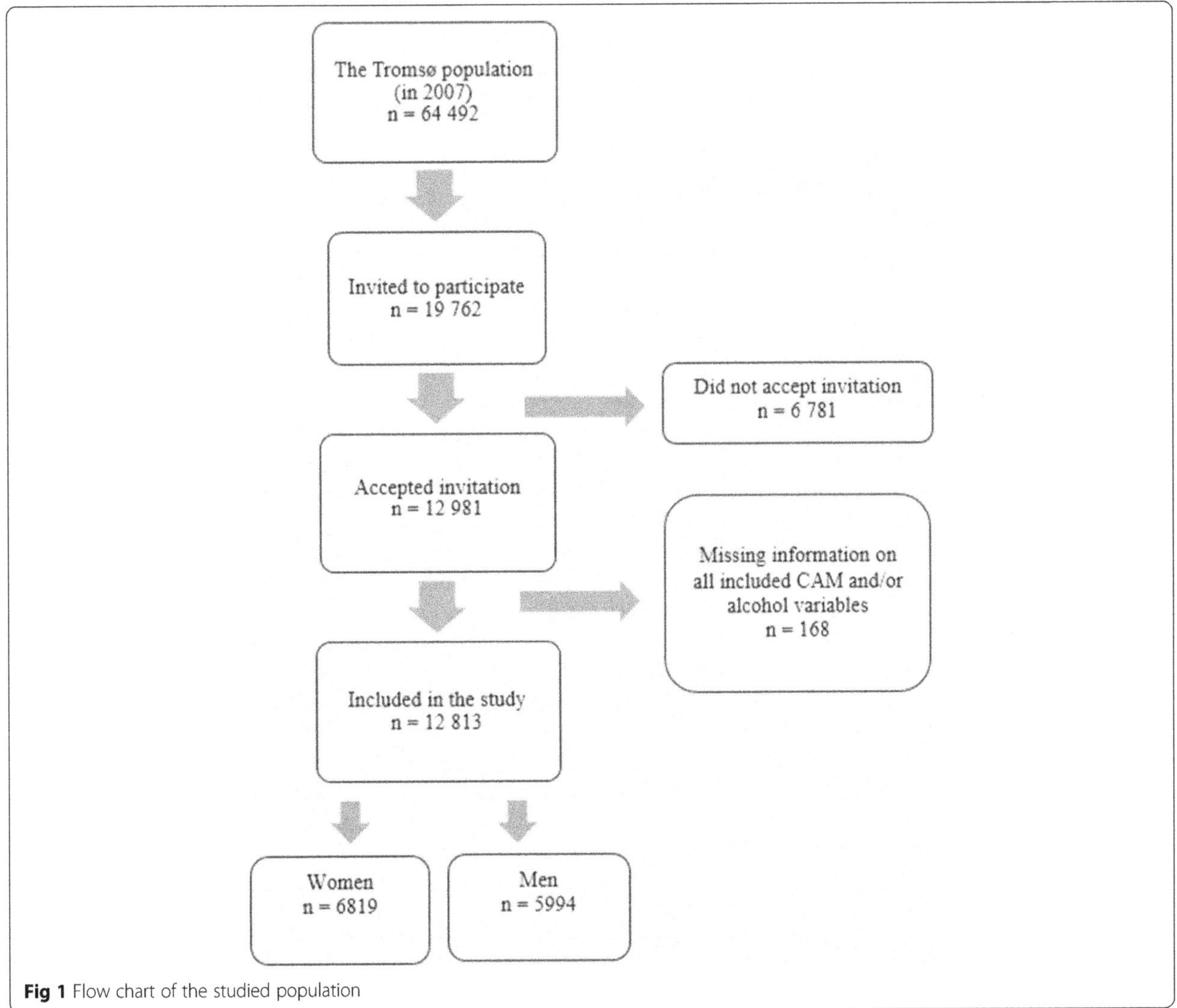

Fig 1 Flow chart of the studied population

In order to get information on the use of CAM, three questions were analysed separately. *"Have you during the past year visited: Alternative medical practitioner (homeopath, acupuncturist, foot zone therapist, herbal medical practitioner, laying of hands practitioner, healer, clairvoyant, etc.)"*, with the two options, *"Yes"* and *"No"*. The participants were also asked: *"In the last 12 months have you used meditation, yoga, qi gong or tai-chi as self-treatment?"* and *"In the last 12 months have you used herbal or "natural" medicine?"* with *"Yes"* and *"No"* as response options. The different CAM variables were not mutually exclusive, as many of CAM users tend to use more than one approach.

Statistical methods

Pearson chi-square tests and independent sample t-tests were used to describe the basic characteristics of the participants and to calculate gender differences regarding these variables. The association between alcohol consumption and the use of CAM was investigated in binary logistic regression models. Each of the CAM approaches (visit to alternative practitioner, use of herbal medicine, and self-treatment) were dichotomised to yes/no and used as a dependent variable in the regression model. We calculated odds ratios (OR) with 95% confidence interval (CI) of having used the three CAM approaches according to alcohol exposure. All the analyses were stratified according to gender. Level of education, household income, age and self-reported health status were included as independent variables in all the adjusted models.

Analyses for each of the outcomes were adjusted for the factors that could have influenced the association between alcohol consumption and the use of CAM [4, 10, 17, 41, 42]. These include level of education (primary, 1–2 years secondary school, vocational school, high secondary school (A-level), college/university less than 4 years, and college/ university 4 years or more), household income (low income (< 200,000 NOK/ 20,000 €), low middle income (201,000–400,000 NOK/20,100–40,000 €), high middle income (401,000–700,000 NOK/40,100–70,000 €), high income (> 701,000 NOK/70,100 €)), age (continuous), and self-reported health status (bad, neither good nor bad, and good).

All the analyses were carried out using the statistical program IBM SPSS, version 24. *P*-values <0.05 were considered statistically significant for all conducted analyses.

Results

Characteristics of the studied participants

The studied population consisted of 6819 women and 5994 men, with the mean age of 57.3 (SD12.9) and 57.4 (SD12.3), respectively. Gender differences was found in regards to education level, household income, self-reported health status, alcohol consumption levels, injuries caused by drinking, and use of all CAM approaches (Table 1). Most of the participants (62%) had middle to high income (> 40,000 €) and good health (66%) and one third of the participants had university education (Table 1).

More women (11%) than men (8%) were teetotallers. Most of the participants (68% of the men and 66% of the women) drank less than five times a month. Only 6% of the men and 4% of the women drank more than 3 times a week. Most of the women (74%) and half of the men (52%) drank 1–2 unites when drinking alcohol. Very few women (4%) drank more than 4 units when drinking (Table 1). More women (42%) than men (24%) had used CAM. Most of the participants had used herbal or "natural" medicine (23%) followed by alternative medical practitioner (12%) and self-treatment with meditation, yoga, qi gong or tai-chi (5%) (Table 1).

Visits to an alternative medical practitioner

We did not find significant associations for men between visits to alternative medical practitioners and any of the three included alcohol consumption variables (Table 2). For women, we found that individuals who had experienced injuries because of their drinking had 1.69 times higher odds (95% CI 1.16–2.47) to have applied an alternative medical practitioner compared to those who never had experienced injuries because of drinking (Table 3).

Use of herbal or "natural" medicine

The odds of using herbal or "natural" medicine were 76% higher (95% CI 1.27–2.44) in women who drank alcohol at least 4 times a week compared to alcohol abstainers (Table 3) The odds for women who drank 2–4 times a month and 2–3 times a week were ORs of 1.43 (95% CI 1.15–1.78) and 1.37 (95% CI 1.08–1.75) respectively compared to teetotallers.

In men, an association was found between the use of herbal or "natural" medicine and injuries caused by drinking. Men who had experienced injuries as a result of their drinking, had a 31% (95% CI 1.03–1.66) higher odds of having applied herbal or "natural" medicine in the previous 12 months compared to those who had not experienced injuries (Table 2). No association was found between the use of herbal or "natural" medicine and other alcohol consumption patterns.

Used self-treatment techniques

An association was found between use of self-treatment (meditation, yoga, qi gong or tai-chi) and frequency of alcohol consumption for women. The odds of having used such self-treatment techniques were highest among those who drank more than 3 times a week, with an odds ratio of 2.62 (95% CI 1.48–4.61) compared to alcohol abstainers (Table 3). We also found a strong positive association for having used self-treatment techniques for

Table 1 Basic characteristics of the studied participants

	Total $n = 12813^a$ (%)	Men $n = 5994^a$ (%)	Women $n = 6819^a$ (%)	*P*-value
Percentage women	53.2			
Age, mean (SD)	57.4 (12.6)	57.4 (12.3)	57.3 (12.9)	0.717[b]
Education, n (%)				
Compulsory	3596 (28.4)	1478 (25.0)	2118 (31.5)	
Middle level	4241 (33.6)	2096 (35.4)	2146 (31.9)	
College/University	4809 (38.0)	2349 (39.7)	2460 (36.6)	< 0.000[c]
Household income, n (%)				
Low to middle income < 400,000 NOK/40,000 €)	4569 (38.5)	1842 (32.0)	2727 (44.6)	
Middle to high income (401,000–700,000 NOK/40,100–70,000 €)	4199 (35.4)	2235 (38.9)	1964 (32.1)	
High income (701,000 NOK / 70,100 € or more)	3093 (26.1)	1668 (29.0)	1425 (23.3)	< 0.000[c]
Self-reported health status, n (%)				
Very bad or bad	686 (5.4)	279 (4.7)	407 (6.0)	
Neither good nor bad	3633 (28.6)	1671 (28.1)	1962 (29.1)	
Good or excellent	8386 (66.0)	4004 (67.2)	4382 (64.9)	0.001[c]
Alcohol frequency of use, n (%)				
Never	1413 (11.2)	454 (7.6)	959 (14.3)	
Monthly or more infrequently	3633 (28.7)	1545 (26.0)	2088 (31.1)	
2–4 times a month	4834 (38.2)	2481 (41.7)	2353 (35.0)	
2–3 times a week	2155 (17.0)	1125 (18.9)	1030 (15.3)	
More that 3 times a week	634 (5.0)	342 (5.8)	292 (4.3)	< 0.000[c]
Units of alcohol consumed when drinking, n (%)				
1–2 units	7095 (63.3)	2858 (52.3)	4237 (73.8)	
3–4 units	3020 (26.9)	1754 (32.1)	1266 (22.0)	
5 or more units	1091 (9.7)	852 (15.6)	239 (4.2)	< 0.000[c]
Injuries because of drinking, n (%)				
Never	10,882 (93.5)	4937 (89.4)	5945 (97.2)	
Yes	752 (6.5)	583 (10.6)	169 (2.8)	< 0.000[c]
Overall use of CAM modalities, n (%)	3730 (33.6)	1259 (24.1)	2471 (42.1)	< 0.000[c]
Alternative medical pratictioner[d]	1423 (11.9)	428 (7.6)	995 (15.9)	< 0.000[c]
Herbal or 'natural' medicine[e]	2677 (23.0)	937 (17.1)	1740 (28.3)	< 0.000[c]
Self-treatment[f]	590 (5.0)	107 (1.9)	483 (7.8)	< 0.000[c]

[a] Due to missing responses on the individual questions, not all number add up to total number of participants. [b] Independent sample t-test. [c] Pearson Chi-square test [d] Answered yes to: Have you during the past year visited: An alternative medical practitioner (homeopath, acupuncturist, foot zone therapist, herbal medicine practitioner, laying on of hands practitioner, healer, clairvoyant etc.)? [e] Answered yes to: In the last 12 months have you used herbal or "natural" medicine? [f] Answered yes to: In the last 12 months have you used meditation, yoga, qi gong or tai-chi as self-treatment?

Table 2 Association between alcohol and CAM for male participants

	Alternative practitioner[a]				Herbal medicine[b]				Self-treatment[c]			
	Unadjusted		Adjusted		Unadjusted		Adjusted		Unadjusted		Adjusted	
	OR (95% CI)	*P*-value	OR (95% CI)	*P*-value	OR (95% CI)	*P*-vaule	OR (95% C)	*P*-value	OR (95% CI)	*P*-value	OR (95% CI)	*P*-value
Alcohol Frequency of use												
Never	1.00		1.00		1.00		1.00		1.00		1.00	
Monthly or more infrequently	1.10 (0.79–1.66)	0.648	0.98 (0.63–1.50)	0.911	0.80 (0.60–1.06)	0.117	0.84 (0.62–1.14)	0.272	0.91 (0.41–2.02)	0.818	0.95 (0.40–2.23)	0.900
2–4 times a month	1.05 (0.70–1.56)	0.807	0.96 (0.63–1.45)	0.834	0.81 (0.62–1.06)	0.122	0.94 (0.70–1.26)	0.686	0.81 (0.38–1.75)	0.590	0.73 (0.31–1.68)	0.454
2–3 times a week	0.91 (0.59–1.40)	0.671	0.86 (0.54–1.40)	0.523	0.84 (0.63–1.13)	0.260	1.01 (0.73–1.38)	0.970	1.33 (0.60–2.95)	0.481	1.21 (0.51–2.87)	0.670
More that 3 times a week	0.82 (0.46–1.46)	0.495	0.86 (0.47–1.57)	0.627	1.10 (0.76–1.58)	0.620	1.19 (0.81–1.77)	0.371	1.09 (0.39–3.05)	0.865	1.1 (0.36–3.17)	0.903
Units of alcohol consumed when drinking												
1–2 units	1.00		1.00		1.00		1.00		1.00		1.00	
3–4 units	1.07 (0.85–1.35)	0.560	1.11 (0.87–1.41)	0.404	0.88 (0.74–1.04)	0.127	0.99 (0.83–1.18)	0.880	1.18 (0.76–1.83)	0.462	1.12 (0.72–1.76)	0.615
5 or more units	1.05 (0.78–1.41)	0.732	0.93 (0.67–1.28)	0.662	0.86 (0.69–1.06)	0.162	1.07 (0.84–1.35)	0.590	1.13 (0.64–1.99)	0.680	0.85 (0.46–1.56)	0.602
Injuries because of drinking												
Never	1.00		1.00		1.00		1.00		1.00		1.00	
Yes	1.08 (0.78–1.50)	0.626	0.98 (0.69–1.37)	0.890	1.12 (0.89–1.40)	0.333	1.31 (1.03–1.66)	0.027	1.65 (0.97–2.79)	0.064	1.23 (0.72–2.12)	0.449

[a] Visited an alternative medical practitioner within the previous year. [b] Used herbal or "natural" medicine within the previous year. [c] Used meditation, yoga, qi gong or tai-chi as self-treatment within the previous year. Adjusted *p*-value, OR and CI were adjusted for health status (cat.), household income (cat.), age (count) and level of education (cat). Cat.: categorical; Cont.: continuous

Table 3 Association between alcohol and CAM for female participants

	Alternative practitioner[a]				Herbal meedicine[b]				Self-treatment[c]			
	Unadjusted		Adjusted		Unadjusted		Adjusted		Unadjusted		Adjusted	
	OR (95% CI)	*P*-value	OR (95% CI)	*P*-value	OR (95% CI)	*P*-value	OR (95% CI)	*P*-value	OR (95% CI)	*P*-value	OR (95% CI)	*P*-value
Alcohol Frequency of use												
Never	1.00		1.00		1.00		1.00		1.00		1.00	
Monthly or more infrequently	0.94 (0.75–1.17)	0.570	0.88 (0.68–1.14)	0.336	1.13 (0.94–1.37)	0.198	1.20 (0.96–1.48)	0.105	2.02 (1.32–3.09)	0.001	1.46 (0.92–2.30)	0.104
2–4 times a month	1.17 (0.94–1.45)	0.161	1.08 (0.84–1.39)	0.555	1.36 (1.14–1.64)	0.001	1.43 (1.15–1.78)	0.001	2.86 (1.89–4.31)	0.000	1.71 (1.09–2.66)	0.019
2–3 times a week	1.04 (0.80–1.34)	0.779	1.02 (0.76–1.37)	0.885	1.30 (1.05–1.61)	0.015	1.37 (1.08–1.75)	0.010	3.69 (2.39–5.69)	0.000	2.07 (1.29–3.31)	0.002
More that 3 times a week	1.09 (0.75–1.58)	0.649	1.13 (0.75–1.71)	0.550	1.60 (1.91–2.16)	0.002	1.76 (1.27–2.44)	0.001	4.16 (2.46–7.03)	0.000	2.62 (1.48–4.61)	0.001
Units of alcohol consumed when drinking												
1–2 units	1.00		1.00		1.00		1.00		1.00		1.00	
3–4 units	1.13 (0.95–1.35)	0.153	1.03 (0.85–1.24)	0.763	1.01 (0.87–1.16)	0.918	1.03 (0.89–1.21)	0.668	1.12 (0.89–1.40)	0.335	0.90 (0.71–1.15)	0.395
5 or more units	1.03 (0.72–1.48)	0.862	0.79 (0.54–1.17)	0.247	0.76 (0.55–1.05)	0.092	0.76 (0.54–1.07)	0.114	1.05 (0.65–1.71)	0.837	0.77 (0.46–1.28)	0.316
Injuries because of drinking												
Never	1.00		1.00		1.00		1.00		1.00		1.00	
Yes	1.94 (1.35–2.79)	0.000	1.69 (1.16–2.47)	0.006	1.45 (1.06–2.00)	0.022	1.38 (0.98–1.93)	0.059	2.85 (1.91–4.24)	0.000	1.95 (1.28–2.96)	0.002

[a] Visited an alternative medical practitioner within the previous year. [b] Used herbal or "natural" medicine within the previous year. [c] Used meditation, yoga, qi gong or tai-chi as self-treatment within the previous year. Adjusted *p*-value, OR and CI were adjusted for health status (cat.), household income (cat.), age (count) and level of education (cat). Cat.: categorical; Cont.: continuous

those who reported drinking 2–4 times a month (OR 1.71, 95% CI 1.09–2.66) and 2–3 times a week (OR 2.07, 95% CI 1.29–3.31) compared to teetotallers. The odds of using self-treatment techniques were 96% higher (95% CI 1.28–2.96) in women who reported injuries caused by their drinking compared to those with no such experience. No significant relationship was found between the use of self-treatment techniques and alcohol consumption patterns in men (Table 2).

Discussion

We found a positive relationship between more frequent alcohol consumption and use of herbal or "natural" medicine and self-treatment techniques in women, but not in men. We also found a positive association between having experienced injuries to themselves or others because of their drinking and CAM use in general among women. For men this association was found only for herbal or "natural" medicine.

CAM use and alcohol consumption

Studies on CAM use and alcohol consumption are limited and are conducted in few countries. The findings on whether and to what extent alcohol consumption is associated with use of CAM is not consistent [1, 9, 12, 23, 28, 43]. Few studies have gender specific analyses despite the fact that both CAM use and alcohol consumption is influenced by gender [1, 10, 22]. In accordance with the men in the present study, several other studies failed to find any significant association between alcohol consumption and CAM use [30–32]. Ever drinkers were, however found to be more likely to have used CAM, compared to lifetime teetotallers in the US [27]. This is in accordance with our findings among women where ever drinkers of alcohol were more likely to have used herbal medicine and CAM self-treatment than the teetotallers. They found, however that those who drank infrequently (less than one alcohol unit a week) had the highest use of CAM, while heavy drinkers (15 or more units a week) were least likely to have used CAM. This is in contrast to the men in the present study where no significant differences were found, and to the women who were more likely to have used herbal medicine and self-help techniques the more frequently they drank. Grey et al. found that CAM users reported a lower overall consumption of alcohol than non-users [29]. One of the reasons for the inconsistency in our findings compared to the findings in these two studies from the US might be different CAM use and alcohol consumption patterns in the two countries [12, 23, 43]. One possibility is that Norwegian women drink more frequently, but when doing so they drink small amounts. This is suspected as 84% of the women who were drinking alcohol more than 3 times a week reported to only drink 1–2 units of alcohol when drinking.

It might also be that the participants used both CAM and alcohol to cope with the same condition. Partner strain, for instance, have been associated with both increased use of CAM [44] and alcohol [42]. Also pain and psychiatric problems [45–49] could contribute to explain the association between CAM use and alcohol consumption in women. CAM users have shown to be more likely to report mental disorders such as major depression and panic disorders compared to non-users [44] and might also drink alcohol to cope with the same issues. Some CAM therapies have also been used as strategies to cope with alcohol craving and dependencies [45–48], which also could explain the association found in this study. The relationship is complex, as many factors in life could influence both on use of CAM and alcohol consumption.

CAM use and injuries caused by drinking

This study revealed an association between having experiences injuries caused by own drinking and use of CAM for both men and women. One possible explanation for the association, could be the Norwegian drinking culture that is characterized by heavy episodic drinking during the weekends [4], causing people without drinking problems to injury themselves or others. Injuries caused by drinking and other discomfort caused by heavy drinking could also increase the need for medical treatment and pain relief, thus increase the use of CAM modalities.

Gender differences

Most of the associations found between CAM modalities and alcohol consumption, was found among the female participants. The only significant association found for men was between use of herbal or "natural" medicine and injuries cause by own drinking. This relationship was, however, not significant for women. The gender differences found are likely due to different associations for use of CAM and different patterns of alcohol consumption for men and women [4, 17, 42, 49]. Men often frame their use of CAM in terms of rationality and have reported treatment of health related issues as their main motivation for CAM use. Women, on the other hand, use in addition CAM to deal with low self-esteem, eating disorders and body image concerns [49]. The association between CAM use and injuries caused by drinking was found only for men. The reason for this might be that men experience such injuries more frequently than women [50]. It is also possible that such drinking behaviour is more accepted among men, leading women to underreport such behaviour.

Strength and limitations

The main strength of this study is the large number of participants ($n = 12{,}981$) representing 20% of the total population of Tromsø [51], and the rather high response rate of 65%.

Populations based studies are considered to be an excellent source of data in research [36], nevertheless, the results should be interpreted in light of some limitations. These data reflects a cross-sectional set of associations with no information on possibly causal events [52]. The experience of injuries caused by own drinking was recoded into ever having had such an experience while the question of CAM use was restricted to use within the last 12 months. Injuries caused by drinking might have happened only once and/or a long time ago and might not be representative for that person's current or general alcohol consumption. Another limitation is that the findings are based on self-reported data that might be influences by the participants' perceptions of right and wrong and misinterpretations of the questions [52, 53]. Both intentionally and unintentionally, people tend to overestimate their healthy lifestyle choices and underestimate unhealthy habits [52]. Hence, questions regarding alcohol consumption and injuries caused by drinking could be especially prone to report bias [53, 54].

The ability to answer accurately and completely could be difficult when describing drinking behaviour in distant past [53]. Injuries might also occur under severe intoxication, when blackouts are not uncommon [55] and it is therefore likely to be under-reported.

Reduced accuracy due to recall bias might also be present for CAM, as participants were asked to report use as far back as 12 months. Men might also be more prone to underreport use of CAM compared to women as CAM use is often associated with feminine qualities and traditional female gender roles [22]. Women on the other hand, might be less inclined to report heavy episodic drinking and injuries caused by drinking due to the same traditional gender roles.

Due to the fact that CAM users often apply more than one CAM approach, the different CAM variables were not mutually exclusive in the analyses. The non-users of one approach might still have applied other CAM modalities. The analyses does therefor not compare CAM users to non-users of CAM in general. This is in line with the aim of the study which was to compare users of the different CAM approaches to non-users of these. Finally, even though we have adjusted for the most important factors, a residual confounding cannot be excluded.

Implication of the findings

The main aim of this study was to address the almost total lack of studies investigating the associations between alcohol consumption and use of different CAM approaches. Knowledge of this association could be important for health care personnel when discussing the patient's health problems and how the patient deal with these problems themselves, and further how approaches like CAM use and alcohol consumption can interact with conventional care. CAM providers can use the findings of this study to discuss their client's use of alcohol and risks of excessive drinking and further, to suggest other, healthier ways to cope with the cause of their drinking.

Future research

The findings from this study cannot fully explain the relationship between alcohol consumption and CAM approaches, and inconsistency in international findings indicate that both CAM and alcohol use vary across cultures and over time. The relationship is likely to be complex, as many factors in life could influence both use of CAM and alcohol consumption. In order to get a clearer picture of the associations between CAM use and alcohol consumption, further research is needed focusing on the underlying causes of use of different CAM modalities and alcohol consumption patterns. There is also a need for research with longitudinal design to explore the causation of the relationship.

Conclusion

In this study we found different associations between CAM use and alcohol consumption than what is found earlier in studies conducted in other countries. This underline the need for local studies since both patterns of CAM use and alcohol consumption varies widely across cultures and regions. The associations between frequent alcohol consumption and injuries caused by drinking and use of CAM in Norway can be useful for both conventional and unconventional health care personnel in meeting with their patients.

Acknowledgements

We thank the people of Tromsø and the Tromsø Study for giving data to this study.

Funding

The publication charges for this article have been funded by a grant from the publication fund of UiT The Arctic University of Norway. No further funding was received.

Authors' contributions

The paper is based on an unpublished master thesis in public health at Uit The Arctic University of Norway by first author KS submitted in 2017, with AEK and ML as supervisors. KS and AEK conceived the study. KS and ML made the analyze strategy and ML supervised KS when conducting the initial and final analyses. KS drafted the initial version of the paper and all authors reviewed subsequent versions, read, and approved the final manuscript.

Competing interests
The authors declare that they have no competing interests.

Author details
[1]Department for drugs – and addiction treatment and A-larm Norway, Hospital of Southern Norway, Kristiansand, Norway. [2]Department of Community Medicine, Faculty of Health Sciences, UiT The Arctic University of Norway, Tromsø, Norway. [3]National Research Center in Complementary and Alternative Medicine (NAFKAM), Department of Community Medicine, Faculty of Health Sciences, UiT The Arctic University of Norway, Tromsø, Norway.

References

1. Global status report on alcohol and health 2014 [Internet] [http://apps.who.int/iris/bitstream/10665/112736/1/9789240692763_eng.pdf], 2014, Accessed: 11.04.2018.
2. Rehm J, Mathers C, Popova S, Thavorncharoensap M, Teerawattananon Y, Patra J. Global burden of disease and injury and economic cost attributable to alcohol use and alcohol-use disorders. Lancet. 2009;373(9682):2223–33.
3. Alcohol sales, Statbank. [Internet] [https://www.ssb.no/statistikkbanken/selecttable/hovedtabellHjem.asp?KortNavnWeb=alkohol&CMSSubjectArea=varehandel-og-tjenesteyting&checked=true], 2016, Accessed: 15.05. 2017.
4. Rusmidler i Norge 2016: Alkohol, tobakk, vanedannende legemidler, narkotika, sniffing, doping og tjenestetilbudet [Internet] [https://www.fhi.no/globalassets/dokumenterfiler/rapporter/rusmidler_i_norge_2016.pdf], 2016, Accessed: 29.06.2017.
5. Hansen-Krone IJ, Braekkan SK, Enga KF, Wilsgaard T, Hansen JB. Alcohol consumption, types of alcoholic beverages and risk of venous thromboembolism - the Tromso study. Thromb Haemost. 2011;106(2):272–8.
6. Sacks JJ, Gonzales KR, Bouchery EE, Tomedi LE, Brewer RD. 2010 national and state costs of excessive alcohol consumption. Am J Prev Med. 2015; 49(5):e73–9.
7. Lim SS, Vos T, Flaxman AD, Danaei G, Shibuya K, Adair-Rohani H, AlMazroa MA, Amann M, Anderson HR, Andrews KG. A comparative risk assessment of burden of disease and injury attributable to 67 risk factors and risk factor clusters in 21 regions, 1990–2010: a systematic analysis for the global burden of disease study 2010. Lancet. 2013;380(9859):2224–60.
8. Stahre M. Contribution of excessive alcohol consumption to deaths and years of potential life lost in the United States. Prev Chronic Dis. 2014;11
9. WHO Traditional Medicine Strategy 2014–2023. Geneva; 2013 [Internet] [http://apps.who.int/iris/bitstream/10665/92455/1/9789241506090_eng.pdf], 2014, Accessed:30.07.2018.
10. Reid R, Steel A, Wardle J, Trubody A, Adams J. Complementary medicine use by the Australian population: a critical mixed studies systematic review of utilisation, perceptions and factors associated with use. BMC Complement Altern Med. 2016;16(1):176.
11. Molassiotis A, Fernadez-Ortega P, Pud D, Ozden G, Scott JA, Panteli V, Margulies A, Browall M, Magri M, Selvekerova S. Use of complementary and alternative medicine in cancer patients: a European survey. Ann Oncol. 2005;16(4):655–63.
12. Use of complementary and alternative medicine in Norway [Internet] [http://nifab.no/content/download/98429/596946/file/NAFKAM-2012.pdf], 2012, Accessed: 30.07.2018.
13. Kristoffersen AE, Norheim AJ, Fønnebø VM: Complementary and alternative medicine use among Norwegian cancer survivors: gender-specific prevalence and associations for use. Evidence-Based Complementary and Alternative Medicine, vol. 2013, Article ID 318781, 10 pages, 2013. doi: https://doi.org/10.1155/2013/318781.
14. Thomas D-A, Maslin B, Legler A, Springer E, Asgerally A, Vadivelu N. Role of alternative therapies for chronic pain syndromes. Curr Pain Headache Rep. 2016;20(5):1–7.
15. Kanodia AK, Legedza AT, Davis RB, Eisenberg DM, Phillips RS. Perceived benefit of complementary and alternative medicine (CAM) for back pain: a national survey. J Am Board Fam Med. 2010;23(3):354–62.
16. Hansen AH, Kristoffersen AE. The use of CAM providers and psychiatric outpatient services in people with anxiety/depression: a cross-sectional survey. BMC Complement Altern Med. 2016;16(1):461.
17. Kristoffersen AE, Stub T, Salamonsen A, Musial F, Hamberg K. Gender differences in prevalence and associations for use of CAM in a large population study. BMC Complement Altern Med. 2014;14(1):463.
18. Harris P, Cooper K, Relton C, Thomas K. Prevalence of complementary and alternative medicine (CAM) use by the general population: a systematic review and update. Int J Clin Pract. 2012;66(10):924–39.
19. Clarke TC, Black LI, Stussman BJ, Barnes PM, Nahin RL. Trends in the use of complementary health approaches among adults: United States, 2002–2012. Natl Health Stat Rep. 2015;79:1.
20. Use of complementary and alternative medicine in Norway [Internet] [http://nifab.no/content/download/101011/632568/file/NAFKAM-2016%20rapport%20_finale.pdf], 2016, Accessed: 30.07.2018.
21. Steinsbekk A, Rise MB, Johnsen R. Changes among male and female visitors to practitioners of complementary and alternative medicine in a large adult Norwegian population from 1997 to 2008 (the HUNT studies). BMC Complement Altern Med. 2011;11(1):61.
22. Keshet Y, Simchai D. The 'gender puzzle'of alternative medicine and holistic spirituality: a literature review. Soc Sci Med. 2014;113:77–86.
23. Barnes PM, Bloom B, Nahin RL. Complementary and alternative medicine use among adults and children. United States. 2007;2008(12):1–23.
24. Li K, Kaaks R, Linseisen J, Rohrmann S. Consistency of vitamin and/or mineral supplement use and demographic, lifestyle and health-status predictors: findings from the European prospective investigation into Cancer and nutrition (EPIC)-Heidelberg cohort. Br J Nutr. 2010;104(07):1058–64.
25. Weathermon R, Crabb DW. Alcohol and medication interactions. Alcohol Res Health. 1999;23(1):40–54.
26. Klein S, Wolf U. Users of complementary medicine generally maintain a healthy lifestyle. Eur J Integrative Med. 2016;8(Suppl1):64.
27. Nahin RL, Dahlhamer JM, Taylor BL, Barnes PM, Stussman BJ, Simile CM, Blackman MR, Chesney MA, Jackson M, Miller H. Health behaviors and risk factors in those who use complementary and alternative medicine. BMC Public Health. 2007;7(1):217.
28. Micke O, Bruns F, Glatzel M, Schönekaes K, Micke P, Mücke R, Büntzel J. Predictive factors for the use of complementary and alternative medicine (CAM) in radiation oncology. Eur J Integrative Med. 2009;1(1):19–25.
29. Gray CM, Tan A, Pronk N, O Connor P. Complementary and alternative medicine use among health plan members. A cross-sectional survey. Effective Clinical Practice. 2002;5(1):17–22.
30. Robinson AR, Crane LA, Davidson AJ, Steiner JF. Association between use of complementary/alternative medicine and health-related behaviors among health fair participants. Prev Med. 2002;34(1):51–7.
31. Cherniack EP, Senzel RS, Pan CX. Correlates of use of alternative medicine by the elderly in an urban population. J Altern Complement Med. 2001;7(3):277–80.
32. Astin JA, Pelletier KR, Marie A, Haskell WL. Complementary and alternative medicine use among elderly persons: one-year analysis. J Gerontol Med Sci. 2000;55:M4–9.
33. Jacobsen BK, Eggen AE, Mathiesen EB, Wilsgaard T, Njølstad I. Cohort profile: the Tromsø study. Int J Epidemiol. 2012;41(4):961–7.
34. The sixth Tromsø Study [Internet] [https://en.uit.no/forskning/forskningsgrupper/sub?sub_id=453665&p_document_id=453582], 2017, Accessed: 20 Apr 2017.
35. Hansen JC, Van Oostdam J: AMAP Assessment 2009: Human Health in the Arctic. In: *Documentation Arctic Monitoring and Assessment program (AMAP)*. Oslo, Norway; 2009.
36. Eggen AE, Mathiesen EB, Wilsgaard T, Jacobsen BK, Njølstad I. The sixth survey of the Tromsø study (Tromsø 6) in 2007–08: collaborative research in the interface between clinical medicine and epidemiology: study objectives, design, data collection procedures, and attendance in a multipurpose population-based health survey. Scandinavian journal of public health. 2013; 41(1):65–80.
37. Questionnaire 1, the sixth Tromsø study [https://uit.no/Content/100349/Q1_t6.pdf], 2014, Accessed: 11th of April 2018.
38. Questionnaire 2, the sixth Tromsø study [https://uit.no/Content/100351/Spoerreskjema_2_t6.pdf], 2014, Accessed: 11th of Apr 2018.
39. Roerecke M, Rehm J. Irregular heavy drinking occasions and risk of ischemic heart disease: a systematic review and meta-analysis. Am J Epidemiol. 2010; 171(6):633–44.
40. Rehm J, Room R, Graham K, Monteiro M, Gmel G, Sempos CT. The relationship of average volume of alcohol consumption and patterns of drinking to burden of disease: an overview. Addiction. 2003;98(9):1209–28.

41. Halkjelsvik T, Storvoll EE. Andel av befolkningen i Norge med et risikofylt alkoholkonsum målt gjennom Alcohol Use Disorders Identification Test (AUDIT). Nordic Stud Alcohol Drugs. 2015;32(1):61–72.
42. Sosial ulikhet i alkoholbruk og alkoholrelatert sykelighet og dødelighet [Internet] [https://helsedirektoratet.no/Lists/Publikasjoner/Attachments/1204/Sosial%20uikhet%20i%20alkoholbruk%20og%20alkoholrelatert%20sykelighet%20og%20d%C3%B8delighet%20IS-2474.pdf], 2016, Accessed: 11th of April 2018.
43. Steinsbekk A, Rise MB, Aickin M. Cross-cultural comparison of visitors to CAM practitioners in the United States and Norway. J Altern Complement Med. 2009;15(11):1201–7.
44. Honda K, Jacobson JS. Use of complementary and alternative medicine among United States adults: the influences of personality, coping strategies, and social support. Prev Med. 2005;40(1):46–53.
45. Reynolds A, Keough MT, O'Connor RM. Is being mindful associated with reduced risk for internally-motivated drinking and alcohol use among undergraduates? Addict Behav. 2015;42:222–6.
46. Murphy CM, MacKillop J. Mindfulness as a strategy for coping with cue-elicited cravings for alcohol: an experimental examination. Alcohol Clin Exp Res. 2014;38(4):1134–42.
47. Roos CR, Pearson MR, Brown DB. Drinking motives mediate the negative associations between mindfulness facets and alcohol outcomes among college students. Psychol Addict Behav. 2015;29(1):176.
48. Stein L, Lebeau R, Colby SM, Barnett NP, Golembeske C, Monti PM. Motivational interviewing for incarcerated adolescents: effects of depressive symptoms on reducing alcohol and marijuana use after release. J. Stud Alcohol Drugs. 2011;72(3):497–506.
49. Brenton J, Elliott S. Undoing gender? The case of complementary and alternative medicine. Sociol Health Illn. 2014;36(1):91–107.
50. Rusmiddelstatistikk: Alkohol. [Internet] [http://norgeshelsa.no/russtat/], 2017, Accessed: 2nd June 2017.
51. Statistikkbanken: Folkemengde og befolkningsendringer [Internet] [https://www.ssb.no/statistikkbanken/SelectVarVal/Define.asp?MainTable=NY3026&KortNavnWeb=folkemengde&PLanguage=0&checked=true], 2017, Accessed: 22 May 2017.
52. Armitage P, Colton T: Encyclopedia of Epidemiologic Methods Chichester John Wiley & Sons ltd; 1999.
53. Del Boca FK, Darkes J. The validity of self-reports of alcohol consumption: state of the science and challenges for research. Addiction. 2003;98(s2):1–12.
54. Ekholm O. Influence of the recall period on self-reported alcohol intake. Eur J Clin Nutr. 2004;58(1):60–3.
55. Hartzler B, Fromme K. Fragmentary blackouts: their etiology and effect on alcohol expectancies. Alcohol Clin Exp Res. 2003;27(4):628–37.

5

Tinospora cordifolia as a potential neuroregenerative candidate against glutamate induced excitotoxicity: an in vitro perspective

Anuradha Sharma and Gurcharan Kaur*

Abstract

Background: Glutamate, the major excitatory neurotransmitter of CNS acts as a neurotoxin at higher concentrations. Prolonged activation of glutamate receptors results in progressive neuronal damage by aggravating calcium influx, inducing mitochondrial damage and oxidative stress. Excitotoxic cell death is associated with the pathogenesis of various neurodegenerative disorders such as trauma, brain injury and neurodegenerative diseases. The current study was designed to investigate the neuroprotective and neuroregenerative potential of *Tinospora cordifolia* against glutamate-induced excitotoxicity using primary cerebellar neuronal cultures as a model system.

Methods: Monosodium salt of glutamate was used to induce neurotoxic injury in primary cerebellar neurons. Four extracts including Hexane extract, Chloroform extract, Ethyl acetate, and Butanol extract were obtained from fractionation of previously reported aqueous ethanolic extract of *T. cordifolia* and tested for neuroprotective activity. Out of the four fractions, Butanol extract of *T. cordifolia* (B-TCE) exhibited neuroprotective potential by preventing degeneration of neurons induced by glutamate. Expression of different neuronal, apoptotic, inflammatory, cell cycle regulatory and plasticity markers was studied by immunostaining and Western blotting. Neurite outgrowth and migration were also studied using primary explant cultures, wound scratch and gelatin zymogram assay.

Results: At molecular level, B-TCE pretreatment of glutamate-treated cultures normalized the stress-induced downregulation in the expression of neuronal markers (MAP-2, GAP-43, NF200) and anti-apoptotic marker (Bcl-xL). Further, cells exposed to glutamate showed enhanced expression of inflammatory (NF-κB, AP-1) and senescence markers (HSP70, Mortalin) as well as the extent of mitochondrial damage. However, B-TCE pretreatment prevented this increase and inhibited glutamate-induced onset of inflammation, stress and mitochondrial membrane damage. Furthermore, B-TCE was observed to promote regeneration, migration and plasticity of cerebellar neurons, which was otherwise significantly inhibited by glutamate treatment.

Conclusion: These results suggest that B-TCE may have neuroprotective and neuroregenerative potential against catastrophic consequences of glutamate-mediated excitotoxicity and could be a potential therapeutic candidate for neurodegenerative diseases.

Keywords: *Tinospora cordifolia*, Neuritogenesis, Neurodegeneration, Neuroprotection, Neurotoxicity, Neuronal plasticity, Cerebellar neurons

* Correspondence: kgurcharan.neuro@yahoo.com
Department of Biotechnology, Medical Biotechnology lab, Guru Nanak Dev University, Amritsar, Punjab 143005, India

Background

The challenging diversity of neurological disorders such as trauma, ischemia, stroke, epilepsy as well as neurodegenerative diseases, although have different initial causes of disease onset but share a common final destructive pathway known as excitotoxicity [1]. L-glutamic acid is a major excitatory amino acid in the CNS, which plays a major role in neurotransmission and is responsible for performing fundamental brain functions such as neuronal circuit formations and synaptic plasticity underlying memory and cognition [2]. Glutamate acts through both inotropic as well as metabotropic receptors and increased extracellular levels of glutamate lead to overactivation of glutamate receptors resulting in neuronal damage [3]. Higher concentration of glutamate released during hypoxia or ischemia causes overstimulation of glutamate receptors and rise in intracellular calcium levels [4]. Higher intracellular calcium further activates various enzymes such as proteases, endonucleases, phospholipases and nitric oxide synthase (NOS), thus enhancing structural degradation, mitochondrial damage, ROS/RNS production, DNA damage and increased expression of inflammatory mediators which lead to increased neuronal damage [5, 6].

The currently available drug therapies for neurodegenerative diseases are palliative with limited effectiveness and adverse side effects [7–9]. The major challenge for the researchers is to develop a therapy that addresses the underlying cause/mechanism of degeneration with improved effectiveness and least side effects. Therapeutic interventions that modify the progression of neurodegeneration may prove useful and plant-based interventions offer various possibilities to modify the disease progression and symptoms [8]. *T. cordifolia*, a Rasayana herb of Indian Ayurvedic system has been reported to possess anti-cancer, anti-oxidative, anti-diabetic, anti-aphrodisiac, adaptogenic, immune stimulant and immune protective activities [10–14]. However, neuroprotective activity of this plant is least explored. Recently, the ethanolic extract of *T. cordifolia* was reported to exhibit neuroprotective activity against 6-OHDA induced Parkinsonism [15]. Recent studies from our lab have reported that 50% aqueous ethanolic extract of *T. cordifolia* (TCE) ameliorated anxiety, improved exploratory behavior and modulated synaptic plasticity in sleep-deprived rats [16]. Various medicinal properties of *T. cordifolia* have been attributed to its phytochemical constituents belonging to different classes such as alkaloids, terpenoids, glycosides, sesquiterpenoids, aliphatic compounds and steroids. Some alkaloids, glycosides and aliphatic compounds are broadly considered responsible for immune modulatory and neuroprotective properties of this herb [17–19]. n-Butanol fraction of *T. cordifolia* extract has been reported to have tinocordifolioside A and tinocordiside as active compounds [20, 21].

The current study was aimed to investigate the neuroprotective potential of Butanol extract of *T. cordifolia* (B-TCE) against glutamate-induced excitotoxicity using primary cerebellar neurons as a model system. Cerebellum constitutes the major neuronal population of the nervous system. A homogenous population of cerebellar granular neuronal cells developed postnatally from new born rats and mice has been widely accepted as a cellular model system to study various aspects of neurogenesis, neuronal development, death and other brain pathologies [22, 23]. Primary cerebellar neuronal cultures were established using 6-day old rat pups and were treated with glutamate, B-TCE alone and B-TCE + glutamate. After initial microscopic observations, we further investigated the interplay between glutamate and B-TCE on the expression of different molecular effectors responsible for neuronal structural integrity, senescence, apoptosis, inflammation and neuronal plasticity.

Methods

Preparation of plant extract

T. cordifolia was collected in last week of January, 2015 from the local forest in Ropar district of Punjab, India and was identified by Dr. Amarjeet Singh Soodan, Herbarium in-Charge of Department of Botanical and Environmental Sciences, Guru Nanak Dev University, Amritsar, India. A voucher specimen of stem and leaves has been deposited in departmental herbarium with reference no. 65 Bot. & Env. Sc. Dated 04-09-2017. Initially, 50% aqueous ethanolic extract was prepared by percolating 1.5 kg dry stem powder in a percolator with 5 L capacity for 4 times. Collected extract was evaporated at 45 °C using rotavapor and lyophilizer yielding 220 g of TCE which was further fractionated with n-Hexane, Chloroform, Ethyl acetate and n-Butanol (SRL, Analytical grade). Each fraction was collected and evaporated to dryness using a rotary evaporator which yielded 1.17 g Hexane extract, 10 g Chloroform extract, 12 g Ethyl acetate extract and 56.2 g Butanol extract (B-TCE). For use in culture, 100 mg/mL stock was prepared in DMSO and diluted in neurobasal medium (Invitrogen, CA, USA) to the final concentration of 20 μg/mL according to experimental requirements.

Primary cerebellar neuronal and explant cultures

Primary cerebellar and neuronal cultures were obtained from 6-day old albino Wistar rat pups. Briefly, rat pups were sacrificed by decapitation and brain was removed out from the skull. Cerebellum was dissected out in chilled 1X PBS and after removal of meninges, it was transferred to Petri dish containing fresh chilled 1X PBS. Three cuts were given in a cerebellum and 1X PBS was replaced with 0.05% Trypsin-EDTA containing DNase I (2 units/mL) (Invitrogen). Trypsinization was carried out for 10 min at 37 °C with 2–3 intermediate gentle shakings, followed by addition of equal volume of neurobasal medium for stopping the digestion. Partially digested tissue was centrifuged for 2 min (1000 rpm) and the pellet was re-suspended in 4 mL chilled neurobasal medium. To obtain single cell population, the pellet was triturated with micropipette (25 strokes) and allowed to settle down for 5–10 min. Leaving the debris undisturbed, the suspension was then collected into a fresh tube and centrifuged for 2 min at 1000 rpm. Obtained pellet was re-suspended in 1 mL neurobasal medium (normalized to room temperature), counted using hemocytometer and seeded on Poly-L-Lysine (PLL) coated coverslips in 12 or 24 well plates according to experiment.

For explant culture, after removing meninges, cerebellum was chopped into very small pieces using scalpel or micro-dissector. These small pieces of the cerebellar tissue were placed onto PLL coated coverslips with the help of micropipette, allowed to attach for few minutes followed by neurobasal medium replenishment in the wells. At least three explants per well were established and the experiment was carried out in triplicates.

Cell culture and treatments

Primary cerebellar neurons were seeded in 12 or 24 well plates containing PLL coated coverslips at a seeding density of 40,000 cells/mL. Four groups were studied 1) Control 2) Glutamate treatment 3) B-TCE alone treatment 4) B-TCE + Glutamate treatment. After 24 h of seeding, group 3 and 4 were treated with 20 μg/mL of B-TCE and group 1 and 2 were given medium change only. After the next 24 h, glutamate was added to group 2 and 4 at a final concentration of 2 mM and incubation was done for another 24 h. Control cultures i.e. group 1 was given only medium change. Cultures were maintained in neurobasal medium containing B27, bFGF supplement (Invitrogen) and were incubated in a humidified 5% CO_2 incubator at 37 °C temperature. From the reported literature, we initially checked 1, 2 and 5 mM concentration of glutamate on primary cerebellar neurons and selected 2 mM concentration as a subtoxic dose [31]. Two different concentrations of B-TCE (10 and 20 μg/mL) were tested against 2 mM glutamate out of which 20 μg/mL was more effective, so it was selected for further experiments (Additional file 1: Fig. S1). Each experiment was carried out in triplicate.

Cellular and nuclear morphological studies

After completion of treatment regime i.e. 72 h of seeding, primary cerebellar neurons were observed and phase contrast images were captured using EVOS FL microscope (Invitrogen). Further, to gain detailed information about the effect of glutamate and B-TCE pretreatment on number of processes or length of processes, morphometric study was carried out. Cells were seeded at a seeding density of 20,000 cells/mL in PLL coated 12 well plates, followed by the treatment regime mentioned above and harvested by fixing in 2.5% glutaraldehyde (in neurobasal medium). After fixing, cells were stained with staining solution containing 1% methylene blue and 1% toluidine blue in 1% sodium tetraborate for 40 min, followed by rinsing with distilled water and then allowed to dry. Images were captured using EVOS FL microscope and analyzed with Image Pro Plus software from media cybernetics version 4.5.1. The experiment was performed in triplicates and 100 cells from each group were analyzed for the study of number and length of processes. For nuclear morphology, cells were stained with a fluorescent stain 4′, 6-diamidino-2-phenylindole (DAPI) (Sigma-Aldrich, MO, USA) which specifically binds to AT-rich regions in DNA.

Immunostaining

Control and treated cells were given a washing with chilled 1X PBS followed by fixation with acetone and methanol (1:1) and permeabilization with 0.3% Triton- X100 in 1X PBS. Cells were then blocked with 2% BSA and incubated with primary mouse monoclonal antibody anti-α-Tubulin (1:500), anti-NF-κB (1:500), anti-MAP-2 (1:250), anti-NF200 (1:500), anti-GAP 43 (1:250), anti-HSP70 (1:500), anti-Mortalin (1:500), anti-Bcl-xL (1:200), anti-Cyclin D1(1:250), anti-NCAM (1:250), rabbit monoclonal anti-AP-1(1:250) (all from Sigma-Aldrich) and mouse monoclonal anti-PCNA (1:250), mouse polyclonal anti-PSA-NCAM (1:250) (from Millipore, MA, USA) for 24 h in humid chamber at 4 °C. No permeabilization was carried out for PSA-NCAM immunostaining. After primary antibody incubation, three washings were given with 0.1% PBST and incubated with secondary antibody (goat anti-mouse/ rabbit IgG/ IgM Alexa Fluor 488/543) for 2 h at RT. Cells were stained with nuclear staining dye DAPI (Sigma-Aldrich) for 15 min, washed with 0.1% PBST and mounted with antifading agent Fluoromount (Sigma-Aldrich). Images were captured with Nikon AIR Confocal Laser Scanning Microscope and analyzed with NIS elements analysis software version 4.11.00 (Nikon Co., Tokyo, Japan). Each experiment was carried out in triplicate.

Western blotting

For total protein extraction, Primary cerebellar neurons were grown and treated in multi-well plates followed by harvesting using chilled PBS–EDTA (1 mM). The cell pellet was homogenized in RIPA buffer (50 mM Tris (pH 7.5), 150 mM NaCl, 0.5% sodium deoxycholate, 0.1% SDS, 1.0% NP-40). Protein concentration was determined by the Bradford method and protein lysate (25 μg) was resolved in 7%, 10% and 12% gels by Sodium dodecyl sulfate- Polyacrylamide gel electrophoresis (SDS-PAGE), followed by semi-dry transfer onto a PVDF membrane (Hybond-P). Further, membranes were incubated with mouse monoclonal anti-α-Tubulin (1:5000), anti-NF-κB (1:5000), anti-MAP-2 (1:2500), anti-NF200 (1:5000), anti-GAP-43 (1:2500), anti-HSP70 (1:5000), anti-Mortalin (1:5000), anti-Bcl-xL (1:2000), anti-Cyclin D1(1:2500), anti-NCAM (1:2500), mouse polyclonal anti-PSA-NCAM (1:2500), and rabbit monoclonal anti-AP-1(1:2500) antibodies for overnight at 4 °C. This was followed by washing with 0.1% TBST and incubation with HRP labeled secondary antibodies for 2 h at RT. Immunoreactive bands were detected by ECL Plus Western blot detection system using LAS 4000 (Amersham Biosciences, GE Healthcare, UK). The final expression of each protein of interest was calculated after normalizing the protein expression with expression of endogenous control α-tubulin in the same sample. The change in expression of the gene of interest was calculated from average of IDV (integrated density values) obtained from at least three independent experiments.

mRNA expression

Total RNA was extracted from the cells by TRI reagent (Sigma-Aldrich) according to manufacturer's instructions and cDNA was synthesized from it. 50 ng of cDNA was used for reaction in 5 μL of reaction mixture in triplicate containing 2.5 μL of 2X TaqMan Master Mix, 0.5 μL of 20X predesigned Primer Probe mix (Applied Biosystem, CA, USA) and 1 μL of water, using amplification Step One Plus Real-Time PCR system (Applied Biosystem). Amplification conditions comprised of initial holding stage of 50 °C for 2 min followed by 95 °C for 10 min, and then cycling stage comprised of 40 cycles of amplification (denaturation at 95°C for 15 sec, further annealing and elongation at 60 °C for 1 min). GAPDH was used as an endogenous control for each gene of interest. The relative gene expression of each candidate gene was calculated by 'Livak method' and represented as $2^{-\Delta\Delta Ct}$ and final gene expression as $2^{-\Delta\Delta Ct}$±SEM. Final results were obtained as average of minimum three different observations for each experimental group.

Pro-inflammatory cytokine ELISA based determination

Media was collected from different wells of all the four different treatment groups and used for determination of pro-inflammatory cytokines using sandwich ELISA based kits from Cayman Chemical Company, USA (TNF-α and IL-6) and Sigma Aldrich, USA (IL-1β). Estimation and calculations were performed as per manufacturer's protocol. The experiment was performed at least three times in triplicate.

Wound scratch assay

To study the effect of B-TCE on migration behavior of primary neurons, primary cerebellar neurons were seeded at a high density and grown to achieve confluency. A straight scratch was given with microtip on all the coverslips containing a confluent monolayer of cells which was followed by treatment with Glutamate (2 mM), B-TCE (20 μg/mL), B-TCE (20 μg/mL) + Glutamate (2 mM). Phase contrast images were captured at zero and 24 h of treatment using EVOS FL microscope. Gap closure was calculated after image analysis by Image-Pro Plus software version 4.5.1 from the media cybernetics. The distance cells migrated into the cell-free area was measured with respect to the initial cell-free area to determine percent gap closure.

Mitotracker staining

To carry out Mitotracker staining, after completion of treatment regime, Mitotracker green FM (Invitrogen) was added to all the treatment groups in multi-well plate at 100 nM final concentration and incubated in CO_2 Incubator at 37 °C. After 45 min of incubation, the medium was discarded, cells were washed with chilled 1X PBS and fixed using chilled acetone and methanol (1:1) solution. Coverslips containing cultures were mounted using antifading medium and captured using Nikon A1R confocal microscope on the same day.

Gelatin zymogram study

In order to study the effect of glutamate and B-TCE on Matrix Metalloproteinases expression, cell culture medium was collected from different treatment groups, briefly spun to remove any floating debris and supernatant samples were separated on 10% SDS–polyacrylamide gels containing 0.1% gelatin. Further, gels were incubated in renaturation buffer (Invitrogen) for 1 h followed by 3 washings with distilled water. Gels were then incubated in developing buffer (Invitrogen) for 72 h at RT on a platform rocker. After 72 h, gels were washed again in distilled water, stained with Coomassie Brilliant Blue (CBB) and destained using buffer containing 10% acetic acid and 50% methanol (*v*/v). Clear white bands in blue stained gel were considered as regions of gelatinolytic activity.

UPLC/MS analysis of B-TCE

In order to determine different compounds present in B-TCE, it was subjected to LC/MS profiling. 10 mg

B-TCE was dissolved in 1 mL methanol, vortexed and passed through 0.22 μm filter. 1 μL sample was subjected to Waters Acquity UPLC system (Waters, MA, USA) with Acquity UPLC BEH C_{18} column (100 mm × 2.1 mm, particle size 1.7 μm) and photodiode array (PDA) detector. The sample was separated using mobile phase solvent gradient consisting of 1% formic acid in water (A) and 1% formic acid in acetonitrile (B). MS was performed using Q-TOF triple Quadrupole Mass Spectrometer attached with Electrospray Ionisation (ESI) source (Waters Micromass, Manchester, UK). LC/MS analysis was performed using Masslynx v4.1.

Statistical analysis

Values are expressed as mean ± SEM from at least three independent experiments. Results were analyzed to determine the significance of means by using one way ANOVA (Holm-Sidak post hoc method), which was performed by Sigma Stat software (Version 3.5) for Windows. Values with $p \leq 0.01$ were considered as statistically significant. Data were compared between control and other groups such as glutamate, B-TCE and B-TCE + glutamate ($^{*}p \leq 0.01$) as well as glutamate alone with B-TCE and B-TCE + glutamate groups ($^{\#}p \leq 0.01$).

Results

B-TCE modulated the effect of glutamate on cellular and nuclear morphology

Effect of glutamate and B-TCE pretreatment was initially studied by phase contrast microscopy followed by confocal imaging for α- tubulin immunostaining. Glutamate exposure was observed to degenerate primary cerebellar neurons, however, B-TCE pretreated culture exhibited healthy morphology with long and stellate processes as seen in control and B-TCE alone treatment groups (Fig. 1a). B-TCE alone treatment promoted defasciculation (Fig. 1a). To study the effect of glutamate and B-TCE on number and length of processes of primary cerebellar neurons, morphometric analysis from toluidine and methylene blue stained cells was carried out. It was observed that number of processes in all the three treatment groups i.e. glutamate, B-TCE alone and B-TCE pretreatment followed by glutamate were although significantly higher than control ($p \leq 0.01$) (Fig. 1b), but the sum length as well as length of individual processes were significantly reduced by glutamate (Fig. 1c). However, B-TCE pretreatment was seen to increase the length of processes significantly ($p \leq 0.01$) (Fig. 1a and c). Further, to observe nuclear condensation, which is considered as induction of apoptosis, nuclei were stained with DAPI. Number of apoptotic cells was calculated in each group and 67% of total population was found to be apoptotic in glutamate-treated group, whereas, only 19.5% and 15.9% cells showed condensed nuclear morphology in control and B-TCE alone group, respectively. B-TCE pretreatment significantly reduced apoptotic cell population to 23.9% ($p \leq 0.01$), thus suggesting that B-TCE suppressed the onset of apoptosis (Fig. 1a and Additional file 1: Fig. S2). As the cultures treated with B-TCE alone showed cellular and nuclear morphology similar to control, it may be suggested that B-TCE did not have any adverse effects on primary cerebellar neurons.

B-TCE suppressed glutamate-induced neuronal degeneration by supporting neuronal differentiation and maturation

To study the molecular basis of glutamate-induced neurodegeneration, immunostaining for neuronal markers MAP-2, GAP-43 and NF200 was carried out in different groups. MAP-2 and NF200 are neuron specific proteins which are responsible for neuronal spindle formation and axonal caliber in dendrites of post-mitotic neurons [24, 25], whereas, GAP-43 has been reported to express at neuronal growth cones during development and axonal regeneration. The decrease was observed in expression of all the three markers after glutamate exposure, but their expression was found comparable to the control group in B-TCE pretreatment and B-TCE alone treatment groups in immunostaining (Fig. 2a). This immunostaining data was further supported by Western blotting results, where glutamate treated group showed a significant decrease in MAP-2, GAP-43 and NF200 expression as compared to control group ($p \leq 0.01$). B-TCE pretreatment significantly normalized the glutamate-induced reduction in expression of these markers ($p \leq 0.01$). B-TCE alone treatment was found to increase MAP-2 and NF200 significantly w.r.t control. MAP-2 has three isoforms MAP-2a, MAP-2b and MAP-2c (280 kDa, 280 kDa and 70 kDa, respectively) out of which MAP-2b and 2c have been reported to be present in new born rat pups brain. In the given blot, these two isoforms were detected by monoclonal mouse anti-MAP-2 antibody (Cat# M9942, Sigma-Aldrich). The histogram for MAP-2 represents combined analysis for both the isoforms (Fig. 2b). These observations suggest that B-TCE pretreatment suppresses glutamate-induced reduction of neuronal protein expression.

B-TCE abolished the onset of inflammation as a result of glutamate-induced excitotoxicity

To further elucidate whether B-TCE pretreatment suppresses glutamate-induced inflammation, expression of inflammatory markers NF-κB and transcription factor AP-1 was studied by immunostaining and Western blotting. A significant increase in NF-κB and AP-1 expression was observed in glutamate-treated cells, whereas, B-TCE pretreatment significantly reduced the expression of these markers as compared to glutamate alone group ($p \leq 0.01$). The immunostaining data was supported by

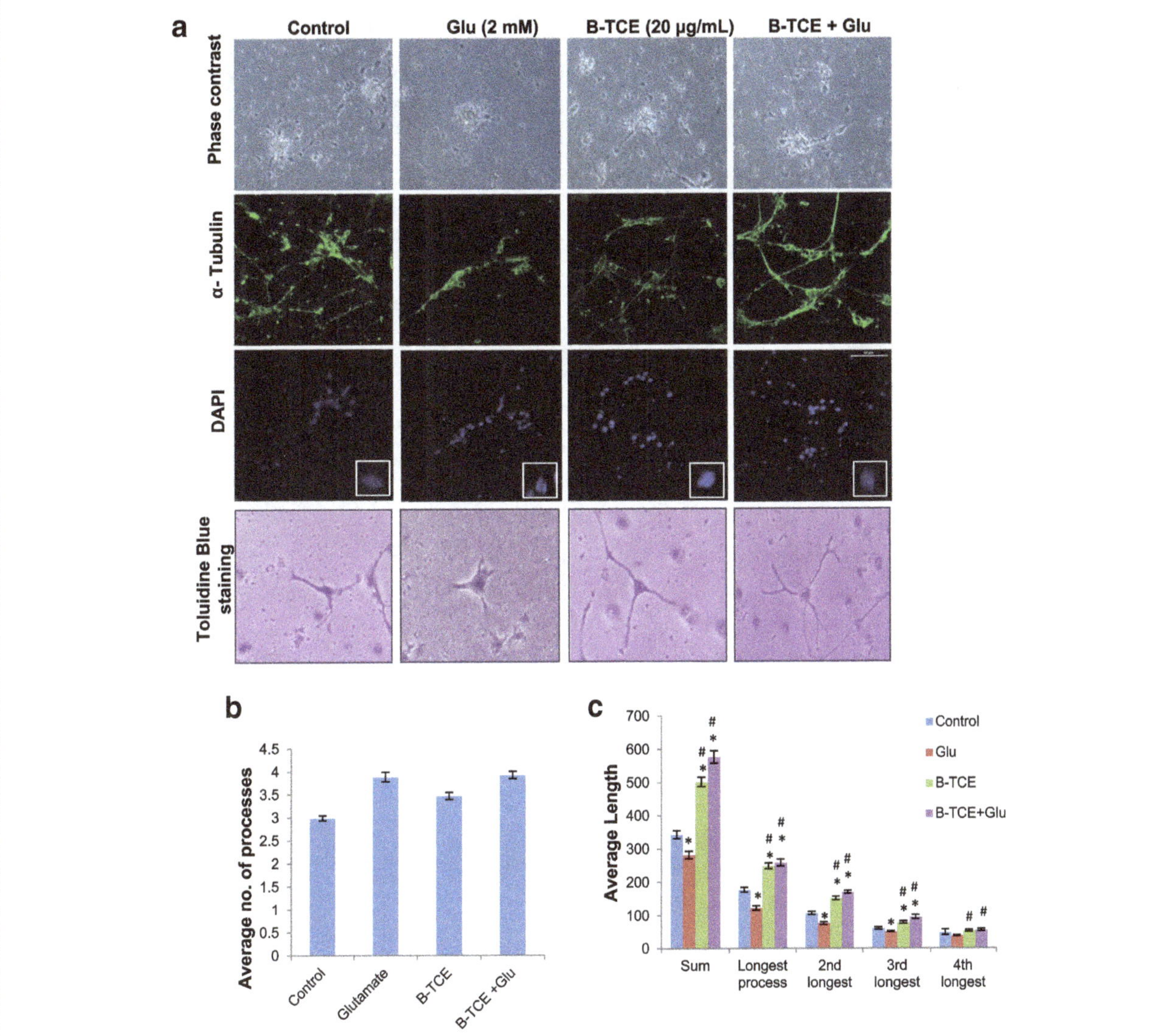

Fig. 1 B-TCE pretreatment inhibited adverse effects of glutamate on cellular and nuclear morphology. **a**) Phase contrast, α-Tubulin immunostained and nuclear staining (DAPI) confocal micrographs and Toluidine blue stained Control, Glutamate (2 mM), B-TCE (20 µg/mL) and B-TCE + Glu treated primary cerebellar neurons. **b**) The histogram represents average number of processes and **c**) average length of processes of primary cerebellar neurons of these four different groups. Data was compared between Control and other groups such as Glutamate, B-TCE and B-TCE + Glu ($^{*}p \leq 0.01$) as well as Glutamate alone with B-TCE and B-TCE + Glu groups ($^{\#}p \leq 0.01$)

Western blotting results (Fig. 3a and b). Secretory levels of pro-inflammatory cytokines TNF-α, IL-6 and IL-1β in culture media were assayed by ELISA. Although no significant change was observed in levels of TNF-α but a pronounced increase was found in IL-6 and IL-1β levels in primary cerebellar neurons exposed to glutamate, which was significantly suppressed in B-TCE pretreated culture ($p \leq 0.01$) (Fig. 3c). Mitochondrial dysfunction and increased oxidative stress are the well-known consequences of glutamate-induced excitotoxicity. Further, to test whether B-TCE pretreatment attenuates the mitochondrial membrane damage and oxidative stress induced by glutamate, Mitotracker green FM staining and iNOS mRNA expression were studied. Change in intensity of mitotracker staining is related to altered mitochondrial activity. Significantly higher intensity of mitotracker was observed in glutamate-treated primary cerebellar neurons indicating higher oxidative stress and membrane damage, which was prevented by B-TCE pretreatment as indicated by intensity of mitotracker staining comparable to control group (Fig. 3d). Glutamate-induced rise in iNOS expression (3.7 fold) at transcriptional level was significantly inhibited by B-TCE pretreatment ($p \leq 0.01$) (Fig. 3e). These observations suggested that B-TCE pretreatment abolished glutamate-induced rise in inflammatory protein expression, secretory levels of pro-inflammatory cytokines, mitochondrial membrane damage and iNOS expression.

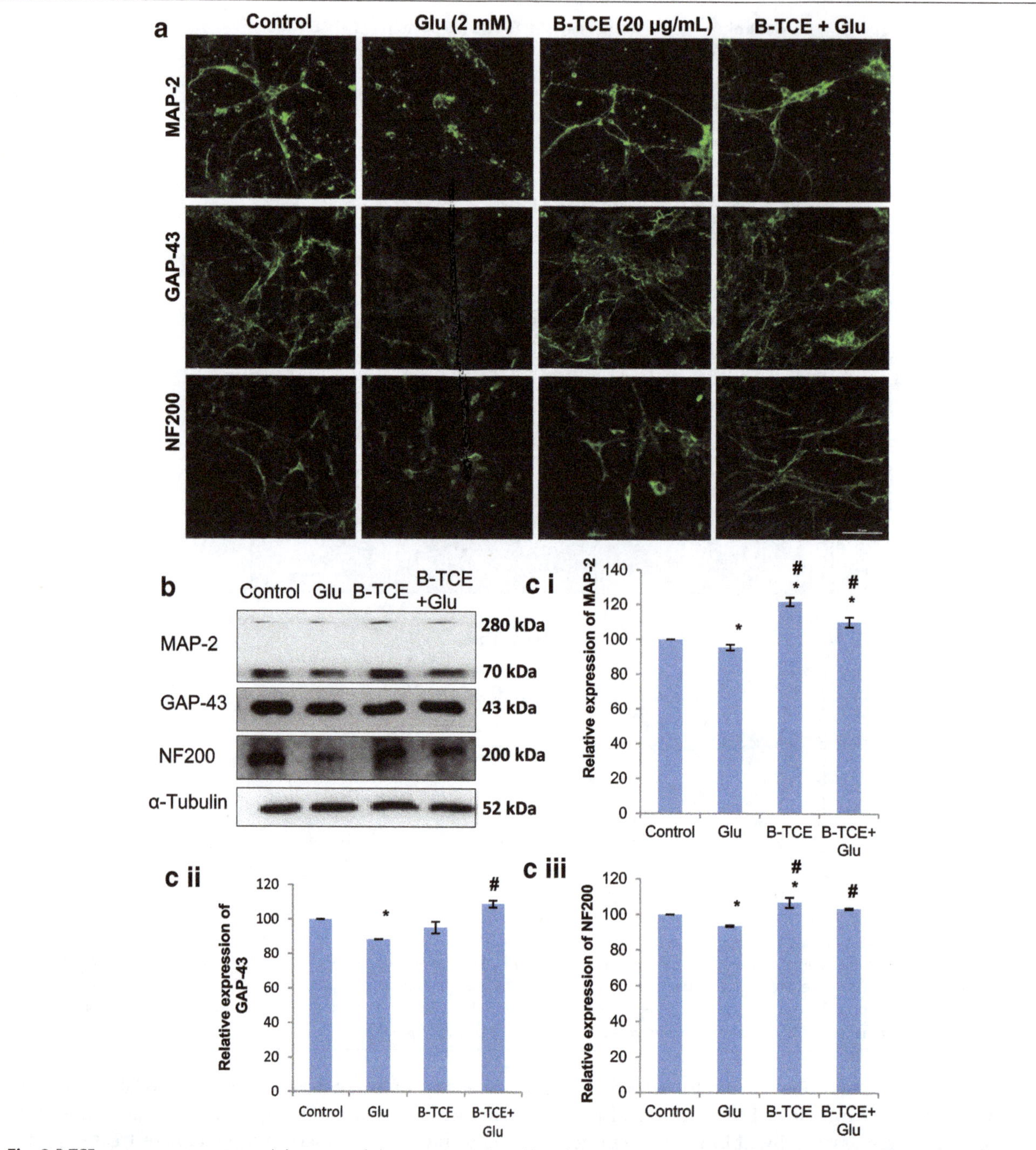

Fig. 2 B-TCE pretreatment suppressed the neuronal degeneration induced by glutamate by modulating the expression of neuronal structural markers. **a**) Confocal micrographs of Control, Glutamate (2 mM), B-TCE (20 μg/mL) and B-TCE + Glu treated primary cerebellar neurons immunostained for MAP-2, GAP-43 and NF200. **b**) Representative immunoblots for MAP-2, GAP-43 and NF200 where α-Tubulin was used as internal control. **c**) Histogram representing relative expression of MAP-2 (i), GAP-43 (ii) and NF200 (iii) obtained from normalized relative optical densities of bands. Data was compared between Control and other groups such as Glutamate, B-TCE and B-TCE + Glu ($^*p \leq 0.01$) as well as Glutamate alone with B-TCE and B-TCE + Glu groups ($^\#p \leq 0.01$). Confocal Images were captured at 60X objective (Scale bar: 50 μm)

B-TCE normalized glutamate-induced enhanced expression of stress chaperone proteins

To investigate the effect of glutamate on stress chaperone proteins expression and whether B-TCE abrogates these changes, expression of stress chaperones, i.e. heat shock protein HSP70 and Mortalin was studied. HSP70 and Mortalin protect neurons from protein aggregation and toxicity. Immunostaining data revealed increase in expression of HSP70 and Mortalin in glutamate exposed group, whereas,

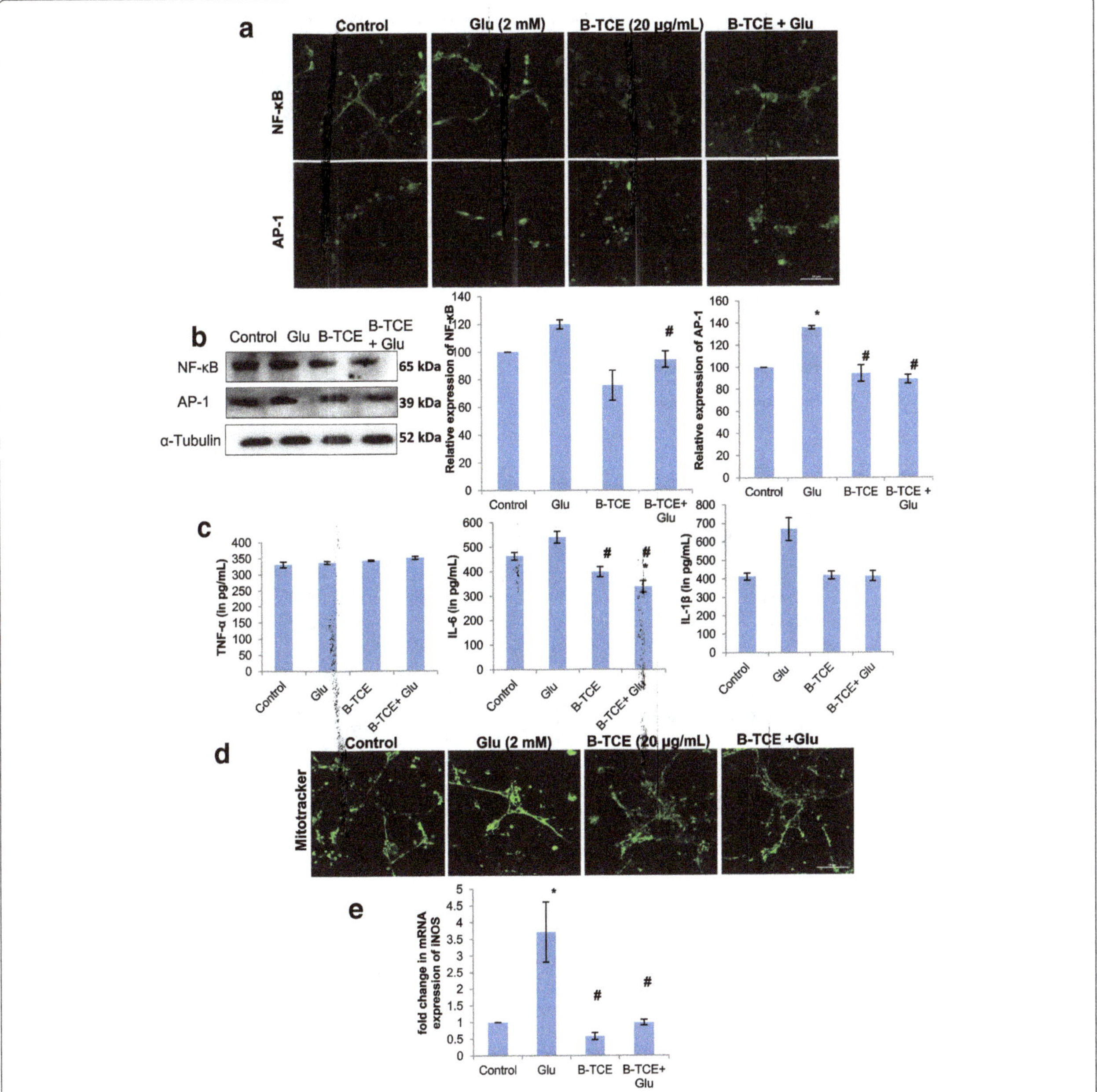

Fig. 3 B-TCE pretreatment abolished the glutamate-induced onset of inflammation. **a**) Confocal micrographs of Control, Glutamate (2 mM), B-TCE (20 μg/mL) and B-TCE + Glu treated primary cerebellar neurons immunostained for NF-κB and AP-1. **b**) Representative immunoblots and histograms showing relative expression of NF-κB and AP-1 where α-Tubulin was used as internal control. **c**) Histograms representing secretory levels of pro-inflammatory cytokines TNF-α, IL-6 and IL-1β (in pg/mL) in the four different treatment groups. **d**) Confocal micrographs of primary cerebellar neurons stained with Mitotracker green FM **e**) Histogram representing fold change in mRNA expression of iNOS in four different treatment groups. Data was compared between Control and other groups such as Glutamate, B-TCE and B-TCE + Glu ($^{*}p \leq 0.01$) as well as Glutamate alone with B-TCE and B-TCE + Glu groups ($^{\#}p \leq 0.01$). Confocal Images were captured at 60X objective (Scale bar: 50 μm)

B-TCE pretreatment suppressed this increase (Fig. 4 Ia). The Western blot data also showed that glutamate treatment enhanced the expression of HSP70, however, the change was not statistically significant (Fig. 4 Ib). B-TCE pretreatment reduced the expression of HSP70 as compared to both control and glutamate treated group. Further, glutamate treated cultures showed significant increase in Mortalin expression ($p \leq 0.01$) as compared to control as well as B-TCE pretreatment group (Fig. 4 Ib). These

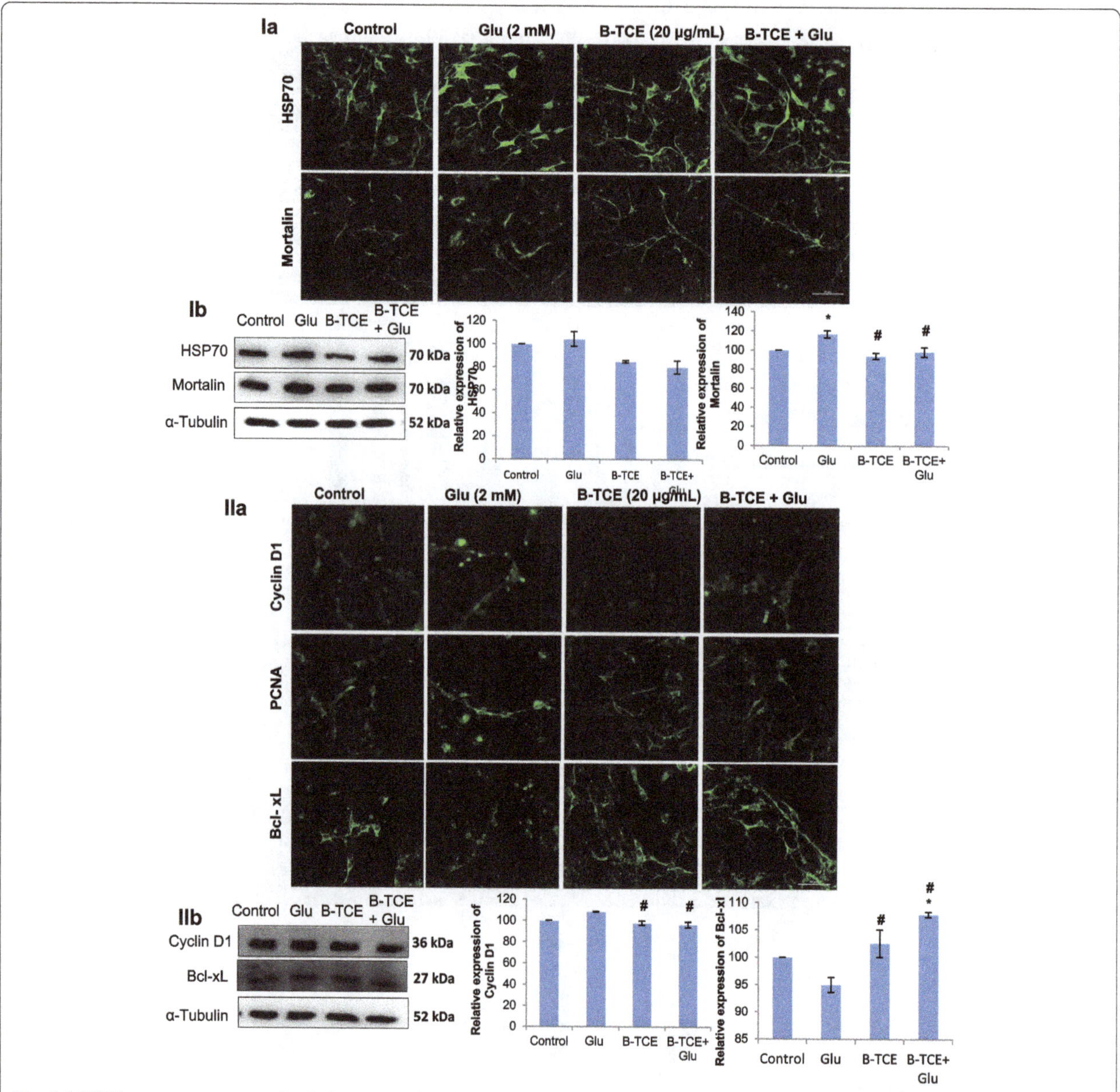

Fig. 4 **I**) B-TCE pretreatment normalized glutamate-induced increase in stress chaperones expression. **a**) Confocal micrographs of Control, Glutamate (2 mM), B-TCE (20 μg/mL) and B-TCE + Glu treated primary cerebellar neurons immunostained for HSP70 and Mortalin. **b**) Representative immunoblots and histograms showing relative expression of HSP70 and Mortalin. **II**) B-TCE pretreatment regulated the expression of cell cycle and pro-apoptotic proteins during glutamate exposure. **a**) Confocal micrographs of Control, Glutamate (2 mM), B-TCE (20 μg/mL) and B-TCE + Glu treated primary cerebellar neurons immunostained for Cyclin D1, PCNA and Bcl-xL. **b**) Representative immunoblots and histograms showing relative expression of Cyclin D1 and Bcl-xL where α-Tubulin was used as internal control. Data was compared between Control and other groups such as Glutamate, B-TCE and B-TCE + Glu ($^{*}p \leq 0.01$) as well as Glutamate alone with B-TCE and B-TCE + Glu groups ($^{\#}p \leq 0.01$). Confocal Images were captured at 60X objective (Scale bar: 50 μm)

results suggest that B-TCE pretreatment protected cells from glutamate-induced increase in stress proteins (Fig. 4 Ia and Ib).

B-TCE regulated glutamate-induced changes in cell cycle proteins and apoptotic marker

Abnormal cell cycle regulation has been reported to be associated with neurodegeneration [26]. To further explore whether B-TCE modulates expression of cell cycle regulators, Cyclin D1 and PCNA expression was studied. Enhanced expression of Cyclin D1 and PCNA was observed in glutamate exposed primary cerebellar neurons. However, B-TCE pretreatment significantly reduced the Cyclin D1 and PCNA expression to near control levels ($p \leq 0.01$) (Fig. 4 IIa). Western blotting for Cyclin D1 also supported these observations (Fig. 4 IIb).

Further, we studied the expression of anti-apoptotic marker Bcl-xL which showed significant downregulation in glutamate-treated culture ($p \leq 0.01$). On the other hand, significantly higher expression of Bcl-xL was observed in B-TCE alone and B-TCE pretreatment followed by glutamate treatment as compared to glutamate treated group ($p \leq 0.01$) (Fig. 4 IIa and IIb). These observations may suggest that glutamate-induced excitotoxicity induced aberrant cell cycle progression of primary cerebellar neurons in cell cycle, reduced the levels of anti-apoptotic protein Bcl-xL which may result in induction of apoptosis, whereas, B-TCE pretreatment inhibited cell cycle reactivation and maintained normal levels of Bcl-xL, thus inhibiting apoptosis induction.

B-TCE promoted plasticity, neurite outgrowth and migration

Glutamate neurotransmission plays an important role in synaptic plasticity, however, abnormal levels of glutamate pose detrimental effects on plasticity development and regulation [27]. The effect of glutamate treatment was also studied on plasticity markers PSA-NCAM and cell adhesion molecule NCAM in primary cerebellar neurons. Glutamate exposure significantly reduced PSA-NCAM and NCAM expression as compared to control cells, whereas, B-TCE pretreated cultures showed expression of these proteins comparable to control group ($p \leq 0.01$). However, a significant difference in expression was observed as compared to glutamate alone treated group ($p \leq 0.01$) (Fig. 5a and b). Immunostaining and Western blotting data are in line with each other. NCAM blot shown two bands of 180 kDa and 140 kDa as due to alternative splicing during RNA processing, three isoforms of NCAM 180 kDa, 140 kDa and 120 kDa exist. The monoclonal anti-NCAM antibody, clone NCAM OB11 (Cat# 9672, Sigma-Aldrich) used for Western blotting detects 180 kDa and 140 kDa bands, justifying the two bands observed in Western blot in Fig. 5b. Further, to study the effect of glutamate on neurite outgrowth and migration, primary cerebellar explant cultures were established. There was no outgrowth observed from glutamate treated explants which also showed low expression of NCAM and PSA-NCAM. However, visible cells with long processes were observed to be migrating from B-TCE pretreated explants with enhanced expression of NCAM and PSA-NCAM (Fig. 5c). To gain more insight into the effect of glutamate exposure and B-TCE treatment, wound scratch assay and Gelatin zymography were performed. A widened gap with negative gap closure (– 94%) was observed in primary cerebellar neuronal cultures treated with glutamate as compared to control cultures (gap closure taken as 100%), whereas, B-TCE and B-TCE + Glutamate treated cells showed almost double percent gap closure (233% and 251%, respectively) (Fig. 6a and b). Furthermore, significantly reduced expression of MMP-2 was also observed in glutamate-treated cells as compared to control, whereas, no change was observed in other two groups ($p \leq 0.01$) (Fig. 6c). These observations suggest that glutamate exposure to cellular explants reduced neuronal plasticity, inhibited neurite outgrowth and migration of primary cerebellar neurons, whereas, B-TCE pre-treatment rescued the primary cerebellar neurons from these adverse effects of glutamate excitotoxicity, maintained plasticity and promoted neurite outgrowth and migration.

Phytochemical characterization of B-TCE by UPLC-MS

T. cordifolia has been reported to consist of a variety of phytochemicals such as alkaloids, glycosides, diterpenoid lactones, steroids, aliphatic compounds and others [17, 28]. Since B-TCE was a butanolic fraction of crude extract of *T. cordifolia* and was observed to show neuroprotective activity, so to study the active compounds UPLC-MS of B-TCE was carried out. Peaks of alkaloids and glycosides were identified on the basis of reported literature for *T. cordifolia*. Peaks of magnoflorine, palmatine, norcoclaurine, cordifolioside A, oblongine, tetrahydropalmatine, 11-hydroxy mustakone and tinocoridiside were identified on the basis of reported mass and mass fragments described in the literature of phytochemical characterization of *T. cordifolia* (Table 1) [29, 30]. [Chromatograms at different wavelengths, TIC and spectra corresponding to retention time are included in supplementary material and identified mass peaks and mass fragments denoted by *(Additional file 1: Fig. S3-S12)].

Discussion

Glutamate-mediated excitotoxicity is the common final destructive pathway in the majority of neurodegenerative diseases and therapeutic strategies inhibiting or providing protection against excitotoxicity induced degeneration are much in the interest of researchers. The current study was aimed to study the neuroprotective potential of Butanol extract of *T. cordifolia* against glutamate-induced excitotoxicity. Initially, our lab has reported anti-proliferative and differentiation-inducing potential of 50% aqueous ethanolic extract of *T. cordifolia*. In an attempt to dissect out the active principle and to find effective lower dose we fractionated TCE with solvents of lower to higher polarity i.e. chloroform, hexane, ethyl acetate and butanol. The Chloroform and Hexane fractions (Chl-TCE and Hex-TCE) were found to exhibit anti-cancer activity against U87MG and IMR-32 cancerous cell lines at a very low dose as compared to TCE. Ethyl acetate fraction exhibited no specific effect on these cell lines, whereas, Butanol fraction exhibited neuroprotective potential. Different doses of Butanol fraction i.e. B-TCE were studied on primary

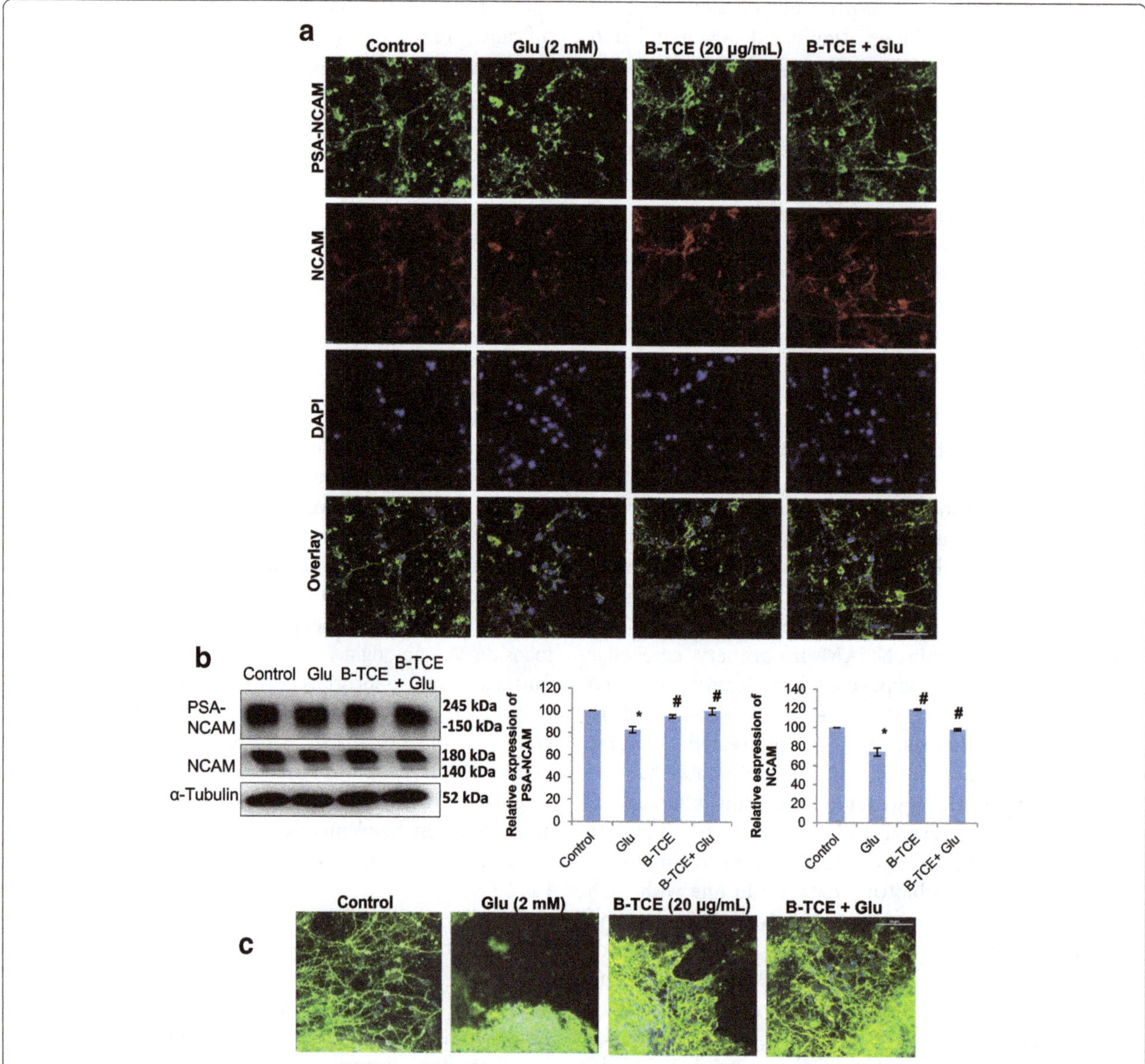

Fig. 5 B-TCE pretreatment promoted plasticity, neurite outgrowth and migration and protected from glutamate-induced excitotoxicity. **a**) Confocal micrographs of Control, Glutamate (2 mM), B-TCE (20 µg/mL) and B-TCE + Glu treated primary cerebellar neurons immunostained for PSA-NCAM and NCAM. Nuclei were stained with DAPI (third panel). The fourth panel represents the overlay of above three panels. **b**) Representative immunoblots and histograms representing relative expression PSA-NCAM and NCAM where α-Tubulin was used as internal control. **c**) Overlay confocal micrographs of primary cerebellar explants stained for PSA-NCAM, NCAM and DAPI. Data was compared between Control and other groups such as Glutamate, B-TCE and B-TCE + Glu ($^{*}p \leq 0.01$) as well as Glutamate alone with B-TCE and B-TCE + Glu groups ($^{\#}p \leq 0.01$). Confocal Images were captured at 60X objective (Scale bar: 50 µm)

cultures in combination with excitotoxic doses of glutamate as reported in the literature and changes in cell viability and morphology were observed. 2 mM concentration of glutamate was selected as toxic concentration against which 20 µg/mL B-TCE was found to exhibit protection. So, 2 mM glutamate and 20 µg/mL of B-TCE were selected for all the experiments. Generally, cerebellar granular cells are characterized by their long processes with defasciculated morphology, which were observed to undergo degeneration under neurotoxic insults.

Increased Ca^{2+} levels due to glutamate excitotoxicity have been reported to induce activation of catabolic enzymes, which causes degradation of majority of neuronal structural proteins including α-Tubulin, neurofilament peptides and microtubule-associated proteins [5]. In the current study, glutamate exposure to primary cerebellar neurons induced structural degradation as was evident from phase contrast micrographs, confocal images of α-Tubulin immunostaining and morphometric studies (Fig. 1). Fasciculated morphology and significantly

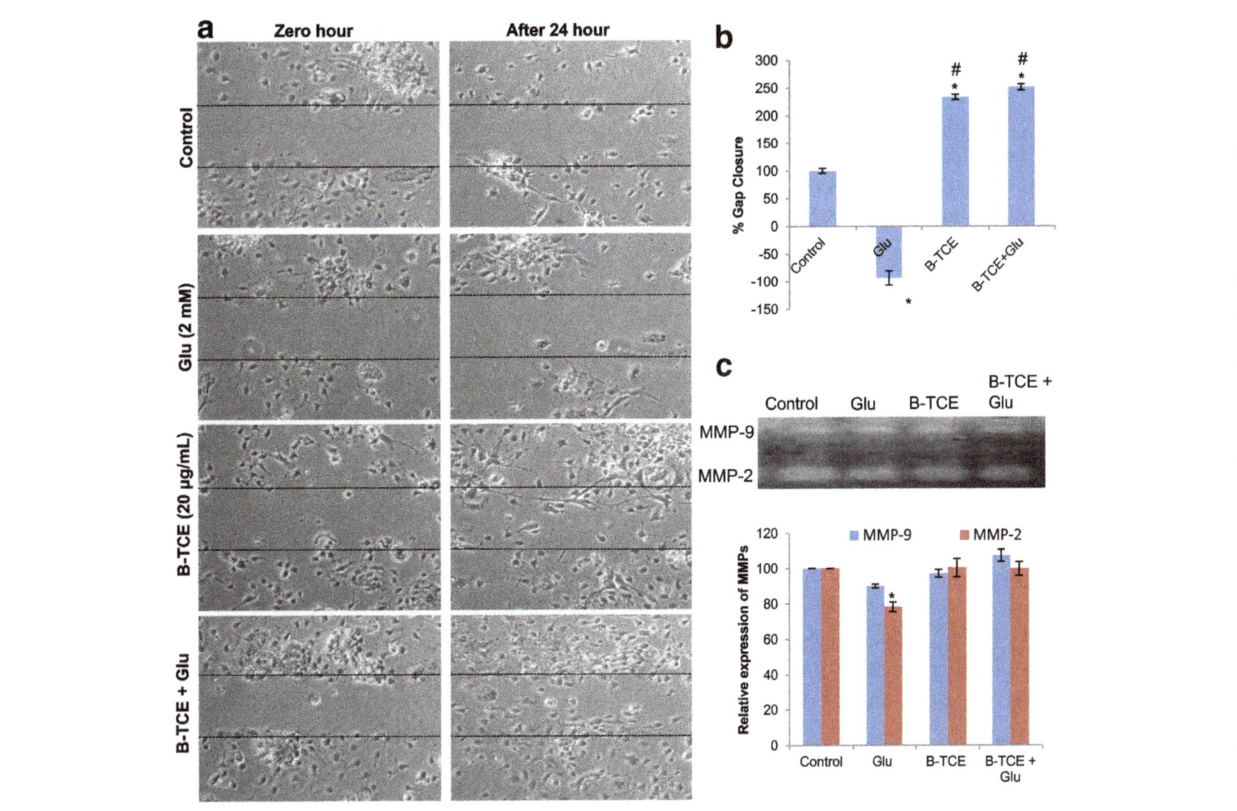

Fig. 6 B-TCE pretreatment promoted migration into the scratched area under glutamate-induced excitotoxic insult. **a**) Phase contrast micrographs of Control, Glutamate (2 mM), B-TCE (20 µg/mL) and B-TCE + Glu treated primary cerebellar neurons captured at 0 and 24 h of treatment. **b**) Representative histogram showing percentage gap closure after 24 h of treatment **c**) Gelatin zymogram showing MMP bands and histogram representing densitometric analysis of corresponding MMP bands. Data was compared between Control and other groups such as Glutamate, B-TCE and B-TCE + Glu ($^{*}p \leq 0.01$) as well as Glutamate alone with B-TCE and B-TCE + Glu groups ($^{\#}p \leq 0.01$). Phase contrast Images were captured at 20X objective

reduced average process length ($p \leq 0.01$) of glutamate-treated primary cerebellar neurons are supported by previously reported reduced dendritic branching and retraction of processes in the presence of toxic concentrations of excitotoxic stimuli [32]. In addition to changes in cellular processes, higher population with nuclear condensation (67%) was also observed which indicates induction of apoptosis by glutamate treatment. However, pretreatment of cerebellar neurons with B-TCE before glutamate exposure suppressed these adverse effects by maintaining structural and nuclear integrity as evident from reduced apoptotic cell population (23.9%) as well as increase in process length. B-TCE alone treatment also promoted defasciculation which allows better axonal branching. Further, toxicity in the neuronal environment has been reported to regulate the expression of neuronal markers [33]. MAP-2 and NF200 are structural proteins of mature neurons which characteristically express in dendrites,

Table 1 UPLC-MS analysis: Observed molecular weight and mass fragments of identified compounds in B-TCE extract

S. No.	Compound	RT	m/z	MS2	Nature	Reference
1.	Magnoflorine	1.135	343.14 $(M+H)^+$	327, 296	Alkaloid	[29, 30]
2.	Palmatine	3.607	353 $(M+H)^+$	337, 308	Alkaloid	[29]
3.	Norcoclaurine	3.701	272 $(M+H)^+$	255, 237	Alkaloid	[30]
4.	Cordifolioside A	3.756	527.25 $(M+Na)^+$	210, 193	Glycoside	[29]
5.	Oblongine	5.597	314 $(M)^+$	269,175	Alkaloid	[30]
6.	Tetrahydropalmatine	6.620	356.18 $(M+H)^+$	340, 164	Alkaloid	[30]
7.	11-Hydroxy mustakone	6.973	235.21 $(M+H)^+$	217, 161, 135	Sesqui-terpenoid	[30]
8.	Tinocordiside	6.973	419.25 $(M+Na)^+$	217, 235	Glycoside	[29]

perikaryon and axons of post-mitotic neurons [25, 34]. Both of these proteins were downregulated by glutamate treatment. GAP-43, the other neuronal growth and plasticity protein which is expressed in growth cones of developing neurons was also found to be downregulated by glutamate exposure [32, 35]. B-TCE pretreated groups showed higher expression of these structural proteins as compared to glutamate treated group. The data may suggest that B-TCE exhibited neuroplastic and neuroprotective response by suppressing the glutamate-induced decrease in MAP-2, GAP-43 and NF200 expression in primary cerebellar neurons. Glutamate treatment has been reported to activate Calpain I (by elevating intracellular Ca^{2+} levels) which in turn downregulated the expression of structural proteins such as MAP-2 and NF200 in primary cortical, motor and hippocampal neurons. These findings were further confirmed by using Calpain I inhibitors which were found to ameliorate alterations in these structural proteins [36–38]. Calpains have also been reported to be involved in proteolysis of GAP-43 [39]. Although we have not studied Calpain I expression in the present work, but based on these literature reports on the glutamate-induced excitotoxicity and its effect on Calpain I activity, it may be suggested that B-TCE suppressed the changes in structural proteins by inhibiting activation of proteases like Calpain I.

Excitotoxic concentrations of glutamate result in oxidative stress and production of inflammatory mediators. Transcription factors NF-κB and AP-1 get activated with the onset of inflammation or stress, get translocated to the nucleus and induce transcription of pro-apoptotic and anti-apoptotic genes depending upon the stimuli. Rel A (P65) subunit of NF-κB has been recently reported to be activated by toxic concentrations of glutamate which further facilitates transcription of pro-apoptotic genes [40]. Pro-apoptotic genes' transcription is also activated by AP-1 under glutamate excitotoxicity [41]. So, the increased levels of NF-κB and AP-1 in glutamate-treated group can be correlated with the onset of inflammation and induction of apoptosis, whereas, B-TCE pretreatment inhibited glutamate-induced activation of these transcription factors. Pro-inflammatory cytokines TNF-α, IL-6 and IL-1β secretion has been reported to increase during glutamate-induced excitotoxicity along with activation of apoptotic p38-MAPK protein [42]. Our data showed enhanced levels of IL-1β and IL-6, but not of TNF-α in glutamate-treated group, thus suggesting that NF-κB may be getting activated through receptors other than TNFR. Enhanced secretion of pro-inflammatory cytokines was also associated with increase in mRNA expression of an inducible form of nitric oxide synthase (iNOS), which may cause increase in synthesis of NO, which plays a major role in glutamate-induced oxidative stress and damage [43]. Further, the mitochondrial membrane was also found to be damaged after glutamate treatment. On the other hand, B-TCE pretreatment prevented the rise in pro-inflammatory cytokines, downregulated iNOS expression and mitochondrial membrane damage as is evident from the current data. These observations collectively suggest that B-TCE pretreatment abolished glutamate-induced onset of inflammation thus inhibiting apoptosis induction.

Neurodegenerative disorders are also known as proteinopathy disorders which involve aggregation and misfolding of proteins [44]. Heat shock proteins (HSP) are induced in response to various injuries such as stroke, trauma, neurodegenerative diseases and epilepsy and act in unison to repair or degrade the aggregated and misfolded proteins [44, 45]. In a previous report from our lab, HSP70, a central component of heat shock proteins was found to increase after glutamate-induced excitotoxicity in retinoic acid treated C6 glioma cells [46]. Upregulation in HSP70 expression has also been reported from animal models of focal ischemia and lithium-induced toxicity [47]. Mortalin, the other member of heat shock protein family is induced by glucose deprivation, metabolic stress, ionophores, ionizing radiation and toxins. Its concentration increases under oxidative stress as it is responsible for cellular homeostasis and tries combating with stress [48]. Under normal conditions, heat shock proteins play anti-apoptotic role, under neurotoxic insults they act as neuroprotective agent and under undealt oxidative stress, Mortalin triggers apoptosis by allowing cytoplasmic p53 activation [48]. These literature reports support upregulated HSP70 and Mortalin expression in glutamate-treated culture in the present study and may suggest that B-TCE pretreatment prevented misfolding of proteins, thus, abrogated the upregulation of expression of these stress chaperones by glutamate treatment.

Several cell culture and human post-mortem tissue studies have suggested the interconnection between activation of cell cycle and neurodegeneration [49]. Differentiated neurons attempt cell cycle re-entry and reactivation under various stress conditions such as nutrient deprivation, CNS injury and oxidative stress [26]. Oxidative stress and excitotoxic stimuli have been reported to induce DNA damage followed by the induction of DNA repair and synthesis, which results in inappropriate cell cycle entry leading to apoptosis and cell death [50]. Glutamate-induced increase in Cyclin D1 and cdk4/6 expression leading to apoptotic cell death in hippocampal and cortical neurons has been reported recently [51]. BDNF deprivation has been reported to show upregulated Cyclin D1 expression and induction of apoptosis in cerebellar granule cells [52]. Both PCNA and Cyclin D1 expression was found to be upregulated in mutant mouse models of trophic factors [53]. B-TCE pretreatment suppressed the increase in Cyclin D1 and PCNA expression after exposure to glutamate, thus, may prevent the glutamate-induced DNA damage and apoptosis induction. The nuclear condensation (as evident from DAPI staining), mitochondrial dysfunction (Mitoctracker staining) and cell cycle deregulation (evident from Cyclin D1 and PCNA) indicated the induction of apoptosis after glutamate treatment. B-TCE pretreatment significantly upregulated Bcl-xL expression ($p \leq 0.01$) and suppressed apoptosis induced by glutamate exposure in primary cerebellar neurons. Previous reports have also suggested that oxidative stress due to high concentration of glutamate induces mitochondrial dysfunction which results in cytochrome c release and activation of downstream molecules involved in apoptosis induction [31]. Overexpression of Bcl-xL, an anti-apoptotic protein of the Bcl-2 family was also shown to delay cytochrome c release from mitochondria in response to Bax in Human embryonic kidney (293 T) cells [54]. In view of these previous reports and our current observations, it may be suggested that upregulated expression of Bcl-xL mitigated the apoptosis induction by suppressing cytochrome c release from mitochondria and activation of downstream activation of apoptosis pathway. A slight increase in Bcl-xL expression in B-TCE alone group may be helping the cells to preserve axonal morphology. Increase in Bcl-xL has also been reported to play important role in functional adaptation and enhanced lifespan of cells by preventing apoptosis as well as by preservation of axonal morphology [55, 56].

We further observed that glutamate exposure downregulated expression of PSA-NCAM and NCAM, whereas, B-TCE pretreatment prevented these changes and maintained the expression of these plasticity proteins to near-control levels. Cell adhesion molecules play important role in cell-cell interactions, migration, plasticity, regeneration and repair [57]. NCAM is a potential neuroprotective protein, and its enhanced expression suggests that B-TCE exerts neuroprotection by upregulating the expression of these neuroprotective plasticity proteins [58, 59]. Polysialated form of NCAM is a characteristic marker of developing, migrating neurons and synaptogenesis of nervous tissue. Application of PSA-NCAM was found to reduce excitotoxic death of cultured hippocampal neurons due to glutamate exposure [60]. In a previous interventional study from our lab, dietary restriction was seen to exert neuroprotection against kainic acid-induced toxicity by upregulating NCAM and PSA-NCAM expression [56]. Further, the neuroprotective activity of Ashwagandha leaf water extract against glutamate-induced excitotoxicity was also reported to upregulate PSA-NCAM and NCAM expression [46]. Neurite outgrowth and migration of glutamate exposed primary cerebellar neurons in the lesioned area was promoted by B-TCE pretreatment which may be attributed to upregulated PSA-NCAM and NCAM expression. Sprouting from organotypic cultures of hippocampal slices in lesion-induced neurite outgrowth model was associated with a pronounced expression of PSA-NCAM [57]. Both of these cell adhesion molecules participate in neurite outgrowth and synaptogenesis and their downregulated expression resulted in glutamate-induced dendritic atrophy in hippocampal neurons [61]. The neurite outgrowth and migration were also accompanied by enhanced MMP-2 and MMP-9 expression which was maintained by B-TCE pretreatment, whereas, glutamate treatment significantly downregulated MMP-2 expression ($p \leq 0.01$). MMP-2 and MMP-9 are major MMPs which play important role in cellular motility and neurite outgrowth across matrix under different pathological and physiological conditions [62]. Depletion of MMP-2 and MMP-9 from culture conditioned media was reported to abolish neurite outgrowth and axonal regeneration from cortical neurons [63]. Based on these observations, it may be suggested that B-TCE pretreatment of primary cerebellar neurons before glutamate exposure promoted migration, neurite outgrowth and enhanced neural plasticity.

We also attempted to characterize eight peaks corresponding to magnoflorine, palmatine, norcoclaurine, cordifolioside A, oblongine, tetrahydropalmatine, 11-hydroxy mustakone and tinocoriside which belong to alkaloids, glycosides and sesquiterpenoids. Our findings are in line with previous reports suggesting cordifolioside A and tinocordiside as active constituents of n-butanol fraction of *T. cordifolia* stem extract [20, 21]. Alkaloids magnoflorine and palmatine were also reported to present in n-butanol fraction of *T. cordifolia* stem extract. The neuroprotective and immune-modulatory activity has been attributed to the presence of alkaloids and glycosides in *T. cordifolia* [17, 63]. Cordifolioside A and B are known to exhibit immunostimulating activity [64, 65]. Further, cordifolioside A has been reported to exert radio and cytoprotective activity [21], whereas, tinocordiside exerted cytotoxicity against cancerous KB and Siha cell lines [66]. Alkaloids palmatine, magnoflorine are reported to possess different biological activities such as anti-cancer, anti-glycemic, whereas, sesquiterpene 11-hydroxymuskatone induced significant proliferation of splenocyte, thus acting as immunomodulatory compound [63]. Levo-tetrahydropalmatine has been reported as a dopamine receptor antagonist, used against drug self-administration and reinstatement behaviour [67, 68]. Presence of dopamine receptor antagonists in *T. cordifolia,* therefore, may explain the basis of anxiolytic, anti-psychotic and neuroprotective effect of extract reported earlier [15, 16, 67, 68].

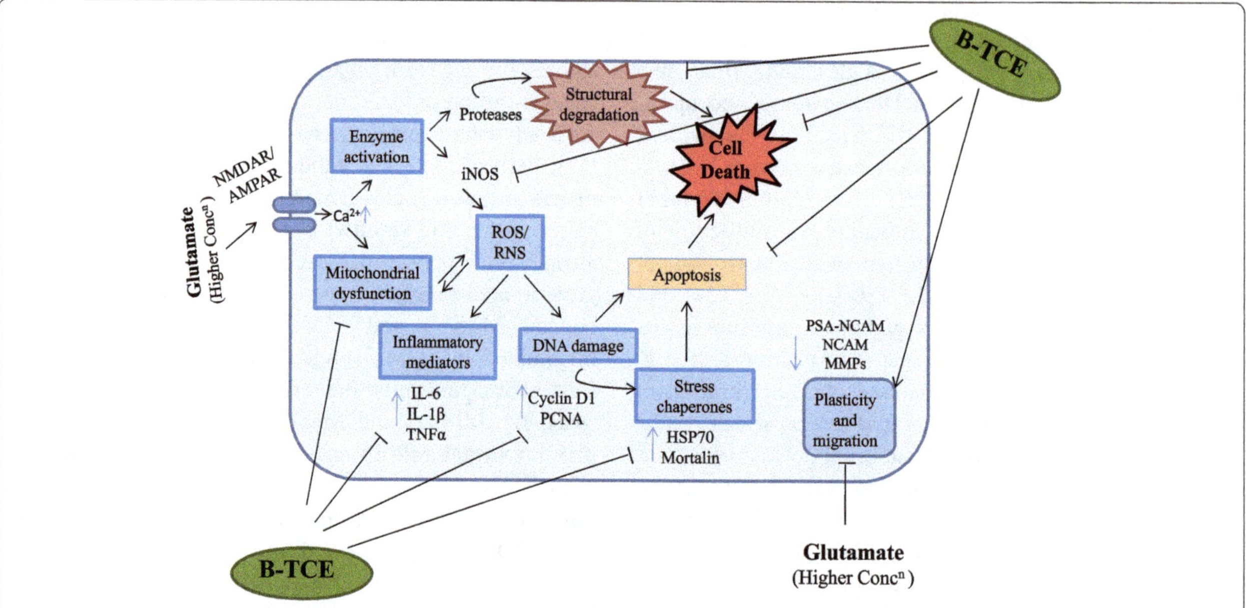

Fig. 7 Representative graphical image presenting the underlying mechanism of glutamate-induced excitotoxicity and how B-TCE pretreatment protects primary cerebellar neurons by modulating the expression of different molecular effectors. Overstimulation of glutamate receptors induced rise in intracellular calcium which leads to mitochondrial dysfunction and activation of enzymes which further results in ROS/RNS generation and structural degradation of neurons. ROS/RNS induce upregulation of inflammatory mediators, DNA damage and stress chaperones thus causing apoptosis and neurodegeneration. In the present study B-TCE pretreatment inhibited glutamate-induced structural degradation (morphometric studies, MAP-2, GAP-43, NF200), mitochondrial dysfunction (Mitotracker green FM), suppressed NO generation (iNOS), secretion of pro-inflammatory cytokines (TNF-α, IL-6 and IL-1β), DNA damage (Cyclin D1 and PCNA) and stress proteins expression (HSP70 and Mortalin), thus inhibited apoptosis induction and neurodegeneration. B-TCE also promoted neuronal plasticity and migration (PSA-NCAM, NCAM expression)

Conclusions

The aim of current study was to investigate the potential benefits of B-TCE in amelioration of glutamate-induced excitotoxicity and it provides the first evidence of neuroprotective and neuroregenerative potential of *T. cordifolia*. Earlier, our lab has tested the crude TCE for its anticancer potential which may be attributed to its hexane and chloroform fraction (effective at much lower concentration), whereas, Butanol fraction showed strong neuroprotective and neuroregenerative potential. Current data may suggest that B-TCE exerted neuroprotection against glutamate-induced excitotoxicity by modulating different pathways such as neuronal differentiation, homeostasis and apoptosis. B-TCE pretreatment prevented glutamate-induced insults on neuronal integrity, promoted neurite outgrowth and cell migration. It also suppressed glutamate-induced onset of inflammation and stress chaperones expression (Fig. 7). The neuroprotective activity may be attributed to immunomodulatory compounds present in this fraction, however, isolation and characterization of single active compounds are being planned in the future study. These findings bestow a stepping stone towards future research aiming to investigate the role of *T. cordifolia* as a candidate for herbal based neuroprotective and neuroregenerative approach against neurodegenerative diseases. B-TCE could be used as a safe and effective non-palliative therapeutic candidate against neurodegenerative diseases.

Abbreviations

6-OHDA: 6-Hydroxydopamine; AP-1: Activator protein-1; Bcl-xL: B-cell lymphoma-extra large; BDNF: Brain-derived neurotrophic factor; B-TCE: Butanol extract of *T. cordifolia*; Chl-TCE: Chloroform extract of *T. cordifolia*; DAPI: 4',6-diamidino-2-phenylindole; ELISA: Enzyme-linked immunosorbent assay; GAP-43: Growth associated protein-43; GAPDH: Glyceraldehyde 3-phosphate dehydrogenase; Hex-TCE: Hexane extract of *T. cordifolia*; HSP70: Heat shock protein 70; IL-1β: Interleukin-1beta; IL-6: Interleukin-6; MAP-2: Microtubule-associated protein 2; MAPK: Mitogen associated protein kinase; MMP: Matrix metalloproteinases; NCAM: Neural cell adhesion molecule; NF200: Neurofilament 200; NF-κB: Nuclear factor-kappa beta; NOS: Nitric oxide synthase; PCNA: Proliferating cell nuclear antigen; PSA-NCAM: Polysialic acid-NCAM; ROS/RNS: Reactive oxygen/ nitrogen species; TNFα: Tumor necrosis factor alpha; UPLC-MS: Ultra performance liquid chromatography-mass spectrometry

Acknowledgments

Infrastructure provided by University grants commission (UGC), India under UPE and CPEPA schemes and DBT under DISC scheme is highly acknowledged. AS is thankful to Department of Science and Technology (DST), New Delhi, India for research fellowship. Dr. Bikram Singh, Retired Chief Scientist, Institute of Himalayan Bioresource Technology and Aarti Sharma are deeply acknowledged for their kind support to characterize the plant extract.

Funding

The funding was provided by the Department of Biotechnology, Ministry of Science and Technology (DBT) to Gurcharan Kaur [BT/PR12200/MED/30/1439/2014]. The funding agency had no role in the design of study, data collection and interpretation, manuscript preparation and decision to publish the study.

Authors' contributions

The study was designed by AS and GK. AS performed experiments and analyzed data. The manuscript was written by AS and GK. Funding to carry out the work reported in the manuscript was provided by GK. Both the authors reviewed and approved the final manuscript.

Ethics approval and consent to participate

All animal experimental protocols were approved by the Institutional Animal Ethical Committee, Guru Nanak Dev University, Amritsar registered to "Committee for the Purpose of Control and Supervision of Experiments on Animals (CPCSEA), GOI" (Registration no. 226/CPCSEA) (permission number 226/CPCSEA/2015/17) and performed in accordance with the relevant guidelines of 'Animal Care and Use' laid down by the same committee. Participation consent is not applicable as this study does not involve any human subjects.

Competing interests

Authors declare no competing financial and nonfinancial interests.

References

1. Mark LP, Prost RW, Ulmer JL, Smith MM, Daniels DL, Strottmann JM, et al. Pictorial review of glutamate excitotoxicity: fundamental concepts for neuroimaging. AJNR Am J Neuroradiol. 2001;22(10):1813–24.
2. Blandini F. An update on the potential role of excitotoxicity in the pathogenesis of Parkinson's disease. Funct Neurol. 2010;25(2):65.
3. Ambrosi G, Cerri S, Blandini F. A further update on the role of excitotoxicity in the pathogenesis of Parkinson's disease. J Neural Transm. 2014;121(8):849–59.
4. Almeida RD, Manadas BJ, Melo CV, Gomes JR, Mendes CS, Graos MM, et al. Neuroprotection by BDNF against glutamate-induced apoptotic cell death is mediated by ERK and PI3-kinase pathways. Cell Death Differ. 2005;12(10):1329.
5. Choi DW. Glutamate neurotoxicity and diseases of the nervous system. Neuron. 1988;1(8):623–34.
6. Perrella J, Bhavnani BR. Protection of cortical cells by equine estrogens against glutamate-induced excitotoxicity is mediated through a calcium-independent mechanism. BMC Neurosci. 2005;6(1):34.
7. Nowacek A, Kosloski LM, Gendelman HE. Neurodegenerative disorders and nanoformulated drug development. Nanomedicine (Lond). 2009;4(5):541–55.
8. Rao RV, Descamps O, John V, Bredesen DE. Ayurvedic medicinal plants for Alzheimer's disease: a review. Alzheimers Res Ther. 2012;4(3):22.
9. Mezeiova E, Korabecny J, Sepsova V, Hrabinova M, Jost P, Muckova L, et al. Development of 2-Methoxyhuprine as novel Lead for Alzheimer's disease therapy. Molecules. 2017;22(8):1265.
10. Mishra R, Kaur G. Aqueous ethanolic extract of Tinospora cordifolia as a potential candidate for differentiation based therapy of glioblastomas. PLoS One. 2013;8(10):e78764.
11. Mishra R, Kaur G. Tinospora cordifolia induces differentiation and senescence pathways in neuroblastoma cells. Mol Neurobiol. 2015;52(1):719–33.
12. Singh B, Sharma P, Kumar A, Chadha P, Kaur R, Kaur A. Antioxidant and in vivo genoprotective effects of phenolic compounds identified from an endophytic Cladosporium velox and their relationship with its host plant Tinospora cordifolia. J Ethnopharmacol. 2016;194:450–6.
13. Rajalakshmi M, Anita R. β-Cell regenerative efficacy of a polysaccharide isolated from methanolic extract of Tinospora cordifolia stem on streptozotocin-induced diabetic Wistar rats. Chem Biol Interact. 2016;243:45–53.
14. Dhama K, Sachan S, Khandia R, Munjal A, Iqbal HMN, Latheef SK, et al. Medicinal and beneficial health applications of Tinospora cordifolia (Guduchi): a miraculous herb countering various diseases/disorders and its Immunomodulatory effects. Recent Pat Endocr Metab Immune Drug Discov. 2016;10(2):96–111.
15. Kosaraju J, Chinni S, Roy PD, Kannan E, Antony AS, Kumar MS. (2014) Neuroprotective effect of Tinospora cordifolia ethanol extract on 6-hydroxy dopamine induced parkinsonism. Indian J Pharmacol. 2014;46(2):176–80.
16. Mishra R, Manchanda S, Gupta M, Kaur T, Saini V, Sharma A, Kaur G. Tinospora cordifolia ameliorates anxiety-like behavior and improves cognitive functions in acute sleep deprived rats. Sci Rep. 2016;6:25564.
17. Saha S, Ghosh S. Tinospora cordifolia: one plant, many roles. Anc Sci Life. 2012;31(4):151–9.
18. Upadhyay AK, Kumar K, Kumar A, Mishra HS. Tinospora cordifolia (Willd.) Hook. f. and Thoms.(Guduchi)–validation of the Ayurvedic pharmacology through experimental and clinical studies. Int J Ayurveda Res. 2010;1(2):112–21.
19. Singh R, Kumar R, Mahato AK, Paliwal R, Singh AK, Kumar S, et al. De novo transcriptome sequencing facilitates genomic resource generation in Tinospora cordifolia. Funct Integr Genomics. 2016;16(5):581–91.
20. Ghosal S, Vishwakarma RA. Tinocordiside, a new rearranged cadinane sesquiterpene glycoside from Tinospora cordifolia. J Nat Prod. 1997;60(8):839–41.
21. Patel A, Bigoniya P, Singh CS, Patel NS. Radioprotective and cytoprotective activity of Tinospora cordifoliastem enriched extract containing cordifolioside-a. Indian J Pharmacol. 2013;45(3):237–43.
22. Contestabile A. Cerebellar granule cells as a model to study mechanisms of neuronal apoptosis or survivalinvivoandinvitro. Cerebellum. 2002;1(1):41–55.
23. Krämer D, Minichiello L. Cell culture of primary cerebellar granule cells. Methods Mol Biol. 2010;633:233–9.
24. Elder GA, Friedrich VL, Kang C, Bosco P, Gourov A, Tu PH, et al. Requirement of heavy neurofilament subunit in the development of axons with large calibers. J Cell Biol. 1998;143(1):195–205.
25. Soltani MH, Pichardo R, Song Z, Sangha N, Camacho F, Satyamoorthy K, et al. Microtubule-associated protein 2, a marker of neuronal differentiation, induces mitotic defects, inhibits growth of melanoma cells, and predicts metastatic potential of cutaneous melanoma. Am J Pathol. 2005;166(6):1841–50.
26. Atabay KD, Karabay A. Pin1 inhibition activates cyclin D and produces neurodegenerative pathology. J Neurochem. 2012;120(3):430–9.
27. Konradi C, Heckers S. Molecular aspects of glutamate dysregulation: implications for schizophrenia and its treatment. Pharmacol Ther. 2003;97(2):153–79.
28. Singh SS, Pandey SC, Srivastava S, Gupta VS, Patro B, Ghosh AC. Chemistry and medicinal properties of Tinospora cordifolia (Guduchi). Indian J Pharmacol. 2003;35(2):83–91.
29. Bala M, Verma PK, Awasthi S, Kumar N, Lal B, Singh B. Chemical prospection of important ayurvedic plant Tinospora cordifolia by UPLC-DAD-ESI-QTOF-MS/MS and NMR. Nat Prod Commun. 2015;10(1):43–8.
30. Bajpai V, Singh A, Chandra P, Negi MPS, Kumar N, Kumar B. Analysis of phytochemical variations in dioecious Tinospora cordifolia stems using HPLC/QTOF MS/MS and UPLC/QqQLIT-MS/MS. Phytochem Anal. 2016;27(2):92–9.
31. Zhang Y, Bhavnani BR. Glutamate-induced apoptosis in primary cortical neurons is inhibited by equine estrogens via down-regulation of caspase-3 and prevention of mitochondrial cytochrome c release. BMC Neurosci. 2005;6(1):13.
32. Juan WS, Huang SY, Chang CC, Hung YC, Lin YW, Chen TY, et al. Melatonin improves neuroplasticity by upregulating the growth-associated protein-43 (GAP-43) and NMDAR postsynaptic density-95 (PSD-95) proteins in cultured

neurons exposed to glutamate excitotoxicity and in rats subjected to transient focal cerebral ischemia even during a long-term recovery period. J Pineal Res. 2014;56(2):213–23.
33. White MG, Wang Y, Akay C, Lindl KA, Kolson DL, Jordan-Sciutto KL. Parallel high throughput neuronal toxicity assays demonstrate uncoupling between loss of mitochondrial membrane potential and neuronal damage in a model of HIV-induced neurodegeneration. Neurosci Res. 2011;70(2):220–9.
34. Rancic A, Filipovic N, Lovric JM, Mardesic S, Saraga-Babic M, Vukojevic K. Neuronal differentiation in the early human retinogenesis. Acta Histochem. 2017;119(3):264–72.
35. Strittmatter SM, Vartanian T, Fishman MC. GAP-43 as a plasticity protein in neuronal form and repair. J Neurobiol. 1992;23(5):507–20.
36. Mahajan SS, Thai KH, Chen K, Ziff E. Exposure of neurons to excitotoxic levels of glutamate induces cleavage of the RNA editing enzyme, adenosine deaminase acting on RNA 2, and loss of GLUR2 editing. Neuroscience. 2011; 189:305–15.
37. Melo CV, Mele M, Curcio M, Comprido D, Silva CG, Duarte CB. BDNF regulates the expression and distribution of vesicular glutamate transporters in cultured hippocampal neurons. PLoS One. 2013;8(1):e53793.
38. Wang W, Zhang F, Li L, Tang F, Siedlak SL, Fujioka H, Liu Y, Su B, Pi Y, Wang X. MFN2 couples glutamate excitotoxicity and mitochondrial dysfunction in motor neurons. J Biol Chem. 2015;290(1):168–82.
39. Zakharov VV, Bogdanova MN, Mosevitsky MI. Specific proteolysis of neuronal protein GAP-43 by calpain: characterization, regulation, and physiological role. Biochem Mosc. 2005;70(8):897–907.
40. Shih RH, Wang CY, Yang CM. NF-kappaB signaling pathways in neurological inflammation: a mini review. Front Mol Neurosci. 2015;8:77.
41. Chen RW, Qin ZH, Ren M, Kanai H, Chalecka-Franaszek E, Leeds P, et al. Regulation of c-Jun N-terminal kinase, p38 kinase and AP-1 DNA binding in cultured brain neurons: roles in glutamate excitotoxicity and lithium neuroprotection. J Neurochem. 2003;84(3):566–75.
42. Chaparro-Huerta V, Rivera-Cervantes MC, Flores-Soto ME, Gomez-Pinedo U, Beas-Zarate C. Proinflammatory cytokines and apoptosis following glutamate-induced excitotoxicity mediated by p38 MAPK in the hippocampus of neonatal rats. J Neuroimmunol. 2005;165(1):53–62.
43. Manucha W. Mitochondrial dysfunction associated with nitric oxide pathways in glutamate neurotoxicity. Clin Investig Arterioscler. 2017;29(2):92–7.
44. Leak RK. Heat shock proteins in neurodegenerative disorders and aging. J Cell Commun Signal. 2014;8(4):293–310.
45. Turturici G, Sconzo G, Geraci F. Hsp70 and its molecular role in nervous system diseases. Biochem Res Int. 2011. https://doi.org/10.1155/2011/618127.
46. Kataria H, Wadhwa R, Kaul SC, Kaur G. Water extract from the leaves of Withania somnifera protect RA differentiated C6 and IMR-32 cells against glutamate-induced excitotoxicity. PLoS One. 2012. https://doi.org/10.1371/journal.pone.0037080.
47. Xu XH, Zhang HL, Han R, Gu ZL, Qin ZH. Enhancement of neuroprotection and heat shock protein induction by combined prostaglandin a 1 and lithium in rodent models of focal ischemia. Brain Res. 2006;1102(1):154–62.
48. Londono C, Osorio C, Gama V, Alzate O. Mortalin, apoptosis, and neurodegeneration. Biomol Ther. 2012;2(1):143–64.
49. Khurana V, Feany MB. Connecting cell-cycle activation to neurodegeneration in drosophila. Biochim Biophys Acta. 2007;1772(4):446–56.
50. Hitomi M, Stacey DW. The checkpoint kinase ATM protects against stress-induced elevation of cyclin D1 and potential cell death in neurons. Cytometry Part A. 2010;77(6):524–33.
51. Negis Y, Karabay A. Expression of cell cycle proteins in cortical neurons—correlation with glutamate-induced neurotoxicity. Biofactors. 2016;42(4):358–67.
52. Sakai K, Suzuki K, Tanaka S, Koike T. Up-regulation of cyclin D1 occurs in apoptosis of immature but not mature cerebellar granule neurons in culture. J Neurosci Res. 1999;58(3):396–406.
53. Herrup K, Busser JC. The induction of multiple cell cycle events precedes target-related neuronal death. Development. 1995;121(8):2385–95.
54. Finucane DM, Bossy-Wetzel E, Waterhouse NJ, Cotter TG, Green DR. Bax-induced caspase activation and apoptosis via cytochromec release from mitochondria is inhibitable by Bcl-xL. J Biol Chem. 1999;274(4):2225–33.
55. Jonas EA, Porter GA, Alavian KN. Bcl-xL in neuroprotection and plasticity. Front Physiol. 2014;5:355.
56. Malik JMI, Shevtsova Z, Bähr M, Kügler S. Long-term in vivo inhibition of CNS neurodegeneration by Bcl-XL gene transfer. Mol Ther. 2005;11:373–81.
57. Muller D, Wang C, Skibo G, Toni N, Cremer H, Calaora V, et al. PSA–NCAM is required for activity-induced synaptic plasticity. Neuron. 1996;17(3):413–22.
58. Sharma S, Kaur G. Dietary restriction enhances kainate-induced increase in NCAM while blocking the glial activation in adult rat brain. Neurochem Res. 2008;33(7):1178–88.
59. Wu W, Guan X, Kuang P, Jiang S, Yang J, Sui N, et al. Effect of batroxobin on expression of neural cell adhesion molecule in temporal infarction rats and spatial learning and memory disorder. J Tradit Chin Med. 2001;21(4):294–8.
60. Hammond MS, Sims C, Parameshwaran K, Suppiramaniam V, Schachner M, Dityatev A. Neural cell adhesion molecule-associated polysialic acid inhibits NR2B-containing N-methyl-D-aspartate receptors and prevents glutamate-induced cell death. J Biol Chem. 2006;281(46):34859–69.
61. Podestá MF, Yam P, Codagnone MG, Uccelli NA, Colman D. Reinés a (2014) distinctive PSA-NCAM and NCAM hallmarks in glutamate-induced dendritic atrophy and synaptic disassembly. PLoS One. 2014. https://doi.org/10.1371/journal.pone.0108921.
62. Ould-Yahoui A, Sbai O, Baranger K, Bernard A, Gueye Y, Charrat E, et al. Role of matrix metalloproteinases in migration and neurotrophic properties of nasal olfactory stem and ensheathing cells. Cell Transplant. 2013;22(6):993–1010.
63. Joshi G, Kaur R. Tinospora cordifolia: a phytopharmacological review. Int J Pharm Sci Res. 2016;7(3):890.
64. Maurya R, Dhar KL, Handa SS. A sesquiterpene glucoside from Tinospora cordifolia. Phytochemistry. 1997;44(4):749–50.
65. Kapil A, Sharma S. Immunopotentiating compounds from Tinospora cordifolia. J Ethnopharmacol. 1997;58(2):89–95.
66. Bala M, Pratap K, Verma PK, Singh B, Padwad Y. Validation of ethnomedicinal potential of Tinospora cordifolia for anticancer and immunomodulatory activities and quantification of bioactive molecules by HPTLC. J Ethnopharmacol. 2015;175:131–7.
67. Yue K, Ma B, Ru Q, Chen L, Gan Y, Wang D, et al. The dopamine receptor antagonist levo-tetrahydropalmatine attenuates heroin self-administration and heroin-induced reinstatement in rats.Pharmacol. Biochem. Behav. 2012;102(1):1–5.
68. Gong X, Yue K, Ma B, Xing J, Gan Y, Wang D, et al. Levo-tetrahydropalmatine, a natural, mixed dopamine receptor antagonist, inhibits methamphetamine self-administration and methamphetamine-induced reinstatement. Pharmacol. Biochem. Behav. 2016;144:67–72.

6

A 12-week evaluation of annatto tocotrienol supplementation for postmenopausal women: safety, quality of life, body composition, physical activity, and nutrient intake

Chwan-Li Shen[1,2,3*], Shu Wang[4], Shengping Yang[1], Michael D. Tomison[1], Mehrnaz Abbasi[4], Lei Hao[4], Sheyenne Scott[4], Md Shahjalal Khan[4], Amanda W. Romero[5], Carol K. Felton[6] and Huanbiao Mo[7]

Abstract

Background: Evidence suggests that tocotrienols may benefit bone health in osteopenic women. However, their safety in this population has never been investigated. This study was to evaluate the safety of a 12-week supplementation of annato tocotrienol in postmenopausal osteopenic women, along with effects of the supplementation on quality of life, body composition, physical activity, and nutrient intake in this population.

Methods: Eighty nine postmenopausal osteopenic women were randomly assigned to 3 treatment arms: (1) Placebo (430 mg olive oil/day), (2) Low tocotrientol (Low TT) (430 mg tocotrienol/day from DeltaGold 70 containing 300 mg tocotrienol) and (3) High tocotrienol (High TT) (860 mg tocotrienol/day from DeltaGold 70 containing 600 mg tocotrienol) for 12 weeks. DeltaGold 70 is an extract from annatto seed with 70% tocotrienol consisting of 90% delta-tocotrienol and 10% gamma-tocotrienol. Safety was examined by assessing liver enzymes (aspartate aminotransferase, alanine aminotransferase), alkaline phosphatase, bilirubin, kidney function (blood urea nitrogen and creatinine), electrolytes, glucose, protein, albumin, and globulin at 0, 6, and 12 weeks. Serum tocotrienol and tocopherol concentrations were assessed and pills counted at 0, 6, and 12 weeks. Quality of life, body composition, physical activity, and dietary macro- and micro-nutrient intake were evaluated at 0 and 12 weeks. A mixed model of repeated measures ANOVA was applied for analysis.

Results: Eighty seven subjects completed the study. Tocotrienol supplementation did not affect liver or kidney function parameters throughout the study. No adverse event due to treatments was reported by the participants. Tocotrienol supplementation for 6 weeks significantly increased serum delta-tocotrienol level and this high concentration was sustained to the end of study. There was no difference in serum delta-tocotrienol levels between the Low TT and the High TT groups. No effects of tocotrienol supplementation were observed on quality of life, body composition, physical activity, and nutrient intake.

(Continued on next page)

* Correspondence: leslie.shen@ttuhsc.edu
[1]Department of Pathology, Texas Tech University Health Sciences Center, Lubbock, Texas, USA
[2]Laura W. Bush Institute for Women's Health, Texas Tech University Health Sciences Center, Lubbock, Texas, USA
Full list of author information is available at the end of the article

(Continued from previous page)

Conclusions: Annatto-derived tocotrienol up to 600 mg per day for 12 weeks appeared to be safe in postmenopausal osteopenic women, particularly in terms of liver and kidney functions. Tocotrienol supplementation for 12 weeks did not affect body composition, physical activity, quality of life, or intake of macro- and micro-nutrients in these subjects.

Trial registration: ClinicalTrials.gov identifier: NCT02058420. Title: Tocotrienols and bone health of postmenopausal women.

Keywords: Vitamin E, Clinical trial, Dietary supplement, Liver function, Women, SF-36

Background

Oxidative stress and low-grade inflammation have been considered to be the central mechanisms underlying the development of osteoporosis in postmenopausal women [1–3]. Recent studies demonstrate that nutritional supplements rich in antioxidants can mitigate the loss of bone matrix and deteriation of bone microstructure in the estrogen-deficient animal model, a model used to represent bone loss in postmenopaual women [4, 5].

Among different types of antioxidants, vitamin E is a collective term for tocotrienols and tocopherols. Tocotrienols and tocopherols each exist in four different forms in nature: alpha (α), beta (β), gamma (γ), and delta (δ) in mixtures of varying compositions [6]. Tocotrienol possesses an unsaturated sidechain, which afford more efficient penetration into cells compared with the completely saturated sidechain of tocopherols [7, 8]. Recently, tocotrienols, especially δ-tocotrienol, has gained an increasing interest due to its higher antioxidant-dependent biological activities in comparions with tocopherols [7, 8]. The order of anti-oxidant potency, as determined by ORAC values, is δ-tocotrienol >> γ-tocotrienol = β-tocotrienol = α-tocopherol > α-tocotrienol > γ-tocopherol = β-tocopherol > α-tocopherol [9, 10].

In a recent comprehensive review, the authors suggested that tocotrienols might reduce bone fracture risk by increasing bone mineral density and supporting osteoblastic activities while suppressing osteoclastic activities in preclinical studies [4]. The osteo-protective effects of tocotrienols are, in part, due to their antioxidant/anti-inflammatory functions [11] and suppressive effect on 3-hydroxy-3-methylglutaryl coenzyme A reductase [12].

Legislation in use of complementary and alternative medicine (i.e., herbal/dietary supplements) is inconsistent and even lacking in many countries. In the US, vitamin E is labeled as a dietary supplement that does not require pre-clinical tests because it is pre-Dietary Supplement Health and Education Act (DSHEA), or already in the market prior to the enactment of the DSHEA of 1994. Most of the published tocotrienol clinical safety studies were either short-term (≤ 2 weeks) [13, 14] or using a mixture of tocotrienol and tocopherol [15, 16]. With a longer study period, only single low dose of tocotrienol was used [16]. A study with high dose tocotrienol had limited safety data related to liver and kidney functions [17]. Furthermore, there is limited clinical information on the safety of δ-tocotrienol supplementation in humans [13, 17, 18]. The limited number of published δ-tocotrienol studies on pharmacokinetics and bioavaiability was either relatively short-term or with a small sample size, and they were not randomized placebo-controlled trial [13, 17, 18]. The detailed safety information at a higher dosage is increasingly important because of mounting interest in clinical studies using tocotrienols. Lacking such safety information hinders research development. Therefore, the present work was the first annatto seed-extract tocotrienol safety report on liver and kidney functions based on two different dosages (300 and 600 mg tocotrienol) with a larger sample size in a 12-week double-blinded placebo-controlled randomized clinical trial. The objective of this paper was to evaluate the safety of tocotrienol supplementation for 12 weeks in postmenopausal osteopenic women. In addition to safety, the effects of treatment arms on quality of life, as assessed by Short Form-36 (SF-36) questionnaires, serum tocotrienol and tocopherol concentrations (as assessed by high pressure liquid chromatography), body composition (as assessed by composition analyzer), physical activity (as assessed by Godin Leisure-Time Exercise Questionaire), and nutrientintake (as assessed by food frequency questionnaires) were also reported.

Methods

Study design and intervention

This was a 12-week, double-blinded, placebo-controlled, randomized intervention trial to investigate the effects of tocotrienol on bone parameters. Participants were randomly assigned to one of the three treatment groups: Placebo group (0 mg tocotrienol/day, 430 mg olive oil), Low tocotrienol (Low TT) group (430 mg DeltaGold 70 containing 300 mg tocotrienol/day), and High tocotrienol (High TT) group (860 mg DeltaGold 70 containing 600 mg tocotrienol/day).

Placebo and tocotrienol supplementof the same lot were supplied by American River Nutrition, Inc., Hadley, MA (US Food and Drug Aministation, Investigational New Drug (IND) number 120,761). Placebo softgels were made of the same size and color as the tocotrienol softgelts for identifical appearance and taste. DeltaGold 70, an extract from annatto seed with 70% purity, consisted of 90% delta-tocotrienol and 10% gamma-tocotrienol. During the 12-week intervention, all participants were provided with 500 mg elemental calcium and 200 IU vitamin D (as cholecalciferol) daily. Trial registration: ClinicalTrials.gov identifier: NCT02058420. Title: Tocotrienols and bone health of postmenopausal women.

Study participants

The complete study protocol was reported in detail previously [19] and only a brief description is provided here. Inclusion criteria were (i) postmenopausal women (at least 1 years after menopause) age 45 and older with osteopenia (mean hip and/or lumbar spine bone mineral density T-score between 1 and 2.5 standard deviation (SD) below the young normal sex-matched areal bone mineral density of the reference database) [12], (ii) normal function of thyroid, liver, and kidney, (iii) serum 25-hydroxy vitamin D ≥ 20 ng/mL, and (iv) no bisphosphonate treatment at least 12 months before study began. Women were excluded if they (i) had a disease condition or were on medication known to affect bone metabolism; (ii) had a history of cancer within the last 5 years; (iii) had hormone/hormone-like replacement therapy within 6 months of the study initation; (iv) had endocrine disease, malabsorption syndrome, cognitive impairment, depression, or other medical/eating disorders; (v) had a history of statin or other cholesterol-reducing drugs within 3 months of the study initiation; (vi) smoked > 10 cigarettes/day, had alcohol intake > 1 drink/day or used non-steroidal anti-inflammatory drugs on a regular basis; (vii) had HbA1c > 7.0; and (viii) were unwilling to accept randomization. Written informed consent was obtained from all the study participants before enrollment. The study was approved by the Texas Tech University Health Sciences Center Institutional Review Board.

Randomization and blinding

To ensure comparable distribution across treatment arms, stratified randomization was applied to eligible participants to balance baseline covariates, including age (≥ 50 or < 50 yr) and body mass index (BMI) (≥ 30 or < 30 kg/m^2). The study participants and investigators were blinded to the group allocation.

Compliance and adverse event monitoring

Adherence/compliance of tocotrienol or placebo study agents was determined as the percentage of all of tocotrienol or placebo softgels ingested throughout the study period. In the course of the 12-week clinical trial, adverse events associated with tocotrienol were self-reported by the participants, and by monitoring liver enzyme activities, aspartate aminotransferase (AST) and alanine aminotransferase (ALT) in particular, through blood analysis. All observed and self-reported adverse events, regardless of suspected causal relationship to the study treatments, were recorded on the adverse event form throughout the study.

Bioavailablity: Serum vitamin E concentration

To evaluate the bioavailability of study agents, the concentations of serum tocotrienol and tocopherol at baseline, 6, and 12 weeks were determined using a high-pressure liquid chromatography (HPLC) system based on our previously published method [19]. Briefly, serum was saponified in 10% KOH solution containing 0.001% of butylated hydroxytoluene acid and 1.1% of ascorbic acid at 95 °C for 30 mintues. *Rac*-Tocol was used as an internal standard. After saponification, vitamin E was extracted using hexane, and dried under a nitrogen evaporator. Tocotrienols and tocopherols were detected using a Waters HPLC system equipped with a silica column (5 μm, 4.6 × 250 mm) and a florescence detector. The mobile phase was composed of hexane and 1–4 dioxane (96:4, volume:volume), and the flow rate was 2.0 mL/min. The excitation and emission wavelengths were 296 nm and 325 nm, respectively.

Data collection and outcome measures

Body composition was measured at baseline and every 6 weeks via bioimpedance measurement (SC-331S Body Composition Analyzer, Tanita Corporation of America, Inc., Arlington Height, IL, USA). Physical activity level, food intake, and quality of life were collected at the baseline and after 12 weeks. Physical activity level was assessed via Godin Leisure-Time Exercise Questionaire. Food nutritent intake was assessed by a semiquantitative Harvard Willett Food Frquency Questionnaire. Quality of life status was assessed with the Medical Outcomes Study 36-item short form Health Survey (SF-36, version 2), which consists of eight dimensions of health (physical function, bodily pain, general health, vitality, mental health, social function, and role of physical and emotional health) in the conduct of daily activity [20].

Laboratory comprehensive metabolic panel including liver function (AST, ALT, bilirubin, and alkaline phosphatase activity (ALP)), kidney function (blood urea nitrogen (BUN), and creatinine), electrocytes (calcium (Ca), sodium (Na), potassium (K), chloride (Cl)), carbon dioxide (CO_2), and others (glucose, total protein, albumin, and globulin) were assessed in overnight fasting blood samples taken at baseline, 6, and 12 weeks. All samples were processed and analyzed in a certified diagnostic laboratory (Quest Diagnostic Laboratory, Dallas, TX).

Statistical analysis

We used power analysis and sample size software (PASS11) to obtain a sample size of 22 in each of the 3 arms (Placebo, Low TT, and High TT) for a power of 80% in our bone biomarker study [11]. Such a sample size was able to detect a clinically significant difference between the group means of urine N-terminal telopeptide (NTX, primary outcome measure in the main study) level at the end of 12 weeks [19]. This calculation is based on an analysis of covariance (ANCOVA), adjusted for three covariates: baseline NTX, age, and body mass index (BMI). With an expected attrition rate of 15%, a total of 78 participants were recruited ($n = 26$ for each group) to start the study.

An "intent-to-treat" principle was adopted in the data analysis. Descriptive statistics were used to describe the characteristics of the study cohort. Categorical variables were summarized as frequencies, and continuous variables were summarized using mean and standard deviation. Participant characteristics were compared to detect differences among the three groups at baseline. Also at each time point, Chi-squared test/Fisher's exact test or one way analysis of variance was used to compare whether there was any difference among the three groups, as appropriate. To compare the differences in change over time among the three groups, a repeated measure ANOVA was used controlling within-subject correlation. Statistical software SAS 9.4 (Cary, NC, USA) was used for all the analyses. A p value less than 0.05 was considered statistically significant.

Results

Participants

A total of 416 participants were prescreened. Among them, 89 were qualified and randomized, and 87 completed the 12-week study. Two participants (1 in the Placebo group and 1 in the Low TT group) withdrew before the end of the study, both due to loss of interest. Baseline characteristics were similar among different treatment groups (Table 1). All subjects were instructed to maintain their pre-existing physical activity, dietary habits, and medications, if any, throughout the study. Based on the results of pill count, the compliance rates were 92.9, 91.7, and 90.5% for the Placbo group, Low

Table 1 Baseline demographic characteristics of study population

Variables	Placebo	Low TT	High TT	*P* value
Number	28	29	30	
Age [y]	59.4±6.3	58.5±6.7	61.2±7.2	0.431
Weight [kg]	74.3±17.9	76.3±14.8	74.3±16.8	0.680
Height [cm]	160.0±6.2	163.7±6.5	155.6±27.1	0.107
Body mass index [kg/m^2]	28.9±6.5	28.5±5.0	28.8±5.8	0.986
Bone mineral density [T-score]				
Femoral Neck	−1.66±0.65	−1.52±0.82	−1.34±1.17	0.795
Trochanter	−1.06±0.95	−1.04±0.79	−0.85±1.30	0.945
Total spine	0.79±0.89	−0.87±0.85	−0.53±1.10	0.654
L1-L4	−0.67±0.99	−0.72±1.17	0.59±1.23	0.919
Serum 25 (OH)D [ng/mL]	35.79±9.13	35.45±9.70	34.27±9.97	0.634
Serum TSH [mIU/L]	2.25±1.01	2.45±1.46	2.52±1.71	0.944
Serum HbA1c [%]	5.66±0.35	5.81±0.34	5.56±0.36	0.011
Medical history [n (%)]				
Broken bone as adult	6 (21.43)	7 (24.14)	8 (26.67)	0.897
Osteoarthritis	3 (12.00)	5 (20.83)	3 (11.54)	0.584
Diabetes	2 (7.14)	2 (6.90)	0 (0.00)	0.331
Asthma	4 (14.29)	3 (10.34)	2 (6.67)	0.636
Use of HRT in the past 2 yr	10 (35.71)	8 (27.59)	6 (20.00)	0.409
Steroid or glucocorticoid use	5 (17.86)	4 (13.79)	3 (10.00)	0.687
Prescribed osteoporosis drugs	1 (3.57)	4 (13.79)	7 (23.33)	0.093

All data are mean ± standard deviation unless otherwise specified

HbA1c hemoglobin A1c, *High TT* tocotrienol supplementation at 860 mg daily (70% purity); *HRT* hormone replacement treatment, *Low TT* tocotrienol supplementation at 430 mg daily (70% purity), *TSH* thyroid stimulating hormone, *25(OH)D* 25-hydroxy-vitamin D

TT group, and High TT group respectively, showing no significant difference among the groups.

Serum tocotrienol and tocopherol concentrations

Table 2 shows the effects of tocotrienol supplementation on blood concentrations of tocotrienol and tocopherol. At the baseline, there was no significant difference in any forms of tocotrienol and tocopherol among the three treatments. Based on the results of repeated ANOVA controlling within-subject correlation, significant difference in the overtime change of serum δ-tocotrienol was found among the three groups (p = 0.042). Compared with the Placebo group, a significant overtime increase in serum δ-tocotrienol concentration was found in Low TT and High TT groups ($p = 0.017$ and $p = 0.048$, respectively).

Blood chemistry profiles

Table 3 depicts the effects of tocotrienol supplementation on blood chemistry at baseline, 6, and 12 weeks. At the baseline, there was no significant difference in any of the blood chemistry parameters among all treatment groups. Based on the results of repeated ANOVA, the levels of serum AST, ALT, and bilirubin (indicators of liver function) were not affected by tocotrienol intervention during the 12-week study period. Similarly, tocotrienol supplementation did not influence kidney function (BUN and creatinine), electrolytes (Ca, Na, K, Cl, CO_2), and any other blood biochemistry parameters (glucose, protein, albumin, and globulin) in the study participants throughout the study period.

Quality of life

Data demonstrating the effects of tocotrienol supplementation on quality of life, including all 8 domains, in postmenopausal osteopenic women are presented in Table 4. There were no significant differences in any domain of quality of life among the Placebo, the Low TT, and the High TT groups at the baseline, 6 weeks, and 12 weeks ($p > 0.05$). Futhermore, throughout the course of the 12-week intervention, there was no statistically significant change in any domain with time in all treatment groups ($p > 0.05$).

Body composition and physical activity

There was no significant difference between baseline and 12 weeks in body weight, % body fat, and BMI among the three groups, and the corresponding p values were 0.574, 0.733, and 0.449, respectively (Table 5). At baseline, the Placebo group had more exercise sessions than those in the High TT group, while there was no difference in estimated exercise time among the Placebo, Low TT, and Hight TT groups. There was no significant difference between baseline and at 12 weeks in physical activity in terms of exercise frequency and exercise time among the three groups (Table 5).

Nutrient intake

Table 6 presents the comparison of the before (0 week) and after (12 weeks) study difference in nutrient intake among the treatments. At baseline, there was no statistical difference in any macro- and micro-nutrients intake among three treatments. As expected, throughout the 12-week study period, no difference in macro- and micro-nutrients intake in study groups was observed ($p > 0.05$) (Table 6).

Discussion

This was the first double-blinded placebo-controlled randomized study to evaluate the safety of 12-week ingestion of annatto seed-extracted tocotrienol in postmenopausal women. This study demonstrated that tocotrienol supplementation of up to 600 mg tocotrienol daily for 12 weeks did not cause any safety concerns with regard to liver function (in terms of AST, ALT, ALP, and bilirubin levels), kidney function (in terms of

Table 2 Concentrations (μmol/L) of tocopherols and tocotrienols in various treatment groups at weeks 0, 6 and 12

VE	Week 0			Week 6			Week 12			Overall P Value
	Placebo[a]	Low TT	High TT	Placebo	Low TT	High TT	Placebo	Low TT	High TT	
α-tocopherol	14.64 (6.89)	14.3 (5.71)	12.38 (6.35)	14.03 (7.4)	13.56 (4.43)	13.67 (5.39)	16.17 (6.44)	15.01 (5.64)	12.42 (6.31)	0.771
β-tocopherol	1.86 (1.86)	3.21 (3.70)	2.72 (2.26)	3.07 (2.49)	2.26 (2.19)	2.50 (1.92)	2.43 (2.35)	2.82 (2.66)	2.57 (2.04)	0.571
δ-tocopherol	1.17 (1.22)	1.59 (2.52)	0.94 (1.31)	1.44 (2.41)	1.64 (2.26)	1.98 (1.43)	1.43 (2.37)	2.38 (3.23)	1.84 (1.25)	0.649
γ-tocopherol	2.58 (2.71)	3.79 (3.32)	3.18 (2.15)	3.13 (2.75)	4.38 (3.13)	3.27 (1.83)	3.79 (3.61)	4.23 (3.49)	2.57 (2.07)	0.189
α-tocotrienol	0.92 (1.69)	1.73 (3.45)	1.82 (2.23)	2.68 (3.73)	1.89 (2.81)	0.96 (1.25)	0.87 (1.84)	1.20 (1.93)	1.79 (2.27)	0.847
β-tocotrienol	0.34 (0.70)	0.11 (0.44)	0.49 (0.97)	0.61 (0.87)	0.59 (0.91)	0.33 (0.61)	0.20 (0.54)	0.12 (0.31)	0.91 (1.40)	0.341
δ-tocotrienol	0.54 (0.92)	1.06 (2.34)	0.77 (1.08)	1.05 (2.39)	1.93 (1.81)	2.32 (1.33)	1.14 (1.84)	3.19 (2.71)	2.59 (2.10)	0.042
γ-tocotrienol	0.40 (0.84)	0.77 (2.61)	1.04 (2.56)	1.58 (4.83)	1.46 (2.99)	1.27 (2.09)	1.08 (2.65)	2.71 (4.25)	1.74 (3.24)	0.307

[a]Values are mean(SD). Repeat measures ANOVA was used to evaluate whether the slopes of change in VE concentration overtime were the same for the three interventions

Table 3 Effect of tocotrienol supplementation on blood parameters in postmenopausal osteopenic women

Variable	Week 0			Week 6			Week 12			Overall P Value
	Placebo[a]	Low TT	High TT	Placebo	Low TT	High TT	Placebo	Low TT	High TT	
AST (U/L)	23.01 (10.68)	20.76 (6.57)	20.77 (4.95)	21.46 (5.53)	20.76 (6.76)	22.07 (7.97)	21 (5.23)	20.21 (9.39)	21.9 (7.63)	0.515
ALT (U/L)	23.75 (11.49)	19.9 (8.35)	19.03 (7.83)	20.82 (8.77)	19.66 (8.88)	20.5 (10.34)	21.14 (8.67)	18.72 (8.65)	19.57 (10.76)	0.494
Bilirubin (mg/dL)	0.53 (0.19)	0.52 (0.14)	0.57 (0.15)	0.46 (0.21)	0.48 (0.13)	0.43 (0.11)	0.5 (0.19)	0.47 (0.15)	0.47 (0.12)	0.583
ALP (U/L)	72.75 (14.68)	79.59 (15.53)	79.23 (22.96)	74.04 (16.95)	76.28 (18.04)	75.23 (16.56)	74.64 (15.6)	75.14 (16.31)	74.4 (16.99)	0.730
BUN (mg/dL)	14.46 (3.48)	16.41 (4.6)	16.57 (4.26)	14.86 (3.33)	15.62 (3.53)	17.07 (4.18)	15.54 (3.96)	16.97 (3.74)	16.67 (4.44)	0.120
Creatinine (mg/dL)	0.79 (0.12)	0.85 (0.13)	0.83 (0.12)	0.82 (0.12)	0.87 (0.15)	0.86 (0.15)	0.82 (0.13)	0.89 (0.17)	0.83 (0.12)	0.111
Ca (mg/dL)	9.62 (0.38)	9.54 (0.37)	9.48 (0.29)	9.44 (0.35)	9.41 (0.36)	9.37 (0.39)	9.57 (0.34)	9.55 (0.53)	9.5 (0.28)	0.607
Na (mmol/L)	138.86 (3.43)	139.72 (1.56)	139.27 (2.33)	139.5 (2.85)	140.03 (2.5)	140.1 (2.17)	139.75 (1.9)	140.48 (2.35)	140.37 (2.51)	0.346
K (mmol/L)	3.99 (0.28)	4.03 (0.36)	4.02 (0.35)	3.83 (0.24)	3.77 (0.29)	3.78 (0.4)	3.84 (0.32)	3.91 (0.31)	3.79 (0.39)	0.986
Cl (mmol/L)	103.71 (3.55)	104.1 (2.55)	104.1 (2.92)	103.61 (2.81)	103.55 (2.32)	104.5 (1.87)	103.29 (2.68)	103.9 (3.02)	104.13 (3.04)	0.314
CO_2 (mmol/L)	21.68 (2.28)	22.48 (2.29)	22.87 (2.61)	19.79 (2.22)	21.1 (1.97)	20.83 (2.35)	20.89 (1.83)	21.45 (1.74)	20.67 (2.92)	0.086
Glucose (mg/dL)	90.61 (10.78)	88.21 (13.91)	85.8 (15.05)	87.43 (11.81)	83.34 (12.29)	83.27 (14.1)	84.75 (11.78)	83.83 (12.74)	83.83 (11.75)	0.282
Protein, total (g/dL)	7.19 (0.41)	7.23 (0.48)	7.17 (0.54)	7.2 (0.37)	7.24 (0.4)	7.2 (0.45)	7.29 (0.33)	7.24 (0.44)	7.31 (0.41)	0.810
Albumin (g/dL)	4.39 (0.26)	4.36 (0.21)	4.35 (0.26)	4.32 (0.24)	4.28 (0.2)	4.26 (0.18)	4.41 (0.19)	4.33 (0.21)	4.38 (0.19)	0.474
Globulin (g/dL)	2.8 (0.35)	2.87 (0.41)	2.82 (0.45)	2.89 (0.3)	2.97 (0.41)	2.95 (0.39)	2.87 (0.28)	2.91 (0.37)	2.94 (0.38)	0.468
Albumin/globulin	1.59 (0.22)	1.55 (0.25)	1.59 (0.26)	1.52 (0.19)	1.48 (0.23)	1.46 (0.21)	1.55 (0.16)	1.52 (0.2)	1.52 (0.22)	0.451

[a]Values are mean(SD). *AST* asparate aminotransferase, *ALT* alanine aminotransferase, *ALP* alkaline phosphatase, *BUN* blood urea nitrogen, *Ca* calcium, *Cl* chloride, CO_2 carbon dioxide, *K* potassium, *Na* sodium

Table 4 Effect of tocotrienol supplementation on quality of life in postmenopausal osteopenic women

Domain	Week 0			Week 12			Overall P Value
	Placebo[a]	Low TT	High TT	Placebo	Low TT	High TT	
Physical function	89.64 (12.24)	83.1 (16.71)	88 (13.68)	77.22 (10.13)	69.29 (16.82)	74.66 (10.93)	0.779
Role-physical	92.19 (11.98)	87.5 (18.3)	89.79 (15.09)	93.75 (11.63)	84.15 (21)	92.71 (12.07)	0.293
Bodily pain	71.43 (16.04)	68.28 (19.65)	71 (13.98)	72.22 (15.77)	71.07 (19.5)	71 (16.26)	0.761
General health	80.18 (16.03)	78.07 (14.7)	83.5 (15.86)	80.56 (17.42)	78.57 (15.76)	83.67 (14.78)	0.754
Vitality	66.29 (16.52)	63.58 (19.7)	66.46 (17.71)	65.97 (16.84)	67.63 (20.2)	73.54 (15.8)	0.079
Social function	94.2 (15.02)	92.24 (14.72)	91.67 (16.52)	93.06 (15.24)	89.29 (23)	94.58 (12.14)	0.167
Role-emotional	89.29 (19.62)	92.24 (14.07)	93.89 (10.48)	90.74 (13.54)	91.67 (16.67)	93.61 (9.71)	0.818
Mental health	80.71 (12.82)	84.31 (12.44)	80.17 (15.51)	82.04 (16.42)	84.82 (14.37)	83.33 (13.22)	0.637

[a]Values are mean(SD)

BUN and creatinine levels), or other blood chemistry parameters. In fact, tocotrienol supplementation seemed to improve liver function by showing reduced ALP in the tocotrienol-treated groups. The findings that tocotrienol supplementation had no adverse effects on liver function is in agreement with a study conducted by Magosso et al. [16]. In Magosso's study, one-year supplementation of mixed tocotrienol isomers (α-tocotrienol, δ-tocotrienol and γ-tocotrienol) and α-tocopherol at 200 mg twice daily did not change blood levels of ALT, AST, glucose, or creatinine in patients with nonalcoholic fatty liver disease [16].

In the present study, we reported that tocotrienol supplementation for 12 weeks did not affect body composition in terms of weight, BMI, and %body fat of study participants. These findings were consistent with Magosso et al. [16], who showed that 1 year of mixed tocotrienol and tocopherol supplementation did not change BMI in patients with nonalcoholic fatty liver disease.

Quality of life is affected by many factors, including physical, social and emotional functions that are in turn modulated by certain chronic conditions such as pain and inflammation. Accumulating evidence suggests the link between mitochondrial dysfunction, oxidative stress and neuropathic pain that could be treated with antioxidants [21]. Oxidative stress and neuroinflammation are among the mechanisms underlying neurodegenerative diseases, adversely affecting mental health and quality of life [22]. This study also evaluated the effect of TT supplementation on the quality of life, and the results showed no adverse effect. There was no evidence supporting that vitamin E (tocopherols) intake benefited the quality of life in patients with amyothrophic lateral sclerosis [23]. Another study found that green tea extract supplementation, also rich in antioxidants, for 24 weeks did not benefit the quality of life in postmenopausal osteopenic women in a randomized placebo-controlled intervention [24]. Although all these supplements (TT, tocopherols, and green tea polyphenols) are considered to be functional in protecting cells from oxidative stress, these published studies along with the present study seem to suggest no impact of these supplements on the quality of life. As expected, tocotrienol supplementation did not influence physical activity or nutrition intake in subjects at 12 weeks (end of study), since the subjects were advised to maintain the same lifestyle. It may be prudent to refrain from interpreting the lack of impact of tocotrienol supplementation on physical activity or

Table 5 Effect of tocotrienol supplementation on body composition and physical activity in postmenopausal osteopenic women

Variable	Week 0			Week 12			Overall P Value
	Placebo[a]	Low TT	High TT	Placebo	Low TT	High TT	
Body Composition							
BMI (kg/m^2)	28.95 (6.47)	28.47 (4.98)	28.77 (5.78)	27.88 (6.44)	28.37 (5.28)	28.95 (6.01)	0.345
Fat (%)	39.13 (7.4)	39.41 (6.89)	39.01 (7.48)	38.97 (7.22)	39.81 (7.28)	39.37 (7.59)	0.959
Weight (kg)	74.26 (17.94)	76.34 (14.76)	74.33 (16.76)	72.87 (16.99)	75.56 (15.25)	74.36 (16.72)	0.504
Physical activity profile							
Exercise frequency (sessions/week)	2.14^a (0.85)	1.96^{ab} (0.88)	1.60^b (0.62)	2.19 (0.62)	2.0 (0.86)	1.75 (0.80)	0.869
Exercise time (min/session)	30.26 (22.53)	31.07 (27.36)	34.30(19.08)	34.74(23.32)	29.69(26.45)	39.83(25.93)	0.318

Within a given row, values that share the same superscript letter (a, b) are not statistically different from each other after adjusting for age and BMI
[a]Values are mean(SD)

Table 6 Effect of tocotrienol supplementation on macro- and micro-nutrient intake in postmenopausal osteopenic women

Variable	Week 0			Week 12			Overall P Value
	Placebo[a]	Low TT	High TT	Placebo	Low TT	High TT	
Total calories (kcal)	1685.9 (624.72)	2399.8 (1549.82)	1928.2 (810.37)	1610.4 (550.15)	2128.6 (1382.71)	2211.9 (1816.89)	0.111
Carbohydrates (g)	199.8 (86.99)	266.5 (169.59)	232.5 (106.84)	190.2 (73.18)	232.9 (159.45)	264.0 (241.36)	0.233
Total sugars (g)	90.7 (52.64)	123.6 (77.6)	112.8 (60.48)	87.2 (42.48)	103.3 (68.72)	124.1 (126.57)	0.192
Total fiber (g)	21.7 (8.99)	27.8(19.94)	24.1 (10.73)	20.7 (8.67)	26.7 (19.18)	29.4 (26.49)	0.252
Total fat (g)	65.9 (26.97)	104.4 (71.73)	72.7 (33.8)	63.3 (24.00)	95.4 (61.70)	84.5 (62.57)	0.215
Cholesterol (mg)	204.5 (99.95)	323.7 (245.7)	297.2 (190.79)	212.5 (95.05)	268.0 (196.27)	309.8 (256.2)	0.278
Saturated fat (g)	20.6 (10.61)	33.5 (25.52)	25.1 (15.02)	19.7 (8.13)	28.0 (18.52)	26.6 (21.59)	0.213
Monounsaturated (g)	25.0 (10.02)	40.2(27.25)	25.90 (11.60)	24.1 (9.04)	38.7 (25.83)	31.8 (21.11)	0.201
Polyunsaturated (g)	14.2 (6.27)	20.9 (14.32)	14.6 (6.66)	13.7 (7.14)	20.2 (14.56)	18.3 (15.28)	0.298
Protein (g)	72.4 (27.83)	101.2 (71.44)	90.0(41.12)	70.5 (23.93)	91.2(74.78)	105.0(97.63)	0.293
Calcium (mg)	1164.1 (587.92)	1277.4 (730.38)	1318.2(792.1)	1184.6 (517.16)	1044.3 (574.77)	1219.5 (1044.16)	0.373
Potassium (mg)	2908.1 (1107.18)	3892.8 (2582.54)	3343.0(1560.48)	2847.1 (972.19)	3463.7 (2495.8)	3970.2 (3551.94)	0.202
Phosphorus (mg)	1211.7 (486.11)	1638.9 (1057.27)	1480.8(655.18)	1217.3 (408.83)	1430.9 (1027.86)	1655.4 (1476.94)	0.309
Sodium (mg)	1849.3 (826.99)	2656 (1860.41)	2337.2(963.73)	1847.2 (719.41)	2355.3 (1609.08)	2609.3 (2047.47)	0.257
Magnesium (mg)	382.1 (183.15)	490.1 (331.28)	413.0(223.5)	363.5 (148.08)	405.1 (273.53)	446.2 (437.75)	0.396
Iron (mg)	12.2 (4.64)	17.2 (11.74)	16.0 (9.24)	12.4 (7.81)	15.5 (12.2)	18.2 (14.12)	0.435
α-Carotene (μg)	703.2 (548.58)	1143.1 (2215.95)	619.2 (475.97)	713.0 (585.51)	1180.0 (2996.32)	1402.5 (2523.89)	0.133
β-Carotene (μg)	5288.3 (3804.98)	6993.7 (9886.87)	5531.6 (3336.1)	5379.9 (4162.6)	7229.7 (11,253.44)	7927.5 (10,896.58)	0.439
Vitamin D (IU)	437.0 (400.57)	443.7 (296.05)	516.0 (403.89)	412.5 (339.19)	286.4 (256.39)	382.7 (371.33)	0.333
Vitamin E (mg)	16.9 (35.42)	29.7 (70.48)	17.2 (19.49)	18.5 (34.65)	61.2 (80.46)	26.3 (46.57)	0.365
Vitamin K1 (μg)	174.1 (132.15)	217.9 (173.9)	228.8 (133.54)	178.5 (130.91)	214.1 (179.3)	253.0 (231.18)	0.805
Vitamin C (mg)	266.4 (351.41)	224.5 (266.92)	163.4 (211.03)	300.2 (410.03)	159.3 (226.95)	209.8 (242.44)	0.058
Thiamine (mg)	3.6 (9.69)	6.5 (14.13)	5.4 (13.11)	5.5 (13.72)	3.5 (10.24)	5.3 (12.86)	0.762
Riboflavin (mg)	4.2 (9.75)	7.2 (14.11)	6.2 (13.35)	6.1 (13.56)	4.0 (10.37)	6.2 (13.17)	0.744
Pyridoxine (mg)	8.1 (29.29)	7.1 (14.19)	13.0 (34.1)	8.0 (16.3)	17.9 (39.61)	11.5 (38.01)	0.255
Vitamin B12 (μg)	46.9 (146.1)	51.5 (137.43)	46.9 (127.98)	70.3 (168.15)	66.1 (168.15)	11.8 (14.73)	0.138
Folic acid (μg)	153.7 (130.66)	277.0 (263.85)	234.0 (301.46)	215.1 (235.85)	161.1 (203.88)	205.6 (191.8)	0.121
Niacin (mg)	25.6 (11.66)	49.7 (57.12)	34.2 (22.63)	47.2 (78.42)	30.3 (25.59)	37.0 (32.63)	0.186

[a]Values are mean(SD)

nutrition intake until further studies since the subjects were advised to maintain the same lifestyle.

In the present study, we measured the concentrations of 4 isomers of tocotrienol and 4 isomers of tocopherol in the overnight-fasting serum of subjects, and we found that only serum δ-tocotrienol concentrations were elevated in the tocotrienol-supplemented groups at 6 weeks and sustained at 12 weeks. The serum δ-tocotrienol concentrations in the tocotrienol-supplemented group reflected the composition of tocotrienol supplement consisting of 90% δ-tocotrienol + 10% γ-tocotrienol. Due to the small amount of γ-tocotrienol in the study supplement, we were not able to observe the difference in serum γ-tocotrienol levels among the three treatment groups. There was neither dose-effect (300 mg in the Low TT group vs. 600 mg in the High TT group) nor time-effect (6 weeks vs. 12 weeks) in tocotrienol-supplemented groups. In addition, we also found serum β-tocotrienol was elevated in tocotrienol-adminstered groups, although the concentration of β-tocotrienol was relative low. Qureshi et al. recently reported the safety and pharmacokinetics of single doses of 750 mg/day and 1000 mg/day of annatto-based tocotrienol, which was the same study agent used in our study, in healthy humans (30–40 year, $n = 3$ per group) by collecting plasma at 0, 1, 2, 4, 6, and 8 h intervals after meal [17]. The authors found (1) the higher single dose of tocotrienol was safe in humans; (2) Tmax was 3–4 h for all isomers of tocotrienol and tocopherol except for α-tocopherol at 6 h; and (3) the plasma levels and areas under curve of all tocotrienol isomers, δ-tocopherol, and β-tocopherol were affected in a dose-dependent fashion. Based on the finidngs of Qureshi et al. [17], it is possible to observe the elevated plasma levels of all tocotrienol isomers, including β-tocotrienol, after supplementation of annatto-based tocotrienol. The reasons why we were not able to observe a dose- and time-dependent manner in our study were (i) because the tocotrienol had cleared the entero-hepatic circulation after 6–8 h, whereas blood draw occurred at 12 h after an overnight fast, and (ii) saturation of tocotrienol [25] after a longer period of intervention (e.g., 6 weeks).

As expected, TT supplementation for 6 weeks significantly increased serum delta-TT levels and this high concentration was sustained to the end of study with continued supplementation. Although the supplement (DeltaGold) is Generally Recognized as Safe (GRAS), it is still worthy to include a follow-up assessment of serum vitamin E concentration and safety in a future study.

Conclusion

Supplementation of 600 mg tocotrienol daily to postmenopausal osteopenic women for 12 weeks did not cause any adverse effects on liver and kidney function, as determined by blood test parameters, and had no influence on quality of life (as assessed by SF-36 questionnaires), body composition, physical activity, and nutritent intake. Based on our findings, tocotrienol at a dose of 600 mg per day for 12 weeks appears to be safe in postmenopausal osteopenic women.

Acknowledgements

We gratefully acknowledge the study participants; without them this study would not have been possible. We thank Jun Cao for the vitamin E method development.

Funding

This study was supported by American River Nutrition, Inc., Hadley, MA. The contents of this manuscript are solely the responsibility of the authors and do not necessarily represent the official views of American Rivier Nutrition. The American River Nutrition declares that they have no competing interests in the design of the study and collection, analysis, and interpretation of data and in writing the manuscript.

Authors' contributions

CLS received the research funding, led the entire study, and drafted the manuscript. SY participated in the design of the study and performed the statistical analysis. SW, MDT, MA, LH, SS, MK made substantial contributions to analysis and interpretation of data for serum vitamin E extraction, HPLC detection of vitamin E, and data collection and analysis of vitamin E 8 isomers. AWR coordinated the study including blood and urine sample collection. CKF participated in recruitment and oversaw participants' medical affairs. HM and SW contributed to the design of this study protocol and the manuscript. All authors have read and approved the manuscript.

Competing interests

American River Nutrition, Inc., Hadely, MA supplied the drugs and funded this study. The authors declare that they have no competing interests.

Author details

[1]Department of Pathology, Texas Tech University Health Sciences Center, Lubbock, Texas, USA. [2]Laura W. Bush Institute for Women's Health, Texas Tech University Health Sciences Center, Lubbock, Texas, USA. [3]Department of Laboratory Sciences and Primary Care, Texas Tech University Health Sciences Center, Lubbock, Texas, USA. [4]Department of Nutritional Sciences, Texas Tech University, Lubbock, TX, USA. [5]Clinical Research Institute, Texas Tech University Health Sciences Center, Lubbock, Texas, USA. [6]Department of Obstetrics and Gynecology, Texas Tech University Health Sciences Center, Lubbock, TX, USA. [7]Department of Nutrition, Georgia State University, Atlanta, GA, USA.

References

1. Cervellati C, Bonaccorsi G, Cremonini E, Bergamini CM, Patella A, Castaldini C, Ferrazzini S, Capatti A, Picarelli V, Pansini FS, Massari L. Bone mass density selectively correlates with serum markers of oxidative damage in post-menopausal women. Clin Chem Lab Med. 2013;51(2):333–8.
2. Yang S, Feskanich D, Willett WC, Eliassen AH, Wu T. Association between global biomarkers of oxidative stress and hip fracture in postmenopausal women: a prospective study. J Bone Miner Res. 2014;29(12):2577–83.
3. Cervellati C, Bonaccorsi G, Cremonini E, Romani A, Fila E, Castaldini MC, Ferrazzini S, Giganti M, Massari L. Oxidative stress and bone resorption interplay as a possible trigger for postmenopausal osteoporosis. Biomed Res Int. 2014;2014:569563.
4. Shen CL, Klein A, Chin KY, Mo H, Tsai P, Yang RS, Chyu MC, Ima-Nirwana S. Tocotrienols for bone health: a translational approach. Ann N Y Acad Sci. 2017;1401(1):150–65. Review
5. Shen CL, Chyu MC. Tea flavonoids for bone health: from animals to humans. J Investig Med. 2016;64(7):1151–7.
6. Ahsan H, Ahad A, Iqbal J, Siddiqui WA. Pharmacological potential of tocotrienols: a review. Nutr Metab (Lond). 2014;11(1):52.
7. Sen CK, Khanna S, Roy S. Tocotrienols: vitamin E beyond tocopherols. Life Sci. 2006;78(18):2088–98. Review
8. Suzuki YJ, Tsuchiya M, Wassall SR, Choo YM, Govil G, Kagan VE, Packer L. Structural and dynamic membrane properties of alpha-tocopherol and alpha-tocotrienol: implication to the molecular mechanism of their antioxidant potency. Biochemistry. 1993;32(40):10692–9.
9. Muller L, Theile K, Bohm V. In vitro antioxidant activity of tocopherols and tocotrienols and comparison of vitamin E concentration and lipophilic antioxidant capacity in human plasma. Mol Nutr Food Res. 2010;54(5):731–42.
10. Palozza P, Verdecchia S, Avanzi L, Vertuani S, Serini S, Iannone A, et al. Comparative antioxidant activity of tocotrienols and the novel chromanyl-polyisoprenyl molecule FeAox-6 in isolated membranes and intact cells. Mol Cell Biochem. 2006;287(1-2):21–32.
11. Shen CL, Yang S, Tomison MD, Romero AW, Felton CK, Mo H. Tocotrienols supplementation suppressed bone resorption and oxidative stress in postmenopausal osteopenic women: a 12-week randomized double-blinded placebo-controlled trial. Osteoporos Int. 2018;29(4):881–91.
12. Mo H, Yeganehjoo H, Shah A, Mo WK, Soelaiman IN, Shen CL. Mevalonate-suppressive dietary isoprenoids for bone health. J Nutr Biochem. 2012; 23(12):1543–51. Review
13. Springett GM, Husain K, Neuger A, Centeno B, Chen DT, Hutchinson TZ, Lush RM, Sebti S, Malafa MP. A phase I safety, pharmacokinetic, and Pharmacodynamic Presurgical trial of vitamin E δ-tocotrienol in patients with pancreatic ductal neoplasia. EBioMedicine. 2015;2(12):1987–95.
14. Meganathan P, Jabir RS, Fuang HG, Bhoo-Pathy N, Choudhury RB, Taib NA, Nesaretnam K, Chik Z. A new formulation of Gamma Delta Tocotrienol has superior bioavailability compared to existing Tocotrienol-rich fraction in healthy human subjects. Sci Rep. 2015;5:13550.
15. Catanzaro R, Zerbinati N, Solimene U, Marcellino M, Mohania D, Italia A, Ayala A, Marotta F. Beneficial effect of refined red palm oil on lipid peroxidation and monocyte tissue factor in HCV-related liver disease: a randomized controlled study. Hepatobiliary Pancreat Dis Int. 2016;15(2): 165–72.
16. Magosso E, Ansari MA, Gopalan Y, Shuaib IL, Wong JW, Khan NA, Abu Bakar MR, Ng BH, Yuen KH. Tocotrienols for normalisation of hepatic echogenic response in nonalcoholic fatty liver: a randomised placebo-controlled clinical trial. Nutr J. 2013;12(1):166.

17. Qureshi AA, Khan DA, Silswal N, Saleem S, Qureshi N. Evaluation of pharmacokinetics, and bioavailability of higher doses of Tocotrienols in healthy fed humans. J Clin Exp Cardiol 2016;7(4).
18. Mahipal A, Klapman J, Vignesh S, Yang CS, Neuger A, Chen DT, Malafa MP. Pharmacokinetics and safety of vitamin E δ-tocotrienol after single and multiple doses in healthy subjects with measurement of vitamin E metabolites. Cancer Chemother Pharmacol. 2016;78(1):157–65.
19. Shen CL, Mo H, Yang S, Wang S, Felton CK, Tomison MD, Soelaiman IN. Safety and efficacy of tocotrienol supplementation for bone health in postmenopausal women: protocol for a dose-response double-blinded placebo-controlled randomised trial. BMJ Open. 2016;6(12):e012572.
20. Pickard AS, Jeffrey AJ, Penn A, et al. Replicability of SF-36 summary scores by the SF-12 in stroke patients. Stroke. 1999;30:1213–7.
21. Carrasco C, Nazıroğlu M, Rodríguez AB, Pariente JA. Neuropathic pain: delving into the oxidative origin and the possible implication of transient receptor potential channels. Front Physiol. 2018;9:95. Review
22. Yusuf M, Khan M, Robaian MA, Khan RA. Biomechanistic insights into the roles of oxidative stress in generating complex neurological disorders. Biol Chem. 2018;399(4):305–19.
23. Galbussera A, Tremolizzo L, Brighina L, Testa D, Lovati R, Ferrarese C, Cavaletti G, Filippini G. Vitamin E intake and quality of life in amyotrophic lateral sclerosis patients: a follow-up case series study. Neurol Sci. 2006;27(3):190–3.
24. Shen CL, Chyu MC, Pence BC, Yeh JK, Zhang Y, Felton CK, Doctolero S, Wang JS. Green tea polyphenols supplementation and tai chi exercise for postmenopausal osteopenic women: safety and quality of life report. BMC Complement Altern Med. 2010;10:76.
25. Qureshi AA, Sami SA, Salser WA, Khan FA. Synergistic effect of tocotrienol-rich fraction (TRF(25)) of rice bran and lovastatin on lipid parameters in hypercholesterolemic humans. J Nutr Biochem. 2001;12(6):318–29.

7

Efficacy of self-management exercise program with spa therapy for behavioral management of knee osteoarthritis

Chloe Gay[1,5*], Candy Guiguet-Auclair[2], Bruno Pereira[3], Anna Goldstein[4], Loïc Bareyre[1], Nicolas Coste[1] and Emmanuel Coudeyre[1]

Abstract

Background: Osteoarthritis (OA) is not limited to joint pain and stiffness, which can lead to disability; it is also linked to comorbidities such as overweight, obesity and fears and beliefs related to the pathology. The knee OA population appears more affected by these risk factors and has a lower physical activity (PA) level than the general population. The key challenge for OA treatment is increasing the PA level to decrease the risk factors.

Methods: We aim to perform a prospective, multicentric, quasi-randomized controlled trial with an alternate-month design (1-month periods). People aged 50–75 years old with symptomatic knee OA (stage I-IV Kellgren and Lawrence scale) with low and moderate PA level will be included in 3 spa therapy resorts. The experimental arm will receive 5 self-management exercise sessions (1.5 h each; education, aerobics, strength training, range of motion) + an information booklet + 18 sessions (1 h each) of spa therapy treatment (STT). The active comparator arm will receive an information booklet + 18 sessions of STT. The primary outcome will be a change at 3 months in PA level (International Physical Activity Questionnaire short form score). Secondary outcomes will be function (WOMAC) pain (numerical scale), anxiety/depression (HAD), fears and beliefs about OA (KOFBeQ) and arthritis self-efficacy (ASES). The barriers to and facilitators of regular PA practice will be assessed by using specific items specifically designed for the study because of lack of any reference scale.

Discussion: The study could demonstrate the impact of a self-management exercise program associated with spa therapy in the medium term by increasing PA level in people with OA. A benefit for ameliorating fears and beliefs and anxiety/depression and improving self-efficacy will also be analysed. The findings could offer new prospects while establishing best clinical practice guidelines for this population.

Trial registration: ClinicalTrials.gov NCT02598804 (November 5, 2015).

Keywords: Knee osteoarthritis, Exercise, Self-management, Education, Spa therapy

* Correspondence: cgay@chu-clermontferrand.fr
[1]Service de Médecine Physique et de Réadaptation, CHU de Clermont Ferrand, INRA, Université Clermont Auvergne, Clermont Ferrand, France
[5]Physical and Rehabilitation Medecine Department, University of Clermont Ferrand, Clermont Auvergne University, France, CHU Hôpital Nord, 61 Rue de Châteaugay – BP 30056, 63118 Clermont Ferrand, Cébazat, France
Full list of author information is available at the end of the article

Background

Osteoarthritis (OA) constitutes the most frequent chronic joint disease. It contributes widely to disability and loss of autonomy in older people [1]. OA localization at the knee, hip and hand are most at risk [2]. According to the World Health Organisation (WHO), in 2020, chronic disease will be the main source of disability. This evolution is related to the increase in life expectancy due to improvements in medical technology [3].

Risk factors are multiple: heredity, overweight and trauma (sports, professional, surgery) [4, 5]. All these factors interact with each other and may contribute to worsened pain and disability and reduced mobility. With lack of any curative treatment, except prosthetic surgery, non-pharmacological treatment is essential [6].

International guidelines such as from the Osteoarthritis Research Society International (OARSI) recommend a non-pharmacological intervention associated with pharmacological treatment for pain for people with knee OA. Non-pharmacological therapies are exercise programs (strength training, aerobic activity, adjunctive range of motion, stretching and increasing physical activity (PA) level), self-management education program and weight loss if necessary [7–9]. Education and self-management exercise have a positive impact on pain, function, exercise level, weight, quality of life, and treatment adherence [10]. Self-management exercise programs have a clinical and behavioral impact [11].

People with OA have less PA level than the general population [12]. Comorbidities and risk of death are increased: history of diabetes, cancer, or cardiovascular disease and the presence of waling disability are major risk factors. People with more concerns are less active. PA practice can have two effects: ameliorating comorbidities and alleviating knee OA symptoms. However, adherence to non-pharmacological treatment is often incomplete. To be fully effective, an exercise program must be accompanied by measures to promote therapeutic adherence. Among these measures, education and information improve guideline adherence [11].

The efficacy of spa therapy in OA has been demonstrated, with good level of evidence for pain and disability, but the effect on behavioral management such as PA level is still unknown [13]. The last OARSI recommendation include spa therapy but restricted spa treatment to a subgroup of patients with generalized OA with comorbidities because of a lack of evidence [7]. Spa therapy effect is well known on pain, physical function [14, 15] and symptomatic drug consumption [16]. Short and long-term efficacy (up to 9 months) were demonstrated [16] on painful symptomatology and functional capacities in knee osteoarthritis people. Average direct costs per patient were higher in the usual treatment than mud-bath therapy in addition to usual care [17]. Mechanisms of action in spa therapy treatment are not fully understood but a combination of factors: mechanical, thermal and chemical seems to be the most evident [18]. Recent research on possible biomarkers showed a significant increase of Carboxy Terminal cross-linked Telepeptides of Type II (CTX-II), two weeks after mud-bath therapy [19]. According to Giannitti [20], mud-bath therapy decrease whole-blood level of miR-155, miR-181a, miR-146a, and miR-223 expression levels for knee osteoarthritis people. Furthermore mud-bath therapy modifies an important mediators of cartilage metabolism, the plasma levels of the adiponectin [21].

SPA therapy resorts, common in Europe, include a large sample of patients with different phenotypes from early to advanced OA stages. The spa treatment context could offer good conditions for behavioral modification and could be a special opportunity for self-management education. The spa resort is the opportunity to meet and interact with other patients and benefit from multidisciplinary medical and paramedical support for ameliorating pain and disability [22]. A combination of spa therapy, physical exercise, and self-management was found to benefit fibromyalgia symptoms [23]. Another study of low back pain, self-management exercise and spa therapy treatment (STT) is under way [24].

We aim to conduct a multicentre, prospective, quasi-randomised study to evaluate the effectiveness of a self-management exercise program associated with STT versus STT alone, on the physical activity level of patient with knee osteoarthritis, at 3 months follow up.

Methods

Aim

This study is aimed at people with knee OA. The main objective is to show a change in PA level 3 months after the self-management education program associated with STT. Secondary objectives are to assess the effectiveness of the self-management exercise program in terms of pain, disability, anxiety, depression, self-efficacy, fears and beliefs and barriers to and facilitators of OA and PA at 3 months, and sarcopenia after treatment (18 days).

Study design and setting

This is a 2-year multicenter, prospective, comparative, and quasi-randomized trial. The population will be randomised according to the alternate-month design method in 2 arms: experimental and active comparator.

The design and conduct of this trial will adhere to the requirements of the Standard Protocol Items: Recommendations for Interventional Trials (SPIRIT) [25]. The results will be reported in accordance with the CONSORT Statement for non-pharmacologic trials [26].

Participants and recruitment

We will recruit 142 participants, male and female, who are 50–75 years old with a diagnosis of mono or bilateral knee OA, in 3 spa therapy resorts, in France. All people already registered for STT will receive an information letter with study notification and eligibility criteria. Posters in each participating spa resort will be used for recruitment. The center is Clermont-Ferrand University Hospital associated with Royat spa center, le Mont Dore spa center and Bourbon-Lancy spa center.

Patient recruitment potential among people with knee OA in spa therapy is important. Indeed, OA represents the main disease treated by spa therapy (250,000 per year in France).

For people who meet the inclusion criteria, the research coordinator will perform the information and consent process and the physician will verify the inclusion criteria.

Eligibility criteria

Inclusion criteria

- People, male or female, 50 to 75 years old
- Mono or bilateral knee OA according to American College of Rheumatology (ACR) criteria [27]
- Radiological score: stage I to IV on Kellgren and Lawrence scale
- Covered under the national health insurance
- Giving informed written consent to participate in the study

Exclusion criteria

- Contraindication to spa therapy
- Unstable angina
- Cardiac failure
- Behavioral disorders or comprehension difficulties making assessment impossible
- High PA level according to International Physical Activity Questionnaire (IPAQ) categorical score [28]

Randomisation

The population was randomized according to the alternate month design method in two arms: experimental and active comparative arm. Weingarten, highlight that's it's possible to avoid contamination between the 2 groups with a therapeutic window between the intervention period and control period [29]. This methodology was previously used with good level of evidence in a self-management education program and low back pain treatment in a spa therapy resort [30]. Individual randomization suggests recruitment difficulties (incomplete intervention group risk) and feasibility, as well as an increase in the number of patients lost to follow-up in the control group.

The randomisation list will be established by the methodologist in charge of the project before starting the trial. Population groups will be assigned to arms by stratified randomization by center: this randomization allows for controlling eligibility and for communicating some information relative to randomisation from the investigator and eventually other actors. A document detailing the procedures for randomisation is kept confidential. Participants will be allocated to one of two arms (Figs. 1 and 2).

Interventions

Both groups will receive 18 sessions of STT over 3 weeks and an education booklet on the benefits of PA practice illustrated with pictures and a detailed description of the exercises to perform (Additional file 1). Only the experimental group will receive the self-management exercise program. The aim is to propose a reinforcement of the STT effect through a self-management exercise program.

The STT and the self-management exercise program will be standardised and designed by expert spa therapy physicians.

Interventions have been designed by a specialist steering committee, standardized and reproducible for the 3 centers. The steering committee consists of investigators, a spa therapist, physician and physiotherapist and the university hospital's medical team (physician, physiotherapist, adapted PA instructor).

Meetings with all members of the steering committee are organized to obtain consensus on the therapeutic protocol describing precisely the content and the organization of the intervention taking into account the context and the expertise of the different centers involved in the study.

Self-management exercise program

The main objective of the self-management exercise program will be to allow people to understand the importance of physical exercise practice and learn when, where and how to practice exercise, in order to adapt their PA practice according to their phenotype and integrate it long term in their daily life.

Each session will consist of 45 min of self-management education and 45 min of PA practice, with aerobic training program, strength training, range of motion and personal feedback. The exercise program will be tailored to each participant. The physiotherapist or adapted PA instructor will drive an experimental arm of 5 to 7 participants. The 5 sessions will take place on days (D) D4, D7, D10, D13 and D16.

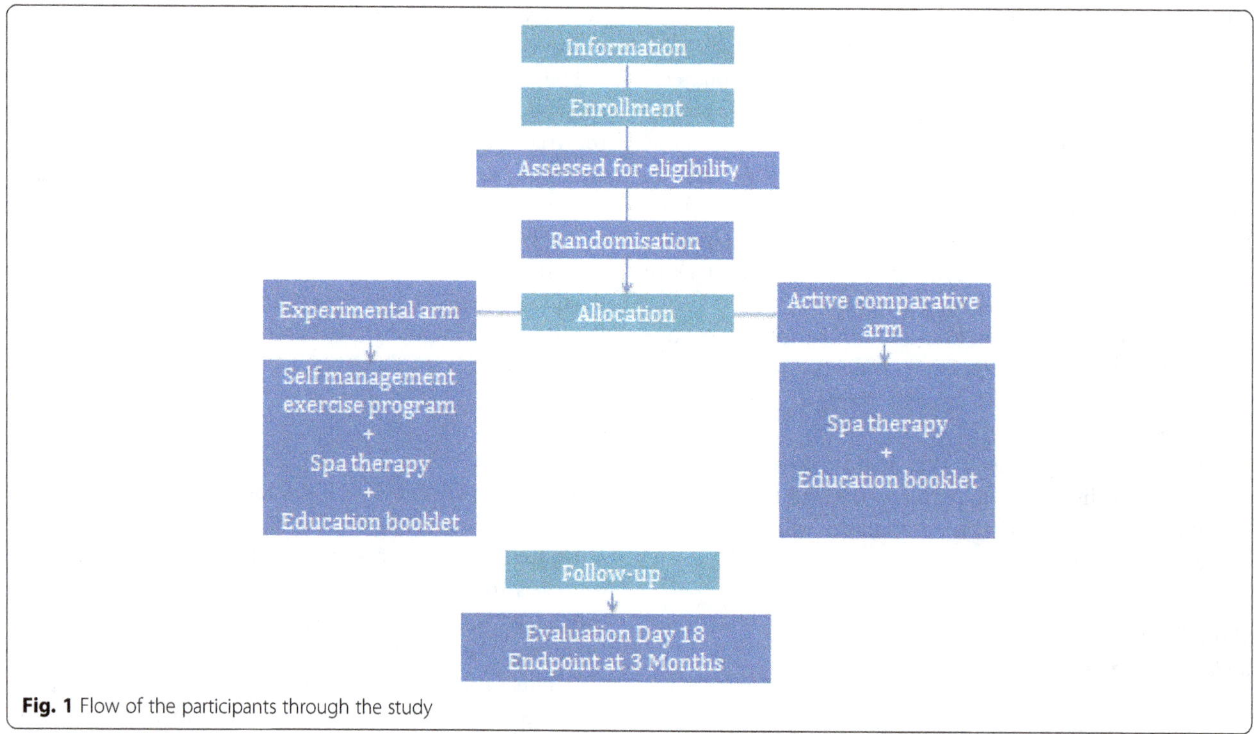

Fig. 1 Flow of the participants through the study

For each workshop, a specific objective and operational objectives are defined, linked to criteria and indicators (Table 1).

To facilitate the workshops, different teaching tools and techniques will be used: paper board, thematic discussion, participative discussion, practical leaflets (Borg scale, deconditioning circle), information booklet, exercise demonstration, feedback, and pain coping skills.

Education booklet

Patients will receive an information booklet containing cards with physical exercises adapted to their pathology

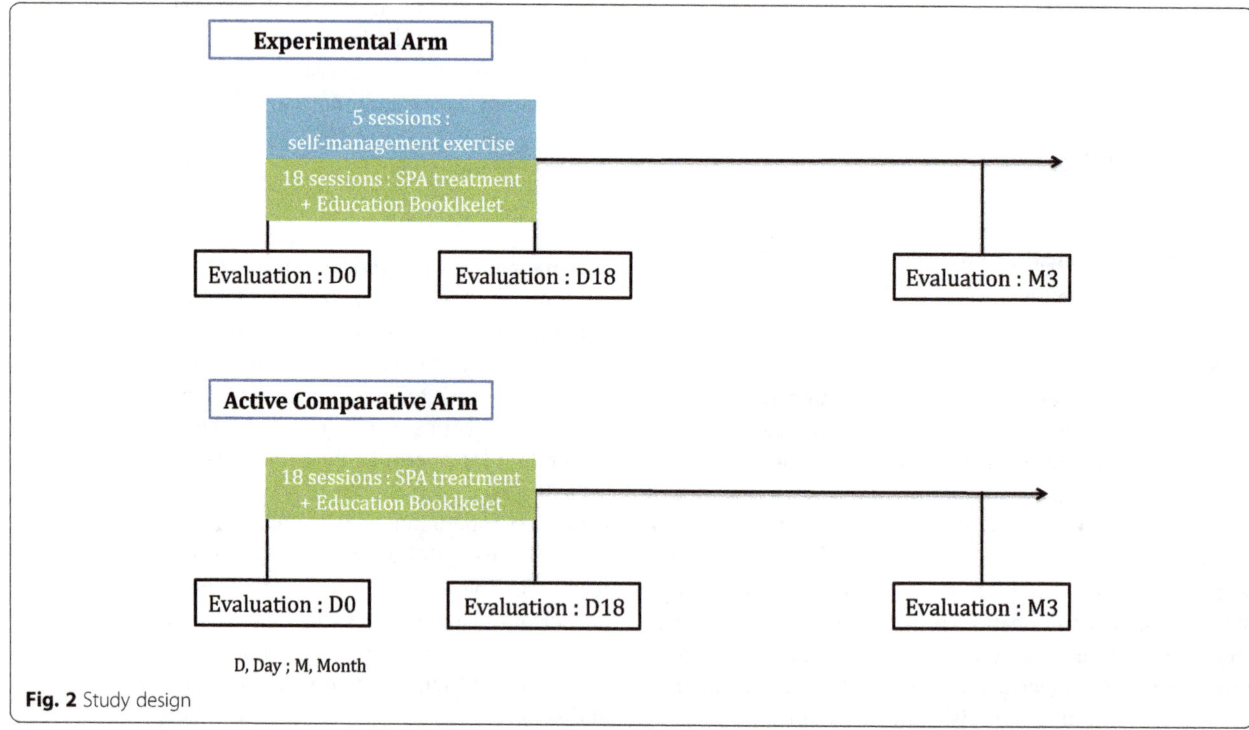

Fig. 2 Study design

Table 1 Self-management education program

Session	Objectives
Session 1: Evaluate the representation of the patient's PA	- Identify the representation of PA - Identify the barriers to and facilitators of regular PA practice -Acquisition of knowledge about OA -Know the methods of the exercise practice
Session 2: Defining the importance of exercise in knee OA	-Name the benefits of PA in the management of knee OA -Identify the normal and abnormal physiological signs during the PA practice - Learn to adapt the exercise according to its knee OA (intensity, duration)
Session 3: Patient engagement in regular PA practice	- Determine where, when and how to exercise throughout the year - Include an exercise program in everyday life - Know the anatomical bases necessary for performing the adapted exercises
Session 4: The consequences of stopping the exercise program	-Know the importance of maintaining exercise program on a regular and long-term basis -Identify factors that could facilitate or limit the continuation of the exercise program -Learn how to build a PA session
Session 5: Knowledge restitution	- Know the means of managing knee OA - Know how to live healthy with knee OA -Set an achievable goal

PA physical activity, *OA* osteoarthritis

to integrate the exercise program into their daily routine. This booklet will contain information about the pathology and PA practice with knee OA and illustrated cards with detailed descriptions of the exercises to be practiced (Additional files 1 and 2).

SPA therapy treatment

Each spa therapy session will comprise a mineral hydrojet session at 37 °C for 15 min, the thigh manipulated under mineral water at 38 °C by a physiotherapist for 10 min, manual massages, the application of mineral-matured mud at 45 °C to the knees for 15 min and supervised general mobilisation in a collective mineral water pool at 32 °C in groups of 8 patients for 15 min of 18 sessions, for 1 h each.

The main component of mineral waters are chloro-barbonated sodium in Royat (63) and Le Mont-Dore (63) spas centers and sodium chlorides in Bourbon Lancy (71).

Both groups will be mixed with the general public in the spa center. The spa therapist will not be aware of which patients will be taking part in the clinical trial.

The experimental and active comparator arms will receive unrestricted non-pharmacological, pharmacological and usual care during the study. Medication taken during or after the intervention will be reported in the follow-up questionnaires.

Measures

At baseline, we will collect data on sociodemographic items (age, Body Mass Index (BMI), marital status, area living, education status), anthropometric measures (Bioimpedance, Short Physical Performance Battery, Handgrip) and co-morbidities association, according to OARSI guidelines [7] (diabetes, hypertension, cardio vascular disease, renal failure; gastrointestinal (GI) bleeding, depression, or physical impairment limiting activity, including obesity).

Primary outcomes

The primary outcome is the proportion of participants varying to one IPAQ class at least (low-moderate or high or moderate-high) at 3 months [28]. The IPAQ short form (International Physical Activity Questionnaire) is a self-administered questionnaire which measures the physical activity level of people in a heterogeneous population as well as knee osteoarthritis people [31].

Secondary outcomes

- The arthritis self-efficacy influence on pain, function and other symptoms is assessed with the Arthritis Self-Efficacy Scale (ASES) [32] validation in French language is in progress NCT: 02977325 [33].
- Fears and beliefs changes are measured by the Knee OA Fears and Beliefs Questionnaire (KOFBeQ) [34].
- Physical function is assessed by the Western and McMaster Universities Osteoarthritis Index (WOMAC subscale for physical function (W-TPFS)) [35, 36].
- Pain intensity during the last 24 h and the worst pain intensity during the last month are measured by a numerical pain scale.

- Overall psychological status is assessed by the Hospital Anxiety and Depression Scale (HAD) [37, 38].
- The barriers to and facilitators of regular PA practice are assessed by 24 independent and specific items designed by a qualitative study [39], specifically for this study because of no reference scale. Each item will be coded from 0 (strongly disagree) to 4 (strongly agree). The prospective validation of this new scale is in progress.
- Use of pharmacological treatment is recorded (paracetamol, opioids, NSAIDs, intra-articular corticoid/hyaluronic acid).

Treatment adherence

Global PA practices, specific exercises and use of the education booklet will be reported in a self-reported questionnaire at 3 months to assess level of adherence to the self-management exercise program [26]. Reasons for low adherence will be explored: therapeutic effect, novelty, social link, global health, body image, habits.

Time-point outcomes

Study outcomes will be collected at baseline and after treatment (18 days) in spa resorts and at 3 months post-randomisation, by mailed self-reporting questionnaires. If needed, the research officer will use a telephone follow-up.

Statistical considerations

Sample size estimation

According to previous works presented in literature [11], we have estimated that a sample size of $n = 65$ patients per randomized group, for a two-sided type I error at 5%, would provide 80% statistical power of detecting an absolute difference of 20% (25% vs 5.) in the primary outcome: proportion of participants varying to one IPAQ class at least (low-moderate or high or moderate-high). Finally, a total of $n = 142$ patients (71 by group) will be considered to take into account lost to follow-up (10%).

Statistical analysis

Statistical analyses will be conducted using SAS software (version 9.3.). A two-sided p-value of less than 0.05 will be considered to indicate statistical significance (except interim analysis).

Concerning the primary outcome, the comparison between groups will be analysed using Chi-squared or Fisher's exact tests. Intention to treat (ITT) analysis will be considered for the primary outcome. Then, the analysis of the primary outcome will be completed by multivariate analysis using a generalized linear mixed model (logistic for dichotomous dependent endpoint) to take into account: (1) fixed effects covariates determined according to univariate results and to clinical relevance (for example gender, age and analgesic treatments), and (2) centre as random-effects (to measure between and within centre variability). Continuous endpoints will be compared between groups using Student's t-test or Mann-Whitney's test. Normality will be studied by the Shapiro-Wilk test and homoscedasticity using the Fisher-Snedecor test. As suggested by Vickers and Altman [40], the comparison between groups will be completed by linear mixed model considering randomization group and baseline values as independent parameters (fixed effects). Other categorical parameters will be analysed as described previously. Longitudinal analyses concerning repeated measures (for example ASES, KOFBeQ, WOMAC, EVA pain, fears and beliefs, assessed at baseline, after intervention and 3 months after intervention) will be studied using random-effect models (linear or generalized linear), to take into account patient as random-effect (slope and intercept), nestled in centre random-effect, while studying the fixed effects group, time and group *interaction x time*.

According to clinical relevance, sub-group analyses depending gender will be proposed after the study of sub-group x randomization group interaction in regression models (for repeated data or not). Secondarily, a per-protocol analysis will be considered. Finally, a sensitivity analysis will be performed and the nature of missing data will be studied (missing at random or not). According to this, the most appropriate approach to the imputation of missing data will be proposed (maximum bias (e.g. last observation carried forward vs. baseline observation carried forward) or estimation proposed by Verbeke and Molenberghs for repeated data). More precisely, concerning the IPAQ score, when participant will mention a number of days, hours or minutes for an activity without checking « yes » or « no » to intense, moderate or walking categories practice, a « yes » response will be imputed to this question. If participant no mentions to the practice of an activity or the number of days, hours or minutes, a « no » response will be imputed to this question.

Discussion

In the context of an aging population, OA is a high-prevalence disease, whose prevalence will increase in the future [41]. In addition, OA is not limited to joint pain and stiffness, and the health care strategy needs to be standardized and personalized with optimized adherence to treatment [42]. This research question is important because OA lacks a cure, and few solutions to the management of knee OA are offered to patients. Treatments will be based on modifiable risk factors, such as pain, function, obesity, comorbidities, intrinsic barriers to PA practice, and sedentary time [43, 44]. The knee OA population appears to be more affected by these risk factors [45, 46], and the most severely affected patients are the less active ones [12]. The key challenge for OA treatment consists in increasing PA level to decrease the risk factors [47].

This quasi-randomized trial will be the first study to compare the effect of a self-management exercise program associated with spa therapy versus spa therapy alone. The non-invasive, adapted, tailored and original character of the intervention is a novel approach for knee OA management.

STT can improve pain and functional capacity of people with knee OA [14]. PA practice must be the key element in managing knee OA symptoms, according to recommendations [8]. However, many obstacles to exercise have been described [48], such as fears and beliefs about pain, treatment and PA [49]. Hence, changing the PA behaviour of people with knee OA is difficult [50]. Education and self-management are based on the bio-psycho-social model, effective strategies for modifying fears and beliefs and increasing adherence to treatment [51].

This protocol has some limitations. The quasi-randomized method could be a limitation, but this method is the most appropriate to avoid contamination biases between groups [29]. When assessing the effectiveness of non-pharmacological treatments such as behavioral therapy the blinding of participants and care providers is frequently impossible [52–54]. Moreover, the success of the treatment often depends on the skill and experience of care providers [26, 55, 56].

The study could demonstrate that self-management exercise programs offer a complementary therapy to the spa therapy effect could reinforce in the medium term increasing PA level and could ameliorate fears and beliefs, self-efficacy and anxiety/depression.

The findings of this trial could offer new perspectives in establishing best clinical practice guidelines for this patient population.

Ethics and dissemination

The study protocol was approved by the medical ethics committee of South-East France (Sud-Est 6), no. 2015/CE38, and was registered at ClinicalTrials.gov (NCT 02598804 on November 5, 2015. The trial will be conducted in compliance with both Good Clinical Practices and the Declaration of Helsinki. In accordance with French law, the ethics committee of South-East France (Sud-Est 6) and the study protocol, all patients will provide written consent to participate in the study after being informed in detail about the study procedures. The written consent will be reported in the medical file. The design and conduct of this trial will adhere to the requirements of the Standard Protocol Items: Recommendations for Interventional Trials (SPIRIT). The results will be reported in accordance with the CONSORT Statement for nonpharmacological trials. The results from this study will be disseminated through peer-reviewed publications and presentations at international scientific meetings.

Abbreviations

ACR: American College of Rheumatology; ASES: arthritis self-efficacy; BMI: Body Mass Index; D: Days; HAD: Hospital Anxiety and Depression Scale; IPAQ: International Physical Activity Questionnaire short form score; ITT: Intention to treat; KOFBeQ: Knee OA Fears and Beliefs Questionnaire; M: month; OA: Osteoarthritis; OARSI: Osteoarthritis Research Society International; PA: Physical Activity; SPIRIT: Standard Protocol Items: Recommendations for Interventional Trials; STT: spa therapy treatment; WHO: World Health Organisation; WOMAC: Western Ontario and McMaster Universities Osteoarthritis Index

Acknowledgements

Nicolas Andant, Christine Levicky, Christine Flouzat: help in study management. Jean-Baptiste Lechauve, Elise Guilley and Anne Plan-Paquet: design the intervention. Patients and employees of Thermal SPA Center.

Funding

This work is financially supported by the "Innovatherm cluster" and "Clermont-Ferrand Communauté". The "Auvergne region" for the "Cluster network research grant" allowed us to recruit a PhD student to carry out this study. The protocol was peer reviewed by the funding committee, prior to funds being granted.

Authors' contributions

CG, EC: conceived the study, designed the study protocol and drafted the manuscript. CGA and BP: designed the statistical analysis. AG: Clinical Trial Registration. LB, CN: contributed to the writing of the protocol and read and approved the final protocol. All authors read and approved the final manuscript.

Ethics approval and consent to participate

The study protocol was approved by the medical ethics committee of South-East France (Sud-Est 6), no. 2015/CE38, and was registered at ClinicalTrials.gov (NCT 02598804 on November 5, 2015. The trial will be conducted in compliance with both Good Clinical Practices and the Declaration of Helsinki. In accordance with French law, the ethics committee of South-East France (Sud-Est 6) and the study protocol, all patients will provide written consent to participate in the study after being informed in detail about the study procedures. The written consent will be reported in the medical file.

Competing interests

The authors declare that they have no competing interests.

Author details

[1]Service de Médecine Physique et de Réadaptation, CHU de Clermont Ferrand, INRA, Université Clermont Auvergne, Clermont Ferrand, France. [2]Service de Santé Publique, CHU de Clermont Ferrand, PEPRADE, Université Clermont Auvergne, Clermont Ferrand, France. [3]Délégation Recherche Clinique et Innovation, CHU de Clermont Ferrand, Université Clermont Auvergne, Clermont Ferrand, France. [4]Délégation Recherche Clinique et Innovation, CHU de Clermont Ferrand, Clermont Ferrand, France. [5]Physical and Rehabilitation Medecine Department, University of Clermont Ferrand, Clermont Auvergne University, France, CHU Hôpital Nord, 61 Rue de Châteaugay - BP 30056, 63118 Clermont Ferrand, Cébazat, France.

References

1. Viton JM, Atlani L, Mesure S, Franceschi JP, Massion J, Delarque A, et al. Reorganization of equilibrium and movement control strategies in patients with knee arthritis. Scand J Rehabil Med. 1999;31(1):43–8.
2. Peat G, McCarney R, Croft P. Knee pain and osteoarthritis in older adults: a review of community burden and current use of primary health care. Ann Rheum Dis. 2001;60(2):91–7.
3. Felson DT, Zhang Y, Hannan MT, Naimark A, Weissman BN, Aliabadi P, et al. The incidence and natural history of knee osteoarthritis in the elderly. The Framingham osteoarthritis study. Arthritis Rheum. 1995;38(10):1500–5.
4. Bijlsma JW, Berenbaum F, Lafeber FP. Osteoarthritis: an update with relevance for clinical practice. Lancet. 2011;377(9783):2115–26.
5. Jordan KM, Arden NK, Doherty M, Bannwarth B, Bijlsma JWJ, Dieppe P, et al. EULAR recommendations 2003: an evidence based approach to the management of knee osteoarthritis: report of a task force of the standing Committee for International Clinical Studies Including Therapeutic Trials (ESCISIT). Ann Rheum Dis. 2003;62(12):1145–55.
6. Coudeyre E, Sanchez K, Rannou F, Poiraudeau S, Lefevre-Colau M-M. Impact of self-care programs for lower limb osteoarthritis and influence of patients' beliefs. Ann Phys Rehabil Med. 2010;53(6–7):434–50.
7. McAlindon TE, Bannuru RR, Sullivan MC, Arden NK, Berenbaum F, Bierma-Zeinstra SM, et al. OARSI guidelines for the non-surgical management of knee osteoarthritis. Osteoarthr Cartil. 2014;22(3):363–88.
8. Bruyère O, Cooper C, Pelletier J-P, Branco J, Luisa Brandi M, Guillemin F, et al. An algorithm recommendation for the management of knee osteoarthritis in Europe and internationally: a report from a task force of the European Society for Clinical and Economic Aspects of osteoporosis and osteoarthritis (ESCEO). Semin Arthritis Rheum. 2014;44(3):253–63.
9. Zacharias A, Green RA, Semciw AI, Kingsley MIC, Pizzari T. Efficacy of rehabilitation programs for improving muscle strength in people with hip or knee osteoarthritis: a systematic review with meta-analysis. Osteoarthr Cartil. 2014;22(11):1752–73.
10. Coleman S, Briffa NK, Carroll G, Inderjeeth C, Cook N, McQuade J. A randomised controlled trial of a self-management education program for osteoarthritis of the knee delivered by health care professionals. Arthritis Res Ther. 2012;14(1):R21.
11. Gay C, Chabaud A, Guilley E, Coudeyre E. Educating patients about the benefits of physical activity and exercise for their hip and knee osteoarthritis. Systematic literature review. Ann Phys Rehabil Med. 2016;59(3):174–83.
12. Rosemann T, Kuehlein T, Laux G, Szecsenyi J. Osteoarthritis of the knee and hip: a comparison of factors associated with physical activity. Clin Rheumatol. 2007;26(11):1811–7.
13. Forestier R, Desfour H, Tessier J-M, Françon A, Foote AM, Genty C, et al. Spa therapy in the treatment of knee osteoarthritis: a large randomised multicentre trial. Ann Rheum Dis. 2010;69(4):660–5.
14. Forestier R, Erol Forestier FB, Francon A. Spa therapy and knee osteoarthritis: a systematic review. Ann Phys Rehabil Med. 2016;59(3):216–26.
15. Tenti S, Cheleschi S, Galeazzi M, Fioravanti A. Spa therapy: can be a valid option for treating knee osteoarthritis? Int J Biometeorol. 2015;59(8):1133–43.
16. Fioravanti A, Iacoponi F, Bellisai B, Cantarini L, Galeazzi M. Short- and long-term effects of spa therapy in knee osteoarthritis. Am J Phys Med Rehabil. 2010;89(2):125–32.
17. Ciani O, Pascarelli NA, Giannitti C, Galeazzi M, Meregaglia M, Fattore G, et al. Mud-Bath therapy in addition to usual Care in Bilateral Knee Osteoarthritis: an economic evaluation alongside a randomized controlled trial. Arthritis Care Res. 2017;69(7):966–72.
18. Fioravanti A, Cantarini L, Guidelli GM, Galeazzi M. Mechanisms of action of spa therapies in rheumatic diseases: what scientific evidence is there? Rheumatol Int. 2011;31(1):1–8.
19. Pascarelli NA, Cheleschi S, Bacaro G, Guidelli GM, Galeazzi M, Fioravanti A. Effect of mud-Bath therapy on serum biomarkers in patients with knee osteoarthritis: results from a randomized controlled trial. Isr Med Assoc J IMAJ. 2016;18(3–4):232–7.
20. Giannitti C, De Palma A, Pascarelli NA, Cheleschi S, Giordano N, Galeazzi M, et al. Can balneotherapy modify microRNA expression levels in osteoarthritis? A comparative study in patients with knee osteoarthritis. Int J Biometeorol. 2017;61(12): pp 2153–2158.
21. Fioravanti A, Cantarini L, Bacarelli MR, de Lalla A, Ceccatelli L, Blardi P. Effects of spa therapy on serum leptin and adiponectin levels in patients with knee osteoarthritis. Rheumatol Int. 2011;31(7):879–82.
22. Bender T, Bálint G, Prohászka Z, Géher P, Tefner IK. Evidence-based hydro- and balneotherapy in Hungary--a systematic review and meta-analysis. Int J Biometeorol. 2014s;58(3):311–23.
23. Zijlstra TR, van de Laar MA, Bernelot Moens HJ, Taal E, Zakraoui L, Rasker JJ. Spa treatment for primary fibromyalgia syndrome: a combination of thalassotherapy, exercise and patient education improves symptoms and quality of life. Rheumatol Oxf Engl. 2005;44(4):539–46.
24. Lanhers C, Pereira B, Gay C, Hérisson C, Levyckyj C, Dupeyron A, et al. Evaluation of the efficacy of a short-course, personalized self-management and intensive spa therapy intervention as active prevention of musculoskeletal disorders of the upper extremities (Muska): a research protocol for a randomized controlled trial. BMC Musculoskelet Disord. 2016;17(1):497.
25. Chan A-W, Tetzlaff JM, Altman DG, Laupacis A, Gøtzsche PC, Krle A-Jerić K, et al. SPIRIT 2013 statement: defining standard protocol items for clinical trials. Rev Panam Salud Publica Pan Am J Public Health. 2015;38(6):506–14.
26. Boutron I, Moher D, Altman DG, Schulz KF, Ravaud P. CONSORT group. Extending the CONSORT statement to randomized trials of nonpharmacologic treatment: explanation and elaboration. Ann Intern Med. 2008;148(4):295–309.
27. Altman R, Asch E, Bloch D, Bole G, Borenstein D, Brandt K, et al. Development of criteria for the classification and reporting of osteoarthritis. Classification of osteoarthritis of the knee. Diagnostic and therapeutic criteria Committee of the American Rheumatism Association. Arthritis Rheum. 1986;29(8):1039–49.
28. Craig CL, Marshall AL, Sjöström M, Bauman AE, Booth ML, Ainsworth BE, et al. International physical activity questionnaire: 12-country reliability and validity. Med Sci Sports Exerc. 2003;35(8):1381–95.
29. Weingarten SR, Riedinger MS, Conner L, Lee TH, Hoffman I, Johnson B, et al. Practice guidelines and reminders to reduce duration of hospital stay for patients with chest pain. An interventional trial. Ann Intern Med. 1994;120(4):257–63.
30. Gremeaux V, Benaïm C, Poiraudeau S, Hérisson C, Dupeyron A, Coudeyre E. Evaluation of the benefits of low back pain patients' education workshops during spa therapy. Jt Bone Spine Rev Rhum. 2013;80(1):82–7.
31. Lee PH, Macfarlane DJ, Lam TH, Stewart SM. Validity of the international physical activity questionnaire short form (IPAQ-SF): a systematic review. Int J Behav Nutr Phys Act. 2011;8:115.
32. Lorig K, Chastain RL, Ung E, Shoor S, Holman HR. Development and evaluation of a scale to measure perceived self-efficacy in people with arthritis. Arthritis Rheum. 1989;32(1):37–44.
33. Bareyre L, Gay C, Coste N, Pereira B, Coudeyre E. French translation and cultural adaptation of the arthritis self-efficacy scale (ASES). Ann Phys Rehabil Med. 2016;59S:e64.
34. Benhamou M, Baron G, Dalichampt M, Boutron I, Alami S, Rannou F, et al. Development and validation of a questionnaire assessing fears and beliefs of patients with knee osteoarthritis: the knee osteoarthritis fears and beliefs questionnaire (KOFBeQ). PLoS One. 2013;8(1):e53886.
35. Bellamy N, Buchanan WW, Goldsmith CH, Campbell J, Stitt LW. Validation study of WOMAC: a health status instrument for measuring clinically important patient relevant outcomes to antirheumatic drug therapy in patients with osteoarthritis of the hip or knee. J Rheumatol. 1988;15(12):1833–40.
36. Faucher M, Poiraudeau S, Lefevre-Colau MM, Rannou F, Fermanian J, Revel M. Assessment of the test–retest reliability and construct validity of a modified WOMAC index in knee osteoarthritis. Joint Bone Spine. 2004;71(2):121–7.
37. Zigmond AS, Snaith RP. The hospital anxiety and depression scale. Acta Psychiatr Scand. 1983;67(6):361–70.
38. Bocéréan C, Dupret E. A validation study of the hospital anxiety and depression scale (HADS) in a large sample of French employees. BMC Psychiatry. 2014;14:354.
39. Gay C, Eschalier B, Levyckyj C, Bonnin A, Coudeyre E. Motivators for and barriers to physical activity in people with knee osteoarthritis: a qualitative study. Jt Bone Spine Rev Rhum. 2018;85(4):481–6.
40. Vickers AJ, Altman DG. Statistics notes: Analysing controlled trials with baseline and follow up measurements. BMJ. 2001;323(7321):1123–4.
41. Zhang Y, Jordan JM. Epidemiology of osteoarthritis. Clin Geriatr Med. 2010;26(3):355–69.

42. Litwic A, Edwards MH, Dennison EM, Cooper C. Epidemiology and burden of osteoarthritis. Br Med Bull. 2013;105:185–99.
43. Palazzo C, Nguyen C, Lefevre-Colau M-M, Rannou F, Poiraudeau S. Risk factors and burden of osteoarthritis. Ann Phys Rehabil Med. 2016;59(3):134-8.
44. Rannou F, Poiraudeau S. Non-pharmacological approaches for the treatment of osteoarthritis. Best Pract Res Clin Rheumatol. 2010;24(1):93–106.
45. Felson DT, Lawrence RC, Dieppe PA, Hirsch R, Helmick CG, Jordan JM, et al. Osteoarthritis: new insights. Part 1: the disease and its risk factors. Ann Intern Med. 2000;133(8):635–46.
46. Kadam UT, Jordan K, Croft PR. Clinical comorbidity in patients with osteoarthritis: a case-control study of general practice consulters in England and Wales. Ann Rheum Dis. 2004;63(4):408–14.
47. Fernandes L, Hagen KB, Bijlsma JWJ, Andreassen O, Christensen P, Conaghan PG, et al. EULAR recommendations for the non-pharmacological core management of hip and knee osteoarthritis. Ann Rheum Dis. 2013;72(7):1125–35.
48. Petursdottir U, Arnadottir SA, Halldorsdottir S. Facilitators and barriers to exercising among people with osteoarthritis: a phenomenological study. Phys Ther. 2010;90(7):1014–25.
49. MacKay C, Jaglal SB, Sale J, Badley EM, Davis AM. A qualitative study of the consequences of knee symptoms: 'It's like you're an athlete and you go to a couch potato'. BMJ Open. 2014;4(10):e006006.
50. Hendry M, Williams NH, Markland D, Wilkinson C, Maddison P. Why should we exercise when our knees hurt? A qualitative study of primary care patients with osteoarthritis of the knee. Fam Pract. 2006;23(5):558–67.
51. Bennell KL, Dobson F, Hinman RS. Exercise in osteoarthritis: moving from prescription to adherence. Best Pract Res Clin Rheumatol. 2014;28(1):93–117.
52. Black N. Why we need observational studies to evaluate the effectiveness of health care. BMJ. 1996;312(7040):1215–8.
53. Boutron I, Tubach F, Giraudeau B, Ravaud P. Methodological differences in clinical trials evaluating nonpharmacological and pharmacological treatments of hip and knee osteoarthritis. JAMA. 2003;290(8):1062–70.
54. Boutron I, Tubach F, Giraudeau B, Ravaud P. Blinding was judged more difficult to achieve and maintain in nonpharmacologic than pharmacologic trials. J Clin Epidemiol. 2004;57(6):543–50.
55. Boutron I, Moher D, Tugwell P, Giraudeau B, Poiraudeau S, Nizard R, et al. A checklist to evaluate a report of a nonpharmacological trial (CLEAR NPT) was developed using consensus. J Clin Epidemiol. 2005;58(12):1233–40.
56. Fourcade L, Boutron I, Moher D, Ronceray L, Baron G, Ravaud P. Development and evaluation of a pedagogical tool to improve understanding of a quality checklist: a randomised controlled trial. PLoS Clin Trials. 2007;2(5):e22.

Complementary and alternative medicine for treatment of atopic eczema in children under 14 years old

Chun-li Lu[1], Xue-han Liu[1], Trine Stub[2], Agnete E. Kristoffersen[2], Shi-bing Liang[3,1], Xiao Wang[1], Xue Bai[1], Arne Johan Norheim[2], Frauke Musial[2], Terje Araek[2], Vinjar Fonnebo[2] and Jian-ping Liu[1,2*]

Abstract

Background: Due to limitations of conventional medicine for atopic eczema (AE), complementary and alternative medicine (CAM) is widely used as an alternative, maintaining, or simultaneous treatment for AE. We aimed to evaluate the beneficial and harmful effects of CAM for children with AE under 14 years old.

Methods: We searched for randomized trials on CAM in 12 Chinese and English databases from their inception to May 2018. We included children (< 14 years) diagnosed with AE, who received CAM therapy alone or combined with conventional medicine. We extracted data, and used the Cochrane "Risk of bias" tool to assess methodological quality. Effect was presented as relative risk (RR) or mean difference (MD) with 95% confidence interval (CI) using RevMan 5.3.

Results: Twenty-four randomized controlled trials involving 2233 children with AE were included. Methodological quality was of unclear or high risk of bias in general. The trials tested 5 different types of CAM therapies, including probiotics, diet, biofilm, borage oil, and swimming. Compared to placebo, probiotics showed improved effect for the SCORAD index (MD 9.01, 95% CI 7.12–10.90; $n = 5$). For symptoms and signs such as itching, skin lesions, CAM combined with usual care was more effective for symptom relief ≥95% (RR 1.47, 95% CI 1.30–1.68; $n = 8$), and for ≥50% symptoms improvement (RR 1.34, 1.25–1.45; $n = 9$) compared to usual care. There was no statistic significant difference between CAM and usual care on ≥95% improvement or ≥ 50% improvement of symptoms. However, swimming, diet and biofilm showed improvement of clinical symptoms compared with usual care. At follow-up of 8 weeks to 3 years, CAM alone or combined with usual care showed lower relapse rate (RR 0.38, 0.28–0.51, $n = 2$; RR 0.31, 0.24–0.40, $n = 7$; respectively) compared to usual care. Twelve out of 24 trials reported no occurrence of severe adverse events.

(Continued on next page)

* Correspondence: Liujp@bucm.edu.cn; Jianping.Liu@uit.no
[1]Centre for Evidence-Based Chinese Medicine, Beijing University of Chinese Medicine, Beijing 100029, China
[2]The National Research Center in Complementary and Alternative Medicine (NAFKAM), Department of Community Medicine, Faculty of Health Science, UiT, The Arctic University of Norway, 9037 Tromsø, Norway
Full list of author information is available at the end of the article

(Continued from previous page)

Conclusions: Low evidence demonstrates that some CAM modalities may improve symptoms of childhood AE and reduce relapse rate. Safety remains unclear due to insufficient reporting. Further well-designed randomized trials are needed to confirm the potential beneficial effect and to establish safety use.

Keywords: Complementary and alternative medicine, CAM, Atopic eczema, Children, Randomized controlled trials, Systematic review, Meta-analysis, Clinical evidence

Background

Eczema, as defined by the World Allergy Organization, encompasses both atopic and non-atopic conditions, and is commonly referred to as atopic eczema (AE) or atopic dermatitis (AD) [1]. AE is a chronically relapsing inflammatory skin disease, often found in children under the age of 14 years. It impairs people's quality of life [2] and the prevalence of AE is estimated to be 15–20% in children worldwide [3]. As one of the most common inflammatory skin diseases, AE has a prevalence exceeding 10% of children in some populations [4]. There is an increasing number of studies focusing on AE, such as clinical trials and systematic reviews [5].

AE can be caused by multiple and complex risk factors such as irritants, contact allergens, food, inhaled allergens, stress or infection [6]. The pathogenesis of eczema is a complex interplay of numerous elements including immune, genetic, infection and neuroendocrine factors and their interaction with the environment [2]. Moreover, the diagnosis of AE relies on the assessment of clinical features because there is no definitive/conclusive test to diagnose the condition. The clinical characteristics are itching, skin inflammation, a skin barrier abnormality, and susceptibility to skin infection [7]. Although not always recognized by health-care professionals as being a serious medical condition, AE can have a significant negative impact on quality of life for children and their parents and care takers [8]. Children with AE may suffer from lack of sleep, irritability, daytime tiredness, emotional stress, lowered self-esteem and psychological disturbance [9]. Moreover, many cases of AE clear or improve during childhood, whereas others persist into adulthood [8]. Thus, there is a substantial need for cure and symptom relief as early as possible. However, despite the common claims for curative interventions, there is currently no known cure for AE in allopathic medicine [9].

Therefore, there is an increasing number of trials studying complementary and alternative medicine (CAM) to treat children with AE. There is a growing interest in CAM as a primary, maintenance, or simultaneous treatment for AE [10]. These studies suggest that CAM may improve health related quality of life of children. In fact, many people rely on these treatments as their primary approach to relieve their illness or at least to improve the duration and quality of symptomatic relief [10]. The most frequently used CAM modalities are herbal medicine, vitamins, Ayurveda, naturopathy, homeopathy, traditional healing [6], and probiotics [11]. However, current literature, published protocols and systematic reviews have not involved or included all kinds of CAM modalities. Moreover, we were not able to find any systematic review focusing on CAM with AE in children (< 14 years). Therefore, we conducted a comprehensive literature search involving CAM for AE in children (< 14 years) to add to current available evidence in order to inform clinical practice further.

Methods

The protocol of the review was registered in PROSPERO (CRD42017071267) on 7th of August 2017 (Available from: http://www.crd.york.ac.uk/PROSPERO/). The content of the review followed the Preferred Reporting Items for Systematic Reviews and Meta-Analyses (PRISMA) [12].

Eligibility criteria

Type of studies

Randomized controlled trials (RCTs) were included in the systematic review.

Type of participants

Children (< 14 years) diagnosed with AE by defined criteria or validated instruments or tools based on either the UK Working Party, Hanifin and Rajka (Hanifin 1980) or explicitly stated provider based diagnostic criteria [13] were included. Trials without clear diagnostic criteria but with detailed description of clinical features to be diagnosed as AE were also eligible for inclusion in a subgroup analysis. The limited age of < 14 years was set because of the maximum age as younger adolescents defined by WHO. No gender or ethnicity limitations were set.

Type of intervention

CAM modalities used alone or in combination with conventional therapies for children (< 14 years) were included. CAM terms have different concepts: If a non-mainstream practice is used together with conventional medicine, it's considered as "complementary". If a non-mainstream practice is used in place of conventional medicine, it is considered "alternative" [14]. Since a separate review on

Traditional Chinese Medicine (TCM) for AE will be prepared due to clinical heterogeneity, we included the following CAM modalities: dietary advices/restriction, dietary supplements, probiotics, prebiotics, psychological interventions, oral evening primrose oil or borage oil, specific allergen immunotherapy, aromatherapy, bath therapy, bioresonance, chromotherapy, homeopathy, hypnotherapy and relaxation techniques in addition to some other CAM modalities that are known to be used for treating AE [10].

However, CAM is different from the new drug to estimate effectiveness, but to focus on its efficacy. So, it is sometimes difficult to to split CAM modalities up into parts to investigate effectiveness and safety of CAM modalities separately, except the placebo-controlled randomized trials [15]. Therefore, from the component level, CAM in the intervention group can be classified as above specific modalities such as probiotics, bath therapy, and so on. And from the system level, CAM can be considered as an integrated "whole system" of intervention.

Type of outcomes

Primary outcomes included clinical disease severity measured by one or more of the following instruments: (1) global improvement in objective AE outcomes as measured by scoring atopic dermatitis index (SCORAD); eczema area and severity index score (EASI); Nottingham eczema severity score (NESS) reported by a clinician; global improvement in subjective AE outcomes as measured by patient oriented eczema measure (POEM); itching visual analogue score (VAS); dermatology life quality index (DLQI) reported by participants or their parents. (2) Frequency of treatment discontinuation due to adverse effects. Secondary outcomes included (1) relapse rate; (2) proportion of participants with ≥50% symptoms and signs improvement in a given outcome as assessed by a clinician; (3) type, frequency, and severity of adverse events.

Search strategy

We conducted systematic literature searches in 12 electronic databases, including 4 Chinese databases (China National Knowledge Infrastructure (CNKI), Wanfang Database, Chinese Scientific Journal Database (VIP), and SinoMed), and 8 English databases: PubMed, EMBASE via OVID, AMED (Allied and Complementary Medicine Database) via OVID, CINAHL (Cumulative Index to Nursing and Allied Health Literature) via EBSCO, PsychoInfo, CAM-QUEST, the GREAT database (the Global Resource for Eczema Trials: www.Greatdatabase.org.uk), and the Cochrane Library from their inception date until May 2018. The filters were English and Chinese language (Additional file 1). We also searched in the grey literature such as conference proceedings and dissertations in CNKI and Wanfang for unpublished trials and trial protocols. References of all included studies were hand searched for additional eligible studies.

Study selection and data extraction

Two authors (CL Lu and SB Liang) independently examined the full text to identify the eligible trials. Four authors in pair (CL Lu, XH Liu, X Wang, and X Bai) extracted data independently from the included studies according to a predesigned data sheet. Any disagreement was resolved by discussion with a third author (JP Liu). Following items were extracted: publication year, study type, funding, inclusion/exclusion criteria, diagnostic criteria, study methodology, demographic characteristics of the participants, details of intervention and controls, outcome measures methods, adverse events, and results.

Quality assessment

Two authors (CL Lu and XH Liu) used the risk of bias tool [16] to assess the methodological quality of the included trials. Seven items including random sequence generation, allocation concealment, blinding of participants and personnel, blinding of outcome assessment, incomplete outcome data, selective reporting and other bias such as pharmaceutical funding, were used to be judged as "low risk", "high risk", or "unclear risk". Any disagreements were resolved by discussion with a third author (JP Liu).

Data analysis

We used RevMan 5.3 software for data analysis. For continuous data, we used mean difference (MD) with 95% confidence intervals (CI), and for dichotomous data we used relative risk (RR) with 95% CI. We performed meta-analyses for trials if the study design, participants, interventions, control, and outcome measures were similar. Bulk data were synthesized quantitatively by descriptive counting. Other data not suitable for pooling analysis were synthesized qualitatively.

We used I-square (I^2) to test the statistical heterogeneity as recommended by the Cochrane Handbook for Systematic Reviews of Interventions (Higgins 2011). We considered I^2 statistic value greater than 50% as a suggestion that there might be substantial heterogeneity [16]. We used random effects model for data pooling with significant heterogeneity ($I^2 \geq 50\%$), otherwise a fixed effect model was applied. If the data were available, we did subgroup analyses for subcategories of CAM modalities.

A sensitivity analysis was conducted to explore the influence of the type of randomized trials (parallel or cross-over randomized) and the quality of trials (high or low) if the data were available. A funnel plot was generated to explore possible publication bias if more than ten trials were included in a meta-analysis.

Results

Description of studies

Our searches identified 4807 citations. After reviewing the titles and abstracts, 3034 citations were excluded due to duplication, reviews, and non RCTs. After scanning the full texts to identify the participants who were over 14 years, we excluded 1648 publications. Among 125 publications that were eligible, three publications were excluded [17–19] due to inappropriate allocation of participants. We excluded 98 trials for the intervention of TCM in separate systematic review. Finally, there were 24 trials [20–43] with a total of 2233 children (< 14 years) included in this review (Fig. 1). Eleven trials [33–43] were published in English, and 13 trials [20–32] were in Chinese. We did not identify any unpublished study. Twenty-two trials [20–41] had two arms with parallel groups, one trial [42] had three arms, and one trial [43] had five arms.

Study characteristics

The details of the 24 trials are presented in Table 1. The sample size of these studies ranged from 15 to 298 participants. The age ranged from 2 months to 13 years. We defined the conventional therapy with more than two modalities (e.g. topical and systemic anti-allergic, and immunomodulatory therapy) as "usual care" in 24 trials [9]. Every trial had more than two modalities of conventional therapy except placebo. Therefore, from the component level, CAM modalities of 22 trials [21, 23–43] in the intervention group could be classified as

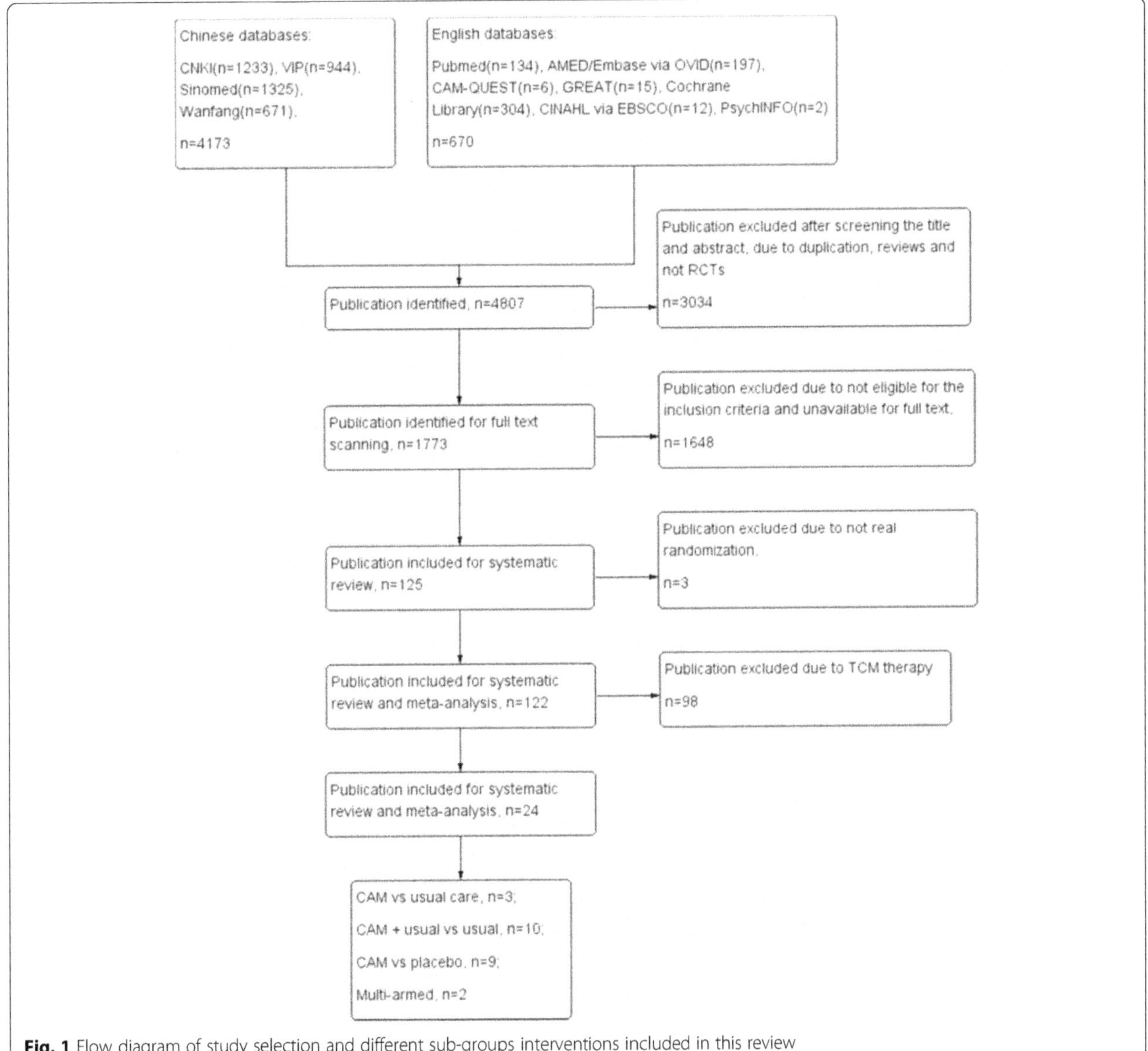

Fig. 1 Flow diagram of study selection and different sub-groups interventions included in this review

Table 1 Characteristics of included randomized clinical trials on CAM therapies for childhood atopic eczema

Study ID	Sample size	Age	Sex M/F	Comparisons	Outcome	Follow up
CAM vs usual care, 3 studies						
Liu CH 2009 [20]	T:150 C:148	T:1-6 m, 80 cases; 6-12 m, 50 cases; 1-2 y, 20 cases C:1-6 m, 83 cases; 6-12 m, 44 cases; 1-2 y, 21 cases	T:88/62 C:86/44	Swimming therapy + Baibu (*Stemona japonica*) lotion (bath) + Tuina vs Cyproheptadine (oral) + Boric lotion (external application with cold lotion)/Hydrocortisone butyrate cream (external use)/ Zinc oxide cream (external use) (7-15d)	Improvement of symptoms and signs and signs; IgG; Relapse (T:26/150, 3 m; 37/150, 6 m C:80/148, 3 m; 96/148, 6 m)	3 m, 6 m
Liu WQ 2016 [21]	T:60 C:60	T:(4.5 ± 3.8) y C:(5.3 ± 4.5) y	T:37/23 C:33/27	Fasting and rotation diet vs Pevisone paste (external use) (3 m)	Improvement of symptoms and signs; IgG; Relapse (T:4/60 C:11/60)	3 m
Wu YQ 2014 [22]	T:74 C:74	T:(6.35 ± 1.36) m C:(5.98 ± 1.23) m	T:41/33 C:31/43	Velvetfeeling lotion (external application) + Moisturizing cream (external use) + Saline water (dipping) vs Boric lotion (external application) + Vitamin E (external use) + Saline water (dipping) (7d)	Improvement of symptoms and signs; CGI-EI	NR
CAM + usual care vs usual care, 10 studies						
Chen DX 2015 [23]	T:20 C:20	T:(3.82 ± 0.7) m C:(2.35 ± 1.3) m	NR	Bifid triple viable capsules (oral) + Hydrocortisone butyrate cream (external use) vs Hydrocortisone butyrate cream (external use) (180d)	Improvement of symptoms and signs	6 m
Chen YL 2015 [24]	T:58 C:58	T:(11 ± 5) m C:(12 ± 5) m	T:31/27 C:30/28	Probiotics (oral) + Chlorphenamine maleate tablets (oral) + Vitamin B6 + Fluocinonide cream (external use) + Calcium supplement (oral) vs Chlorphenamine maleate tablets (oral) + Vitamin B6 + Fluocinonide Cream (external use) + Calcium supplement (oral) (28d)	Improvement of symptoms and signs; CGI-EI; Interleukin; Interferon; Relapse (T:9/58 C:29/58)	NR
Guo YH 2015 [25]	T:90 C:90	T:2 m-3 y C:2 m-3 y	total: 98/82	Tetralogy of viable bifidobacterium tablets (oral) + Usual care (Calamine lotion/ Zinc oxide cream/ Loratadine syrup/ Mometasone furoate cream) vs Usual care (Calamine lotion/Zinc oxide cream/Loratadine syrup/Mometasone furoate cream) (30d)	Improvement of symptoms and signs; IL-4, IL-10, IFN-γ, IgE, Th1/Th2; Relapse (T:24/90 C:62/90)	3 m
Jiang YX 2013 [26]	T:65 C:60	T:2 y C:2 y	total: 72/53	Velvetfeeling lotion (external application) + Usual care (eg. Chlorphenamine maleate tablets) vs Usual care (eg. Chlorphenamine maleate tablets) + Boric lotion (external application) (28d)	Improvement of symptoms and signs	NR
Li DY 2012 [27]	T:32 C:30	T:(7.15 ± 2.06) m C:(6.89 ± 2.54) m	T:17/15 C:16/14	Bifid triple viable capsules (oral) + Zinc oxide cream (external use) + Boric lotion (external application) vs Zinc oxide cream (external use) + Boric lotion (external application) (14d drugs for external use/28d Oral bifid-triple viable capsule)	Improvement of symptoms and signs; Relapse (T:6/32 C:20/30)	NR
Mao HX 2013 [28]	T:50 C:50	T:2 m-5 y C:2 m-5 y	T:24/26 C:28/22	Probiotics (oral) + Antihistamines (oral) + Calcium supplement (oral) + Skincare cream (external use) vs Antihistamines (oral) + Calcium supplement (oral) + Skincare cream (external use)	Improvement of symptoms and signs; Relapse (T:2/50 C:12/50)	NR
Wei MX 2010 [29]	T:38 C:36	T:(6.78 ± 2.62) m C:(7.14 ± 2.10) m	T:22/16 C:19/17	Viable *Bacillus coagulans* tablets (oral) + Boric lotion (wash-out) + Zinc oxide cream (external use) vs Boric lotion (wash-out) + Zinc oxide cream (external use) (28d)	Improvement of symptoms and signs; Relapse (T:7/38 C:24/36)	6 m
Ye CQ 2017 [30]	T:48 C:48	T:(6.9 ± 2.4) m C:(6.8 ± 2.6) m	T:27/21 C:28/20	Condensation living bacterium bacillus (oral) + Boric lotion (wash-out) + Zinc oxide cream (external use) vs Boric lotion (wash-out) + Zinc oxide cream (external use) (28d)	Improvement of symptoms and signs; Relapse (T:6/48 C:28/48)	6 m

Table 1 Characteristics of included randomized clinical trials on CAM therapies for childhood atopic eczema *(Continued)*

Study ID	Sample size	Age	Sex M/F	Comparisons	Outcome	Follow up
Zhang MH 2013 [31]	T:35 C:35	T:(5 ± 3) m C:(6 ± 3) m	T:27/8 C:25/10	Bifico lriple viable (oral) + Boric lotion (wash-out) + Zinc oxide cream (external use) + Cetirizine hydrochloride drops (oral) vs Boric lotion (wash-out) + Zinc oxide cream (external use) + Cetirizine hydrochloride drops (oral) (30d)	IFN-γ; Interleukin; T-Cell; Relapse (T:6/35 C:16/58)	6 m
Zhang XN 2013 [32]	T:36 C:34	total:(7.06 ± 3.48) y	total:32/38	Velvetfeeling lotion (external application) + Butyl flufenamate ointment (external use) + Antihistamine (oral) vs Saline water (external application) + Butyl flufenamate ointment (external use) + Antihistamine (oral) (14d)	Improvement of symptoms and signs; CGI-EI	NR
CAM vs placebo, 9 studies						
D. Sistek 2006 [33]	T:30 C:29	T:3.8 y C:4.4 y	T:15/14 C:17/13	Probiotics (oral) vs Placebo (oral) (12w)	Improvement of symptoms and signs	4w
Hyeon-Jong Yang 2014 [34]	T:50 C:50	T:(58.7 ± 29.9) m C:(47.4 ± 28.1) m	T:29/21 C:24/26	Probiotics (oral) vs Placebo (oral) (6w)	Improvement of symptoms and signs; Fecal cell counts; IL-4; TNF-α	NR
Reza 2011 [35]	T:19 C:21	T:(28.68 ± 40.86) m C:(22.76 ± 34.03) m	T:11/8 C:14/7	Synbiotic (oral) vs Placebo (oral) (8w)	Improvement of symptoms and signs Mononuclear cells	NR
S Weston 2017 [36]	T:28 C:28	T:(11.5 ± 4.2) m C:(10.3 ± 3.2) m	T:14/14 C:16/12	VRI-003 PCC freeze dried powder probiotics (oral) vs Placebo (oral) (8w)	Improvement of symptoms and signs; total IgE levels; radioallergosorbent test	8w
Sergei V. Gerasimov 2010 [37]	T:48 C:48	T:(25.6 ± 7.7) m C:(24.1 ± 6.3) m	T:28/15 after withdrew C:28/19 after withdrew	Probiotics (oral) vs Placebo (oral) (8w)	Improvement of symptoms and signs; Quality of life; Total IgE; Eosinophil count	NR
Shoko 2007 [38]	T:16 C:16	T:4.44 y C:5.56 y	T:9/7 C:12/4	Borage oil (undershirts coated with oil) vs Placebo (non-coated undershirts) (2w)	Improvement of symptoms and signs; Changes of transepidermal water loss	NR
Wu YJ 2017 [39]	T:33 C:33	T:(1.5 ± 1.1) m C:(7.14 ± 2.10) m	T:25/8 C:19/14	Probiotics (Lactobacillus rhamnosus) (oral) vs Placebo (oral) (8w)	Improvement of symptoms and signs; Quality of Life (Infant Dermatitis Quality of Life Questionnaires and Dermatitis Family Impact Questionnaires);	NR
Yavuz 2012 [40]	T:20 C:20	total:1-13 y	total: 23/17	Probiotic bacteria (oral) vs Placebo (oral) (8w)	Improvement of symptoms and signs; cytokine analyse/IgE/Eosinophil cationic protein	10w
Youngshin 2012 [41]	T:58 C:60	T:(4.6 ± 3.3) y C:(5.1 ± 3.3) y	T:34/24 C:35/25	Probiotics (*L. plantarum* CJLP133) (oral) vs Placebo (oral) (12w)	Improvement of symptoms and signs; total IgE levels/specific IgE	2w
Multi-armed trials, 2 studies						
Pasi E. Kankaanpa 2002 [42]	T1:5 T2:5 C1:5	T1:(4.5 ± 2) m T2:(5.7 ± 2.2) m C1:(5.6 ± 2.1) m	T1:2/3 T2:3/2 C1:2/3	Probiotics (Lactobacillus GG) (oral) vs Probiotics (Bifidobacterium Bb12) (oral) vs placebo (oral) (①4.4 ± 1.7 m ②7.3 ± 0.7 m ③5.7 ± 2.0 m)	Fatty acid analysis	≥36 m follow until panticipants at the age of 3 years

Table 1 Characteristics of included randomized clinical trials on CAM therapies for childhood atopic eczema *(Continued)*

Study ID	Sample size	Age	Sex M/F	Comparisons	Outcome	Follow up
C. Gore 2011 [43]	T1:45 T2:45 C1:47 C2:22 C3:49	T1:19 [16-23] w T2:20.5 [17-23] w C1:20 [16-23] w C2:15 [13-19.5] w C3:19 [15-21.5] w	T1:28/17 T2:24/21 C1:28/19 C2:16/6 C3:25/24	Probiotics (Lactobacillus paracasei) (oral) vs Probiotics (Bifidobacterium) (oral) vs Placebo (oral) vs Exclusively breastfed vs Standard formula-fed (12w)	Improvement of symptoms and signs; Quality of life; Stool; GI-Permeability; Specific serum IgE; Urinary EPX	NR

T treatment group, *C* control group, *y* year, *m* month, *d* day, *w* week, *NR* not report

probiotics, diet, biofilm, and borage oil (undershirts coated with oil) (more in Table 2). Moreover, two trials [20, 22] had their main modality referring to swimming and biofilm while accompanying other modalities. So, we considered for three different comparisons in the two-arm trials from system level: CAM versus usual care [20–22], CAM plus usual care versus usual care [23–32], and CAM (probiotics) versus placebo [33–41]. For the two trials with three or more arms [42, 43], probiotics was compared with other formula of probiotics, placebo, usual care, or observation with no intervention.

Risk of bias of included trials

The trials only reporting that the study was "randomized" were defined as "unclear" risk of bias, while the trials describing a specific method of randomized sequences generation, allocation concealment, and blinding as "low" risk of bias. Other bias accessed the funding scheme. Trials supported by non-commercial funding were defined as "low" risk of bias, trials funded by pharmaceutical companies were classified as "high" risk of bias, no information as "unclear" risk of bias. Eight trials [22, 24, 29, 31, 33, 34, 37, 41] reported the random allocation by random number table or computer generated-list. Only five trials [33, 34, 37, 38, 40, 41] reported the allocation concealment by using computer-generated random numbers or randomization software, which can conceal the allocation automatically. Ten trials [33, 34, 36–43] reported double blinding. Eight trials [33–37, 39, 41, 43] reported the drop out in both intervention group and control group, and only four trials [33, 39, 41, 43] used intention-to-treat (ITT) to analyze for all outcome [33, 39, 41] and primary outcome [43], and the other four trials [34–37] analyzed data by per-protocol (PP) and reported the data of available participants. Besides, two trials [39, 41] analyzed by both ITT and PP. We considered one trial [34] as high risk of incomplete data for loss to follow up without ITT analysis because of 13 withdrawals in intervention group and 16 withdrawals in control group among the 100 participants in the trial. Four trials [33, 39, 41, 43] were considered as low risk of bias and the others as unclear. Eleven trials [21, 25, 29, 33, 35–37, 40–43] mentioned non-commercial funding. Three trials [33, 39, 43] reported that probiotic manufacturers produced the drugs used. We considered these three trials [33, 39, 43] as high risk of bias for conflict of interest (Fig. 2). Sample size calculation was reported in five trials [33, 35, 37, 41, 43] according to disease prevalence [33], symptoms and signs reduction in treatment group by 30% [34, 41], 34% [37] and in placebo group by 15% [34], 17% [37], 10% [41], and symptoms and signs scale of SCORAD for a standard deviation increments of 7.65 [43]. The other trials did not report any detail of sample size calculation. We considered the other bias of power calculation as unclear.

Effects of interventions

The 24 trials tested five CAM interventions: combination of probiotics (72%, $n = 18$) [23–25, 27–43], biofilm (12%, $n = 3$) [22, 26, 32], diet (8%, $n = 2$) [21, 43], swimming (4%, $n = 1$) [20], and undershirts coated with borage oil (4%, $n = 1$) [38] (Table 2).

Twenty-two two-arms trials [20–41] involved CAM modalities, including probiotics, swimming, diet, borage oil, and biofilm. Three different comparisons were summarized: CAM versus placebo, CAM versus usual care, and CAM plus usual care versus usual care alone. In addition to this, two multi-arm trials [42, 43] used different probiotic formulae in different groups to compare with placebo, observation with no intervention or diet. Table 3 showed the detailed results of the effect estimation.

Global improvement (symptoms and signs improvement ≥95%, such as itching, skin lesions, swelling, and papula)

Global improvement was better for CAM (probiotics) compared with placebo in five trials [35, 37, 39–41] including 323 participants (MD 9.01, 7.12–10.90; $I^2 = 37\%$). Three trials [20–22] with 566 participants showed no difference between CAM alone (swimming, diet, or biofilm) and usual care (RR 1.43, 0.82–2.48; $I^2 = 91\%$). Eight trials [23–27, 29, 30, 32] involving 763 participants showed better effect from CAM plus usual care (RR 1.47, 1.30–1.68; $I^2 = 11\%$) compared with usual care.

Apart from statistical heterogeneity, the interventions in three trials [20–22] were totally different, including swimming [20], diet [21], biofilm [22], and one trial [20] investigated swimming in combination with Chinese herbal medicine lotion and tuina (Chinese massage for children). We conducted a qualitative description on these three trials. One trial [20] tested swimming, Chinese herbal medicine lotion and tuina compared to usual care. The intervention group showed more symptom reduction than the control group, however, not at a significant level. One trial [21] compared fasting and rotation diet with Pevisone paste, and reported beneficial effects of diet on symptom improvement. Another trial [22] showed statistically significant effects of Velvetfeeling Lotion (biofilm) on symptom improvement when compared with usual care.

Relapse rate

CAM showed lower relapse rate compared to usual care (RR 0.38, 0.28–0.51; $n = 2$, 418 participants) [20, 21]. CAM plus usual care showed lower relapse rate compared to usual care (RR 0.31, 0.24–0.40; $n = 7$, 698 participants) [24, 25, 27–31]. Nine trials [33–41] with 622 participants compared probiotics with placebo, but did not report the relapse, and rest of two trials [22, 23] with 188 participants did not report the relapse either.

Table 2 Description and trials numbers of different CAM therapies

Therapy	Administration	Dosage	Frequency	Detail	Formula	Trials numbers	%(/22)
Probiotics	oral	depend on formula	2–3/d	Oral probiotics preparation	The probiotic formulation was a mixture of Lactobacillus acidophilus DDS-1 and Bifidobacterium lactis UABLA-12 with fructo-oligosaccharide in a rice maltodextrin powder.	18	72%
Diet	oral	None	3 m	To avoid to severe and moderate intolerant food, and take mild intolerant food per 6 days	None	2	8%
Biofilm	external application	appropriate amount	2–3/d	The main ingredient is chitosan with low polymer (OPC). External application help form a protective film on the skin.	Velvetfeeling	3	12%
Borage oil	undershirts coated withoil	498 mg of GLA per 100 g of cotton)	2 w	Borage oil was chemically bonded to the cotton fibers of the undershirts that made of pure organic cotton. The borage oil was gradually released from the cotton fibers and absorbed into the skin. The undershirts were designed such that the sutures did not touch and stimulate the skin directly.	Borage oil	1	4%
Swimming	Passively by nurse; Autonomous swimming	None	1/d	Trained nurse helps baby to stretch the limb as passively swimming or baby swim autonomously.	None	1	4%

m month, *d* day, *w* week

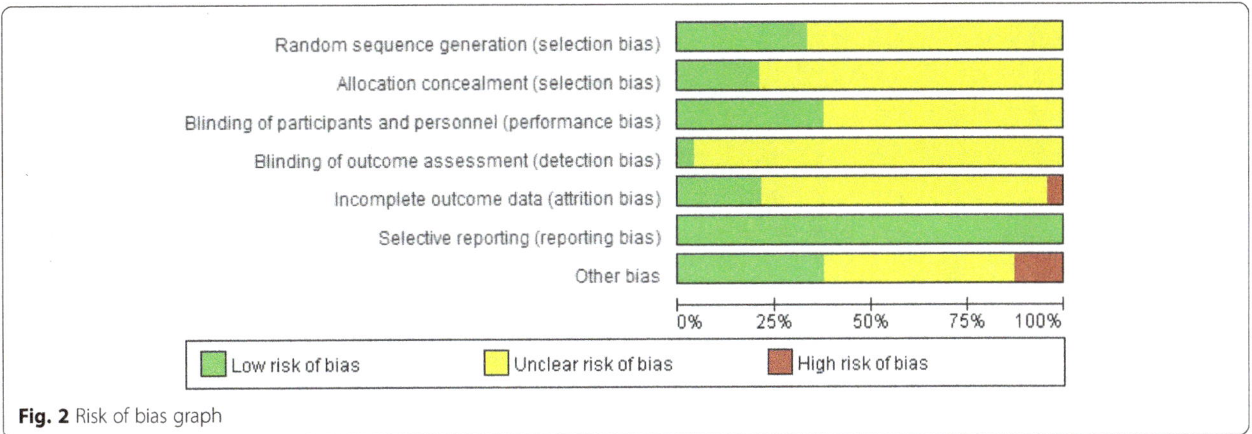

Fig. 2 Risk of bias graph

≥50% improvement of symptoms and signs (such as itching, skin lesions, swelling, and papula)

Three trials [20–22] with 566 participants showed no difference between CAM alone (RR 1.20, 0.90–1.60; I^2 = 92%) and usual care. Nine trials [23–27, 29–32] with 833 participants showed improvement from CAM (RR 1.34, 1.25–1.45; I^2 = 35%) in addition to usual care compared with usual care alone. Nine trials [33–41] with 622 participants compared probiotics with placebo reported as continuous data resulting in unavailable outcome for ≥50% improvement of symptoms.

Apart from statistical heterogeneity, three trials had clinical heterogeneity for different CAM modalities [20–22]. One trial [20] showed that swimming had more children with improvement of symptoms and signs of ≥50% than the control group, but not at a significant level. One trial [21] showed significant effects of diet. Another trial [22] reported the positive effect of biofilm compared with usual care.

Adverse events

Only 12 trials (50%) [20, 22, 24, 25, 29, 30, 32, 35–37, 39, 43] reported the outcome of adverse events. Among these, four trials [27, 29, 35, 36] reported no occurrence of adverse events in either groups, and one trial [39] reported no relation between adverse events and the tested product without any details about adverse events, while seven trials [20, 22, 24, 30, 32, 37, 43] reported that children (< 14 years) with adverse events gradually adapted to treatments without extra treatment or that the adverse events was not related to the medications under investigation (Table 4). No severe adverse event such as death or hospitalization were reported. The reported adverse events included crying, irritability, and worsening of skin lesions (reddening) (Table 4).

Additional analysis

Since the fact that each comparison did not include more than 10 trials, we were not able to conduct meaningful funnel plot analysis in order to identify the publication bias. Due to the same quality and the type of randomized trials, we could not conduct sensitivity analysis in this aspect. Besides, significant heterogeneity in two outcomes with two comparisons was more than 50% (I^2 ≥ 50%), so we conducted a subgroup meta-analysis or a meaningful sensitivity analysis.

The global improvement (≥95% improvement) and ≥ 50% improvement of symptoms and signs in probiotics compared with usual care in three trials with 566 participants [20–22] showed I^2 as 91 and 92%. The interventions were very heterogeneous in the trials including swimming [20], diet [21], and biofilm [22]. One trial [20] investigated not only swimming but also Chinese herbal medicine lotion and tuina. We conducted a sensitivity analysis, which showed improvement from CAM both for global improvement ≥95% improvement) (RR 1.77, 1.36–2.31; n = 2) and ≥ 50% improvement of symptoms and signs (RR 1.33, 1.16–1.52; n = 2).

Discussion

Summary of findings

This review identified 24 RCTs involving 2233 children (< 14 years) with AE. The findings suggest that some of the CAM modalities used alone or in combination with usual care may relieve the symptoms and signs of AE with ≥95% and ≥ 50% improvement, such as itchiness, skin lesions, swelling, and papula, in addition to reduce relapse of eczema. Moreover, some CAM modalities (such as probiotics) showed significant effect compared with placebo. The evaluated modalities appear to be safe and tolerated for lower relapse rate in CAM modality group. In spite of unclear pathogenesis of AE, CAM modalities may reduce symptoms and signs, and relapse of AE compared to conventional therapies.

The majority of trials had unclear risk of bias in many domains such as allocation concealment, blinding, missing data, and sample size calculation. Due to the unclear risk of bias of included trials, we could not come to firm

Table 3 Summary of findings of CAM for childhood atopic eczema in randomized controlled trials

Study ID	Sample size	Main intervention	Estimate effect [95% CI]	Outcome	*P*
CAM vs usual care					
Liu CH 2009 [20]	T:150 C:148	Swimming therapy	RR 1.01 [0.92, 1.11] RR 1.01 [0.96, 1.07] RR 0.38 [0.28, 0.52]	Clinical effectiveness rate 50% Improvement of symptoms and signs Relapse rate	$P = 0.8318$ $P = 0.5671$ $P < 0.00001$
Liu WQ 2016 [21]	T:60 C:60	Fasting and Rotation diet	RR 1.57 [1.04, 2.38] RR 1.32 [1.09, 1.60] RR 0.36 [0.12, 1.08]	Clinical effectiveness 50% Improvement of symptoms and signs; Relapse rate	$P = 0.0323$ $P = 0.0049$ $P = 0.0681$
Wu YQ 2014 [22]	T:74 C:74	Velvetfeeling lotion (external application)	RR 1.92 [1.36, 2.72] RR 1.33 [1.10, 1.61]	Clinical effectiveness rate 50% Improvement of symptoms and signs	$P = 0.0002$ $P = 0.0031$
CAM + usual care vs usual care					
Chen DX 2015 [23]	T:20 C:20	Bifid Triple Viable capsules (oral)	RR 1.63 [0.87, 3.04] RR 1.73 [1.15, 2.60]	Clinical effectiveness rate 50% Improvement of symptoms and signs	$P = 0.1283$ $P = 0.0088$
Chen YL 2015 [24]	T:58 C:58	Probiotics (oral)	RR 1.21 [0.87, 1.68] RR 1.19 [0.99, 1.42] RR 0.31 [0.16, 0.60]	Clinical effectiveness rate 50% Improvement of symptoms and signs Relapse rate	$P = 0.2659$ $P = 0.0624$ $P = 0.0004$
Guo YH 2015 [25]	T:90 C:90	Tetralogy of viable bifidobacterium tablets (oral)	RR 1.37 [1.01, 1.85] RR 1.27 [1.04, 1.55] RR 0.39 [0.27, 0.56]	Clinical effectiveness rate 50% Improvement of symptoms and signs Relapse rate	$P = 0.0400$ $P = 0.0172$ $P < 0.00001$
Jiang YX 2013 [26]	T:65 C:60	Velvetfeeling lotion (external application)	RR 1.85 [0.90, 3.79] RR 1.91 [1.46, 2.50]	Clinical effectiveness rate 50% Improvement of symptoms and signs	$P = 0.0947$ $P < 0.00001$
Li DY 2012 [27]	T:32 C:30	Bifid Triple Viable capsules (oral)	RR 1.36 [1.03, 1.79] RR 1.32 [1.06, 1.65] RR 0.28 [0.13, 0.60]	Clinical effectiveness rate 50% Improvement of symptoms and signs; Relapse rate	$P = 0.0295$ P = 0.0151 $P = 0.0011$
Mao HX 2013 [28]	T:50 C:50	Probiotics (oral)	RR 0.17 [0.04, 0.71]	Relapse rate	$P = 0.0151$
Wei MX 2010 [29]	T:38 C:36	Viable Bacillus Coagulans tablets (oral)	RR 1.33 [1.05, 1.68] RR 1.30 [1.07, 1.58] RR 0.28 [0.14, 0.56]	Clinical effectiveness rate 50% Improvement of symptoms and signs; Relapse rate	$P = 0.0189$ $P = 0.0089$ $P = 0.0004$
Ye CQ 2017 [30]	T:48 C:48	Condensation living bacterium bacillus (oral)	RR 1.57 [1.21, 2.02] RR 1.31 [1.10, 1.55] RR 0.21 [0.10, 0.47]	Clinical effectiveness rate 50% Improvement of symptoms and signs; Relapse rate	$P = 0.0005$ $P = 0.0019$ $P = 0.0001$
Zhang MH 2013 [31]	T:35 C:35	Bifico Lriple Viable (oral)	RR 1.15 [0.91, 1.46] RR 0.38 [0.17, 0.85]	50% Improvement of symptoms and signs; Relapse rate	$P = 0.2371$ $P = 0.0180$
Zhang XN 2013 [32]	T:36 C:34	Velvetfeeling lotion (external application)	RR 6.61 [1.62, 26.96] RR 1.25 [1.00, 1.56]	Clinical effectiveness rate 50% Improvement of symptoms and signs	$P = 0.0084$ $P = 0.0542$
CAM vs placebo					
Reza 2011 [35]	T:19 C:21	Synbiotic (oral)	MD 19.10 [7.60, 30.60]	Clinical effectiveness scores	$P = 0.0017$
Sergei V. Gerasimov 2010 [37]	T:48 C:48	Probiotics (oral)	MD 6.40 [2.71, 10.09]	Clinical effectiveness scores	$P = 0.0009$
Wu YJ 2017 [39]	T:33 C:33	Probiotics (Lactobacillus rhamnosus) (oral)	MD 10.85 [3.82, 17.88]	Clinical effectiveness scores	$P = 0.0035$
Yavuz 2012 [40]	T:20 C:20	Probiotic (oral)	MD 10.20 [7.45, 12.95]	Clinical effectiveness scores	$P < 0.00001$
Youngshin 2012 [41]	T:58 C:60	Probiotics (L. plantarum CJLP133) (oral)	MD 7.30 [2.63, 11.97]	Clinical effectiveness scores	$P = 0.0029$

***CAM* complementary and alternative medicine, *RR* risk ratio, *MD* mean difference, *CI* confidence interval**

Table 4 Adverse events of CAM for childhood atopic eczema in randomized controlled trials

Study ID	Total sample num	Sample num in intervention group	Sample num in control group	Adverse events cases	Intervention group	Control group	Treatment for adverse event
C. Gore 2011 [43]	208	137	71	T: 42/137 C: NR	green loose stools; increased vomiting; feed-refusal; colic	NR	24/137 (17.5%) participants stopped the study formula.
Chen YL 2015 [24]	116	58	58	T: 1/58 C: 2/58	1 for dizzy.	1 for dizzy; 1 for drowsy.	NR
Liu CH 2009 [20]	298	150	148	T: 0/150 C: 57/148	None	21 for facial flushing; 18 for dry skin; 8 for partial facial skin thinning; 10 for facial skin with mild pigmentation; Unclear for other hormonal dermatitis symptoms.	NR
Sergei V. Gerasimov 2010 [37]	96	48	48	T: 26/48 C: 24/48	11 for upper respiratory tract infections; 4 for lower respiratory tract infections; 7 for herpetic stomatitis; 3 for diarrhea; 6 for constipation; 5 for abdominal colic; 2 for burn and croup with severe adverse events.	10 for upper respiratory tract infections; 5 for lower respiratory tract infections; 5 for herpetic stomatitis; 2 for diarrhea; 6 for constipation; 4 for abdominal colic; 3for head injury, food poisoning with severe adverse events.	None was related to the medications under investigation.
Wu YQ 2014 [22]	148	74	74	T: 2/74 C: 5/74	2 for crying and mildly red skin lesions on the 2nd day.	5 for crying, irritability, and red skin lesions.	Without any treatment, to ease soon and symptoms disappearance.
Ye CQ 2017 [30]	96	48	48	T:3/48 C:14/48	1 for diarrhea; 2 for constipation.	6 for diarrhea; 8 for constipation.	NR
Zhang XN 2013 [32]	70	36	34	T: 1/36 C: 2/34	1 for mild skin irritation after using Velvetfeeling Lotion	2 forskin lesions reddening after using Butyl Flufenamate Ointment.	Without any treatment, to ease soon and symptoms disappearance.

***T* treatment group, *C* control group, *NR* not report**

conclusions from the evidence of the included trials in this review.

Comparison with previous studies

By searching the Cochrane Library with "AE", "AD", and "CAM", there are 19 Cochrane reviews and 11 other reviews published, and after scanning, 9 reviews [13, 44–51] with CAM related to children (< 14 years) for treating or preventing. These reviews or protocols included both children and adults, and even pregnant women to prevent, cure and explore the pathogenesis of AE. We found only one protocol [44] similar to our review, but was withdrawn as the author gave up the title "Complementary and alternative medicine treatments for AE". In addition, the previous studies did not exclude the allergic diseases (such as asthma, and intestinal diseases) to focus on AE. Our review included children (< 14 years) suffering only from AE. Moreover, most reviews investigated the specific treatment like probiotics, based on pathological mechanisms but ignoring the complex and unclear pathogenesis of AE. The findings of our review are based on the symptom relief of AE and we included more comprehensive trials involving CAM for children (< 14 years).

Strengths and limitations

Although great effort was made to retrieve all trials, we still cannot confirm that we were able to cover all the evidence due to non identified unpublished data. Besides, selecting and extracting data may also lead to some bias. We included only children under the age of 14 as this is the maximum age as younger adolescents defined by WHO, which may exclude some studies due to unavailable data for their participants over the age of 14 years. In addition, due to the various treatment for AE with an integrated "whole system" of care approach, we considered the control group with usual care as the system effect. The intervention group with CAM for a specific modality as the component efficacy, which cannot be used to document or disprove the effectiveness of a "whole system" treatment approach [15]. Additionally, in terms of the statistical heterogeneity and the variability in the CAM modalities, we were not able to conduct a subgroup meta-analysis, meaningful sensitivity analysis and funnel plot analysis. These factors limit the conclusiveness and robustness of this systematic review.

Implications for research

In fact of the limitations of this review, future trials should be designed as multi-center, double-blind placebo controlled trials with sufficient power, and reported according to the CONSORT (Consolidated Standards for Reporting Trials) Statement [52]. In addition, trials should record the relapse with sufficient length of follow-up. Besides, it is important to provide the definite safe treatments to the patients. Thus, adverse events in each group should be reported respectively so that we could retrospect the reason of different modalities and be easy to estimate the safety of CAM modalities.

Conclusion

Based on evidence from this systematic review we found some promising effect of CAM modalities on reducing symptoms and signs, and relapse of AE. However, it is still premature to recommend the therapy in clinical practice due to the limited number of trials and general low methodological quality of the included trials. Further rigorously double-blind, placebo-controlled trials are warranted to confirm efficacy of the CAM modalities for AE.

Abbreviations

< 14 years: Under 14 years old; AD: Atopic dermatitis; AE: Atopic eczema; CAM: Complementary and alternative medicine; CHM: Chinese herbal medicine; CI: Confidence interval; CNKI: China National Knowledge Infrastructure; DLQI: Dermatology life quality index; EASI: Eczema area and severity index score; I^2: I-square; ITT: Intention-to-treat; MD: Mean difference; NESS: Nottingham eczema severity score; POEM: Patient oriented eczema measure; PP: Per-protocol; RCTs: Randomized clinical trials; RR: Relative risk; SCORAD: Scoring atopic dermatitis index; SMD: Standardized mean difference; VAS: Itching visual analogue score; VIP: Chinese Scientific Journal Database

Acknowledgements

Much appreciation goes to Xun Li and Li-qiong Wang for their advice about data analysis.

Funding

This work was supported by the Capacity Building in Evidence-based Chinese Medicine and Internationalization Project by Beijing University of Chinese Medicine (No. 1000061020008).

Authors' contributions

JPL and VF conceived the review. CLL drafted the protocol and searched literature to identify eligible trials, extracted and analyzed data, and drafted the manuscript. XHL extracted and analyzed data. SBL did searches to identify eligible trials and revised on the tables in the drafted manuscript. XW and XB extracted the data. TS, AEK, AJN, FM, TA, VF, and JPL revised and commented on the drafted protocol and manuscript. All authors approved the final manuscript.

Competing interests

The author JPL is the associate editor of the journal, but all authors declare that they have no competing interests.

Author details

[1]Centre for Evidence-Based Chinese Medicine, Beijing University of Chinese Medicine, Beijing 100029, China. [2]The National Research Center in Complementary and Alternative Medicine (NAFKAM), Department of Community Medicine, Faculty of Health Science, UiT, The Arctic University of Norway, 9037 Tromsø, Norway. [3]School of Basic Medicine, Shanxi University of Chinese Medicine, Taiyuan 030000, China.

References

1. Helen N, Alan M, Williams HC. Mapping randomized controlled trials of treatments for eczema-The GREAT database (The Global Resource of Eczema Trials: a collection of key data on randomized controlled trials of treatments for eczema from 2000 to 2010). BMC Dermatol. 2011;11(1):10.
2. Manjra AI, Du PP, Weiss R, et al. Childhood atopic eczema consensus document. S Afr Med J. 2005;2:435.
3. Nutten S. Atopic dermatitis: global epidemiology and risk factors. Ann Nutr Metab. 2015;66:8–16.
4. Shaw TE, Currie GP, Koudelka CW, et al. Eczema prevalence in the United States: data from the 2003 national survey of children's health. J Investig Dermatol. 2011;131(1):67–73.
5. Genuneit J, Seibold AM, Apfelbacher CJ, et al. Overview of systematic reviews in allergy epidemiology. Allergy. 2017;72:849–56.
6. Silverberg JI, Lee-Wong M, Silverberg NB. Complementary and alternative medicines and childhood eczema: a US population-based study. Dermatitis. 2014;25(5):246–54.
7. McAleer MA, Flohr C, Irvine AD. Management of difficult and severe eczema in childhood. BMJ. 2012;345:e4770.
8. NICE. Atopic eczema in under 12s: diagnosis and management. 2016.
9. Leung TN, Hon KL. Eczema therapeutics in children: what do the clinical trials say? Hong Kong Med J. 2015;21(3):251.
10. Jadotte YT, Santer M, Vakirlis E, et al. Complementary and alternative medicine treatments for atopic eczema (Protocol). Cochrane Database Syst Rev. 2014; https://doi.org/10.1002/14651858.CD010938.pub2.
11. Fuchs-Tarlovsky V, Marquez-Barba MF, Sriram K. Probiotics in dermatologic practice. Nutrition. 2016;32:289–95.
12. Moher D, Liberati A, Tetzlaff J, et al. Preferred reporting items for systematic reviews and meta-analyses: the PRISMA statement. PLoS Med. 2009;6(7): e1000097.
13. Gu S, Yang AWH, Xue CCL, et al. Chinese herbal medicine for atopic eczema. Cochrane Database Syst Rev. 2013; https://doi.org/10.1002/14651858.CD008642.pub2.
14. National Center for Complementary and Alternative Medicine (NCCAM). Complementary, alternative, or integrative health: what's in a name? http://nccam.nih.gov/health/whatiscam. Accessed 7 June 2017.
15. Fønnebø V, Grimsgaard S, Walach H, et al. Researching complementary and alternative treatments-the gatekeepers are not at home. BMC Med Res Methodol. 2007;7(1):7.
16. Higgins JPT, Green S. Cochrane handbook for systematic reviews of interventions version 5.1.0.2011. https://training.cochrane.org/handbook. Accessed 7 June 2017.
17. Wang LH, Zhou LB. Clinical observation on 648 cases of infantile allergic eczema treated by "heat-clarifying and dampness-removing mixture". J Shanghai Univ Tradit Chin Med. 2002;16(1):26–7.
18. Zhang YZ. Clinical observation on 1840 cases of infantile allergic eczema treated by qibaixiaoruan ointment. Chin Community Doct. 2013;15(1):211.
19. Cheng XM. Observation on the curative effect of Yinyanjing on infantile eczema. Pract Prev Med. 2005;12(3):680.
20. Liu CH, Fu R, Wan H, et al. The clinical study of swimming therapy, Tuina and Baibu Heji lotion to treat infantile eczema. Hubei J Tradit Chin Med. 2009;31(12):21–3.
21. Liu WQ, Luo DJ, Teng LZ, et al. Clinical effect observation of diet taboos combined with alternative therapy in childhood eczema with food intolerance. Med Innov China. 2016;13(10):133–6.
22. Wu YQ, Zhao WQ, Pan JS. Assessment of therapeutic effect of medical skin healing biological film combined with moisturizer on infantile acute eczema. China J Lepr Skin Dis. 2014;30(1):38–9.
23. Chen DX. Clinical effect of oral probiotics and butyric acid hydrocortisone cream in the treatment of infantile eczema. Chin Foreign Med Res. 2015;10:21–3.
24. Chen YL. The clinical efficacy and safety of probiotics to treat infantile eczema. China J Pharm Econ. 2015;11:37–8.
25. Guo YH, Mou YD, Wang HS, et al. Clinical effect of microecologics as an adjuvant therapy on infants' eczema. J Dalian Med Univ. 2015;6:571–573,588.
26. Jiang YX. Velvetfeeling lotion to treat 125 cases of infantile eczema. Health Horiz. 2013;6:583–4.
27. Li DY. The efficacy observation of bifid-triple viable capsule to treat infantile eczema. Public Med Forum Mag. 2012;29:3860–1.
28. Mao HX, Hu XH. Clinical observation of supplement the intestinal probiotics as an adjuvant therapy to treat 50 cases of infant eczema. J Aerospace Med. 2013;24(3):337–8.
29. Wei MX, Yan R, Luo HB, et al. The clinical observation of bacillus coagulans tablets to treat 36 cases of infantile eczema. Chin J Pract Pediatr. 2010; 25(12):943–5.
30. Ye CQ. Observation of curative effect on 48 cases of infant eczema treated by coagulative bacillus granulosa bioactive tablets. China Prac Med. 2017; 12(18):120–1.
31. Zhang MH. The study of adhibition and the influence of intestinal flora, immunologic function and cytokines of probiotics to treat infantile eczema. Chin J Clin Ration Drug Use. 2013;6(6):13–4.
32. Zhang XN. Observation of efficacy and safety of the velvetfeeling combined with butyl flufenamate ointment in the treatment of child eczema. China Pract Med. 2013;8(25):26–7.
33. Sistek D, Kelly R, Wickens K, et al. Is the effect of probiotics on atopic dermatitis confined to food sensitized children? J Brit Soc Allergy Clin Immunol. 2006;36(5):629–33.
34. Yang HJ, Min TK, Lee HW, et al. Efficacy of probiotic therapy on atopic dermatitis in children: a randomized, double-blind, placebo-controlled trial. Allergy, Asthma Immunol Res. 2014;6(3):208–15.
35. Reza F, Hamid A, Farahzad J, et al. Effect of a new synbiotic mixture on atopic dermatitis in children: a randomized-controlled trial. Iran J Pediatr. 2011;21(2):225–30.
36. Weston S, Halbert A, Richmond P, et al. Effects of probiotics on atopic dermatitis: a randomised controlled trial. Arch Dis Child. 2005;90(9):892–7.
37. Gerasimov SV, Vasjuta VV, Myhovych OO, Bondarchuk LI. Probiotic supplement reduces atopic dermatitis in preschool children: a randomized, double-blind, placebo-controlled, clinical trial. Am J Clin Dermatol. 2010; 11(5):351–61.
38. Kanehara S, Ohtani T, Uede K, et al. Clinical effects of undershirts coated with borage oil on children with atopic dermatitis: a double-blind, placebo-controlled clinical trial. J Dermatol. 2007;34(12):811–5.
39. Wu YJ, Wu WF, Hung C-W, et al. Evaluation of efficacy and safety of lactobacillus rhamnosus in children aged 4-48 months with atopic dermatitis: an 8-week, double-blind, randomized, placebo-controlled study. J Microbiol Immunol Infect. 2017;50:684–92.
40. Yeşilova Y, Ömer C, Akdeniz N, et al. Effect of probiotics on the treatment of children with atopic dermatitis. Ann Dermatol. 2012;24(2):189–93.
41. Han Y, Kim B, Ban J, et al. A randomized trial of lactobacillus plantarum CJLP133 for the treatment of atopic dermatitis. Pediatr Allergy Immunol. 2012;23(7):667–73.
42. Kankaanpää PE, Yang B, Kallio HP, et al. Influence of probiotic supplemented infant formula on composition of plasma lipids in atopic infants. J Nutr Biochem. 2002;13(6):364–9.
43. Gore C, Custovic A, Tannock GW, et al. Treatment and secondary prevention effects of the probiotics Lactobacillus paracasei or Bifidobacterium lactis on early infant eczema: randomized controlled trial with follow-up until age 3 years. Clin Exp Allergy. 2012;42(1):112–22.
44. Jadotte YT, Santer M, Vakirlis E, et al. Complementary and alternative medicine treatments for atopic eczema (Protocol). Cochrane Database Syst Rev. 2017; https://doi.org/10.1002/14651858.CD010938.pub2.
45. Küster D, Spuls PI, Flohr C, et al. Effects of systemic immunosuppressive therapies for moderate-to-severe eczema in children and adults (Protocol). Cochrane Database Syst Rev. 2015; https://doi.org/10.1002/14651858.CD011939.
46. Kramer MS, Kakuma R. Maternal dietary antigen avoidance during pregnancy or lactation, or both, for preventing or treating atopic disease in the child. Cochrane Database Syst Rev. 2012; https://doi.org/10.1002/14651858.CD000133.pub3.
47. Osborn DA, Sinn JKH. Probiotics in infants for prevention of allergic disease and food hypersensitivity. Cochrane Database Syst Rev. 2007; https://doi.org/10.1002/14651858.CD006475.pub2.
48. Kramer MS. Maternal antigen avoidance during lactation for preventing atopic eczema in infants. Cochrane Database Syst Rev. 1996; https://doi.org/10.1002/14651858.CD000131.
49. Bath-Hextall FJ, Delamere FM, Williams HC. Dietary exclusions for established atopic eczema. Cochrane Database Syst Rev. 2008; https://doi.org/10.1002/14651858.CD005203.pub2.
50. Bamford JTM, Ray S, Musekiwa A, et al. Oral evening primrose oil and borage oil for eczema. Cochrane Database Syst Rev. 2013; https://doi.org/10.1002/14651858.CD004416.pub2.
51. Ersser SJ, Cowdell F, Latter S, et al. Psychological and educational interventions for atopic eczema in children. Cochrane Database Syst Rev. 2014; https://doi.org/10.1002/14651858.CD004054.pub3.
52. CONSORT Statement 2001-Checklist: items to include when reporting arandomized trial. 2001. http://www.consort-statement.org. Accessed 7 June 2017.

Pharmacokinetics and tissue distribution of monotropein and deacetyl asperulosidic acid after oral administration of extracts from *Morinda officinalis* root in rats

Yi Shen[1,2], Qi Zhang[1,2], Yan-bin Wu[1], Yu-qiong He[3], Ting Han[3], Jian-hua Zhang[3], Liang Zhao[4], Hsien-yeh Hsu[5], Hong-tao Song[6], Bing Lin[6], Hai-liang Xin[3*], Yun-peng Qi[3*] and Qiao-yan Zhang[1,2,3*]

Abstract

Background: Iridoid glycosides (IGs), including monotropein (MON) and deacetyl asperulosidic acid (DA) as the main ingredients, are the major chemical components in *Morinda officinalis* How. (MO) root, possessing various pharmacological properties including anti-osteoporosis, anti-inflammation and anti-rheumatism activities.The aim of the present study was to further elucidate the pharmacological actions of MO by investigating the pharmacokinetics and tissue distribution of IGs in MO.

Methods: An ultra high performance liquid chromatography-tandem mass spectrometry (UHPLC-MS) method was developed and validated for simultaneous determination of MON and DA levels in plasma and various tissues of Wistar rats. MON, DA and acetaminophen (ACE) as the internal standard (IS) were extracted from rat plasma and tissue samples by direct deproteinization with methanol. The rats were administered orally at 1650 mg/kg MO and 25, 50 and 100 mg/kg MO iridoid glycosides (MOIGs) or intravenously at MOIG 25 mg/kg for pharmacokinetic study of MON and DA. In addition, 100 mg/kg MOIG was administered orally for tissue distribution study of MON and DA. Non-compartmental pharmacokinetic profiles were constructed. Tissue distributions were calculated according to the validated methods.

Results: Significant differences in the pharmacokinetic parameters were observed in male and female rats. The AUC_{0-t}, C_{max} and bioavailability of MON and DA in female rats were higher than those in male rats. MON and DA mainly distributed in the intestine and stomach after oral administration, and noteworthily high concentrations of MON and DA were detected in the rat hypothalamus.

Conclusion: The results of the present study may shed new lights on the biological behavior of MOIGs in vivo, help explain their pharmacological actions, and provide experimental clues for rational clinical use of these IGs extracted from the MO root.

Keywords: *Morinda officinalis*, Iridoid glycosides, Pharmacokinetics, Tissue distribution, UPLC-MS/MS

* Correspondence: hailiangxin@163.com; qiyunpeng@hotmail.com; zqy1965@163.com
[3]School of Pharmacy, Second Military Medical University, No. 325 Guohe Road, Yangpu District, Shanghai 200433, People's Republic of China
[1]School of Pharmacy, Fujian University of Traditional Chinese Medicine, No. 1 Qiuyang Road, Shangjie Town, Minhou County, Fuzhou 350122, People's Republic of China
Full list of author information is available at the end of the article

Background

The root of *Morinda officinalis* How (MO), also named as "Bajitian" in traditional Chinese medicine [1], has long been used as a tonic or nutrient supplement to prevent and treat multiple diseases including osteoporosis, depression, rheumatoid arthritis, impotence and Alzheimer disease in China, South Korea, Japan and Southeast Asia [2–6]. These pharmacological properties are believed to be mainly attributed to oligosaccharides, polysaccharides, iridoid glucosides, antharaquinines and volatile oil as the main chemical constituents in the MO root [7–9]. Monotropein (MON) and deacetyl asperulosidic acid (DA), the two major MO iridoid glycosides (MOIGs), accounts for more than 2% in the root of MO. Previous investigations showed that MON possessed anti-nociceptive, anti-inflammatory and anti-osteoporotic activities [3, 8, 10–12]. For example, MON could protect against chondrocyte apoptosis and catabolism induced by Interleukin 1β (IL-1β), and improve inflammatory medium of RAW 264.7 macrophages and dextran sulfate sodium (DSS)-induced colitis via the NF-κB pathway [11, 12]. In our previous work on chemical compounds of the MO root [13], we extracted MOIGs from the MO root by using an optimal technical method and found that content of MON and DA was greater than 60%, suggesting potential therapeutic applications of MOIGs in the treatment of inflammatory and bone diseases such as osteoarthritis, rheumatoid arthritis and inflammatory bone loss.

Some recent studies [14, 15] used a new LC-MS/MS method to determine the plasma concentrations of MON and DA for pharmacokinetic study in rats. However, there are scant studies to describe the absorption properties, tissue distribution and oral bioavailability of MON and DA in vivo, and there is little knowledge about the pharmacokinetics and target organs/tissues of these two compounds. The primary goal of this study is to clarify the in vivo distribution and action mechanism of the two compounds by analyzing the pharmacokinetics and tissue distribution. Firstly, MON and DA levels in the plasma and tissue of Wistar rats were simultaneously detected by using ultra high performance liquid chromatography-tandem mass spectrometry (UHPLC-MS), knowing that it is a simple, rapid and reliable assay. Secondly, the pharmacokinetic, tissue distribution and bioavailability of MON and DA were determined in both sexes of Wistar rats after oral and intravenous administration of MOIG and MO ethanol extracts, hoping that the results could provide useful information for the research and development of IGs extracted from the MO root.

Methods

Chemicals, reagents and animals

MON and DA were purchased from Shanghai Yuanye Biological Technology Co., Ltd. The purity was more than 98%, and their chemical structures were verified by NMR, MS and HPLC. ACE ($C_8H_9NO_2$, purity > 98%) purchased from the National Institute for the Control of Pharmaceutical and Biological Products (Beijing, China) was used as internal standard (IS). The chemical structures for MON, DA and ACE are shown in Fig. 1. HPLC grade acetonitrile, methanol and formic acid were obtained from Merck Company (Darmstadt, Germany). All the other reagents were of analytical-grade purity, and purchased from Sinopharm Chemical Reagent Co. Ltd. Deionized water was generated by a Milli-Q system from Millipore (Milford, MA, USA).

The MO root was collected from Zhangzhou of Fujian Province of China in October 2017, and identified by Professor Qiao-yan Zhang of the Department of Pharmacognosy, the Second Military Medical University School of Pharmacy (Shanghai, China). The voucher specimen (MO 20171008) was deposited in the herbarium of this Department. MOIG and MO ethanol extracts were prepared in our laboratory. Briefly, 2.0 kg powder MO root was extracted under permeation with 32.0 L solution of ethanol-water (70:30, *v*/v) for 20 h, and then filtrated. The combined filtrate was concentrated under reduced pressure to obtain the MO extract. Then, the MO extract was diluted with water to obtain 1.0 g crud drug /mL working solution. The MO extract (1.0 g crud drugs /mL) was adsorbed to XDA-1 macroporous adsorption resin, and eluted with water and 10% ethanol. The 10% ethanol elute collected was centrifuged to obtain MOIGs. The yield of MOIGs was 2.4%, and the content of MON and DA in MOIGs was 38.6% and 23.6%, respectively. The content of MON and DA in the MO extract was 1.27% and 0.65%, respectively.

Thirty-six male and 36 female healthy Wistar rats (200-220 g) aged 8 weeks were purchased from Sippur Will Kay Company and housed at the Experimental Animal Center of the Second Military Medical University (Certificate No. SCXK 2013–0016). The rats were acclimatized for a week on a 12 h light-dark cycle under a temperature of 24 ± 0.5 °C and humidity of $47.5 \pm 2.5\%$ before drug administration. All animals were fasted for 12 h before initiation of the experiment, with free access to water during the course of the experiment.

UHPLC-MS/MS equipment and method

An Agilent series 1290 UHPLC system (Agilent, USA) was used in this study. An Agilent ACE3C_{18}-PFP column (3.0×150 mm, 3.0 μm) was used as the stationary phase and the column temperature was maintained at 35 °C. The mobile phase (A) was methanol containing 0.1% formic acid and 5 mM ammonium formate, and mobile phase (B) was water containing 0.1% formic acid and 5 mM ammonium formate. The program of gradient elution was as follows: 6% B phase at 0–2 min, 6–60% B at 2–3 min, 60–60% B at 3–6 min with a flow rate of 0.4 mL/min. The auto-sampler was conditioned at 4 °C and the injection volume was 1 μL.

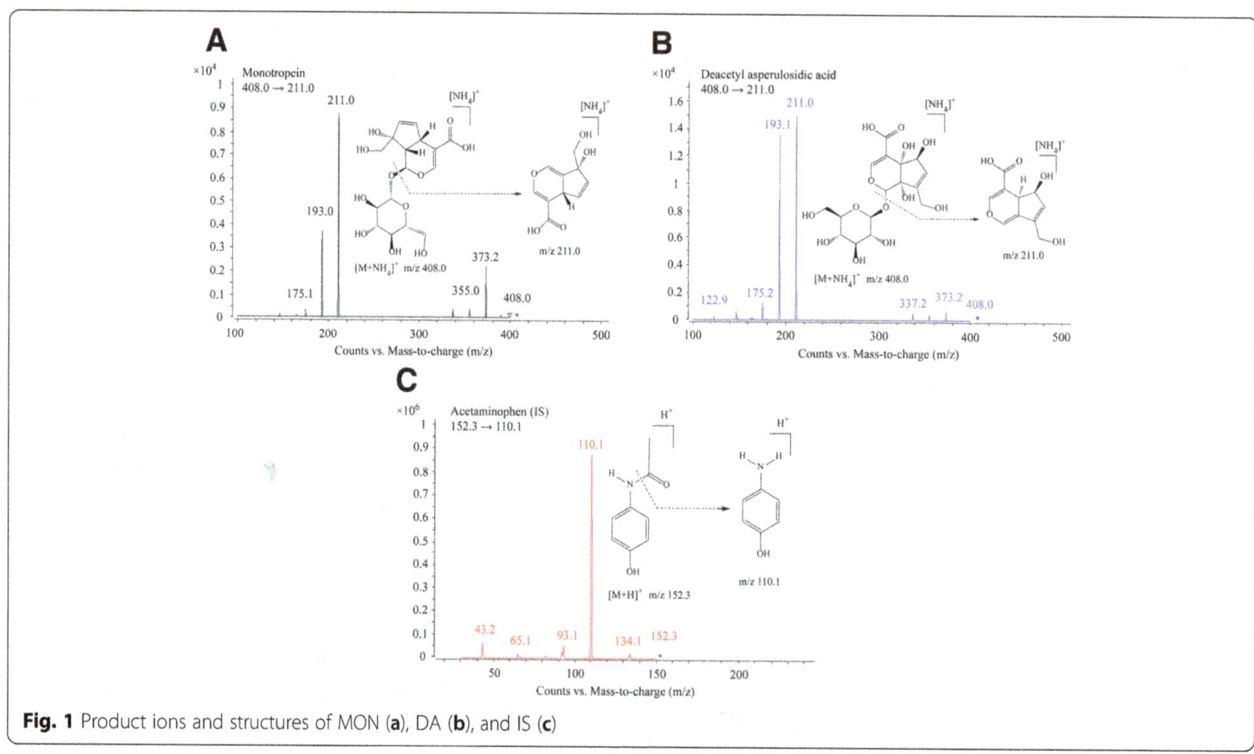

Fig. 1 Product ions and structures of MON (**a**), DA (**b**), and IS (**c**)

The MS detector was composed of an Agilent 6470 tandem mass spectrometer (Agilent technologies, USA) combined with an Agilent Jet Stream Technology (AJS) electrospray source interface (ESI). The mass spectrometric detection was optimized in the positive ion detection mode by multiple reaction monitoring (MRM). The main working parameters of the mass spectrometer are summarized as follows: capillary 4000 V, nebulizer 40 p.s.i., drying gas 10 L/min, gas temperature 350 °C and fragmentor 110 V for analyte and IS, sheath gas temperature 350 °C, sheath gas flow 11 L/min, collosion energy 10 eV for analyte and 20 eV for IS, fragmentation transitions were m/z 408 → 211 for analyte and m/z 152.3 → 110.1 for IS. Data acquisition and analysis were performed using Agilent Mass Hunter Work Station version B.07.00.

Preparation of calibration standards and quality control samples

Stock solutions (1.0 mg/mL) of MON and DA were prepared in water. The two standard stock solutions were mixed at a high concentration. The mixed solutions were diluted with methanol to obtain the final linearity concentrations of 2–5000 ng/mL for MON and DA, respectively. The IS stock solution (1.0 mg/mL) was also prepared in methanol and diluted to a final working concentration of 10 ng/mL. Quality control (QC) samples were also prepared similarly at the concentrations of 5, 1000 and 4000 ng/mL. All working solutions were stored at 4 °C before use.

Sample preparation

The plasma or tissue homogenate was thawed to room temperature 25 °C. 50 μL plasma or tissue homogenate with 100 μL IS solution (10 ng/mL) and 50 μL methanol were added into an 1.5 mL eppendorf tube, and mixed using vortex for 30 s. The mixture was centrifuged (11,000×g) at 4 °C for 10 min. Then, 100 μL of the supernatant was transferred into the sample bottle and 1 μL of the supernatant was injected into the UHPLC-MS/MS system for analysis.

Method validation

Linearity, sensitivity, specificity, accuracy, precision, recovery, matrix effect and stability of the method were validated under the guidelines set by the United States of Food and Drug Administration (FDA) [16] and European Medicines Agency (EMA) [17].

Specificity and sensitivity

The specificity of the method was evaluated by comparing the chromatograms of blank samples (plasma/tissue homogenate) with blank samples spiked with MON, DA, and real samples after oral administration of the MO extract. Endogenous interference was identified by analyzing six individual blank samples.

Linearity of calibration curves and LLOQ

Calibration curve samples were prepared in triplicate as previously described and analyzed. The linear curve was generated by plotting the peak area versus the theoretical concentrations of the calibration standard. The lower limit of quantification (LLOQ) was defined with a signal-to-noise ratio of 10:1 with precision and accuracy below 20%.

Accuracy and precision

Three QC samples on the same day ($n = 5$) were detected to evaluate the intra-day precision and accuracy. The inter-day precision and accuracy along with the standard calibration curve ($n = 15$) were determined at the same procedure for 3 consecutive days. The intra-day and inter-day precisions were evaluated by RSD, and the accuracy was evaluated by RE. The accuracy (RE%) and precision (RSD%) should be within ±15%.

Extraction recovery and matrix effect

The extraction recoveries of MON and DA were estimated by comparing the observed peak areas of the prepared QC samples with those of non-processed samples at six replicates. The matrix effect (ME) was evaluated by comparing the peak areas of the post-extracted blank plasma/tissue homogenate samples with those of analytes from neat standard samples at three different QC concentrations.

Stability

The stability was evaluated by the RE of analysis in plasma samples at three levels of QC during storage and handling conditions: three freeze/thaw cycles, 6 h stability at room temperature, auto-sampler for 24 h and storage at – 80 °C for 30 days. The accuracy (RE) should be below 15%.

Carry-over and dilution

The upper limit of quantification (ULOQ) was detected by the double-blank sample in order to evaluate carry-over. And the peak area of the double-blank sample should be less than 15% of LLOQ, while the IS should be lower than 5%.

Dilution integrity was evaluated by diluting the samples with the 10-fold concentration of ULOQ to 10, 20 and 40 μg/mL for the standard plasma by blank samples matrix (dilution has already covered the concentration range of actual samples). And five parallel processing samples of every dilution level were verified. Finally, the accuracy (RE) and precision (RSD) should be below 15%.

Pharmacokinetic study

All animal treatments in this study were approved by the Administrative Committee of Experimental Animal Care and Use of the Second Military Medical University in accordance with the National Institute of Health guidelines on the ethical use of animals. According to the results of the previous pharmacodynamic experimental study, 30 rats of both sexes were equally randomized to five groups and orally administered with 25, 50 and 100 mg/kg MOIG and 1650 mg/kg MO extract (the quantities of MON and DA are equal to those in 50 mg/kg MOIG) and administered intravenously with 25 mg/kg MOIG, all of which were dissolved in physiological saline for administration. 0.4 mL heparinized plasma samples were collected from the ophthalmic venous plexus with a sterile capillary tube at pre-administration (time = 0) and oral post-administration (time = 0.167, 0.333, 0.5, 0.75, 1, 1.5, 2, 2.5, 3, 5, 7, 10 and 24 h), and intravenous post-administration (time = 0.033, 0.083, 0.167, 0.333, 0.5, 0.75, 1, 2, 3, 5, 7, 10, 12 and 24 h), respectively. At the end of the experiment, all rats were sacrificed by cervical dislocation. The samples were timely centrifuged at 11,000×g at 4 °C for 10 min, and then 100 μL aliquot of supernatant plasma was transferred into another tube and stored at – 20 °C until analysis.

Tissue distribution study

Forty-two rats of both sexes were randomized to seven groups and orally administered with 100 mg/kg MOIG. The rats were sacrificed by cervical dislocation, and various kinds of tissue samples, including the small intestine, large intestine, stomach, spleen, ovary, uterus, heart, kidney, marrow, liver, lung, thymus, hypothalamus and testis were collected at 0.5, 1, 2, 4, 8, 12 and 24 h (6 rats at each time point) and washed with normal saline solution, blotted on filter paper, and then weighed. The tissue samples were homogenized with 10 times of the normal saline solution (*w*/*v*). Then the homogenates were centrifuged at 11,000×g at 4 °C for 10 min, then 1.0 mL aliquot of supernatant homogenates was transferred into another tube and stored at – 20 °C until analysis.

Data analysis

The pharmacokinetic parameters, including area under the plasma concentration-time curve ($AUC_{0\text{-}t}$), the area under the plasma concentration-time curve from zero to time infinity ($AUC_{0\text{-}\infty}$), mean residence time (MRT), half-life ($t_{1/2}$), peak time (T_{max}), peak concentration (C_{max}), body clearance (CL), and apparent volume of body distribution (V_d) were calculated using PK Solver 2.0 of Microsoft Excel under the non-compartmental model. The absolute oral bioavailability (F_{oral}) of MON and DA from MOIG and MO extracts after oral administration was calculated using the following formula:

$$F_{oral} = (AUC_{oral} \cdot Dose_{i.\,v.})/(AUC_{i.\,v.} \cdot Dose_{oral}) \times 100\,\%.$$

Results

Method development

Knowing that it is very important to efficiently eliminate protein and potential interferences in bio-samples before UPLC-MS/MS analysis, the effects of acetonitrile, acetonitrile-methanol (1:1, *v*/v) and methanol were evaluated on protein elimination. Finally, methanol was found to be superior to the other solutions and therefore used as the precipitation reagent. The matrix effect was between 85 and 110% for the bio-samples treated with methanol precipitation.

MRM is very powerful for pharmacokinetic study due to high sensitivity, selectivity and specificity. In this work, the predominant ions of MON ($[M+NH_4]^+$), DA ($[M+NH_4]^+$) and IS ($[M+H]^+$) in the Q1 spectrum were used as the precursor ion to obtain the product ion spectra. The most sensitive mass transitions were m/z 408 → 211 for MON and DA, and m/z 152.3 → 110.1 for IS (Fig. 1). The working parameters of MS/MS were optimized to maximize the analyte response. Under these conditions, the retention time was 3.7 min (MON), 4.2 min (DA), and 5.2 min (IS) in the real samples, and no endogenous interference was observed in the real samples.

Method validation

Specificity

The specificity of the method was determined by comparing the typical chromatograms with UPLC-MS of blank plasma/tissue homogenates, black samples spiked with MON, DA and IS. The actual plasma samples after oral administration of MOIGs are shown in Fig. 2. The retention time of MON, DA and IS was 3.7, 4.2 and 5.2 min, respectively. Due to the high specificity of MRM mode, no significant endogenous interference was observed.

Calibration curve and LLOQ

A linear regression was used to evaluated the linearity by the 1/concentration (1/X) weighting analysis in the given concentration ranges of 2–5000 ng/mL for MON and DA in plasma and tissue samples. The calibration curves, coefficients and linear ranges of MON and DA in plasma and each tissue are listed in Additional file 1: Table S1. The calibration curves for all matrices showed good linearity (R >0.99) over the concentration ranges. The LLOQs of MON and DA were both 2 ng/mL for plasma and tissue samples, with accuracy less than 20.0% and the precision within ±15%.

Precision and accuracy

As shown in Additional file 2: Table S2, the intra-day accuracy ranged from − 9.14% to 4.28% for MON and

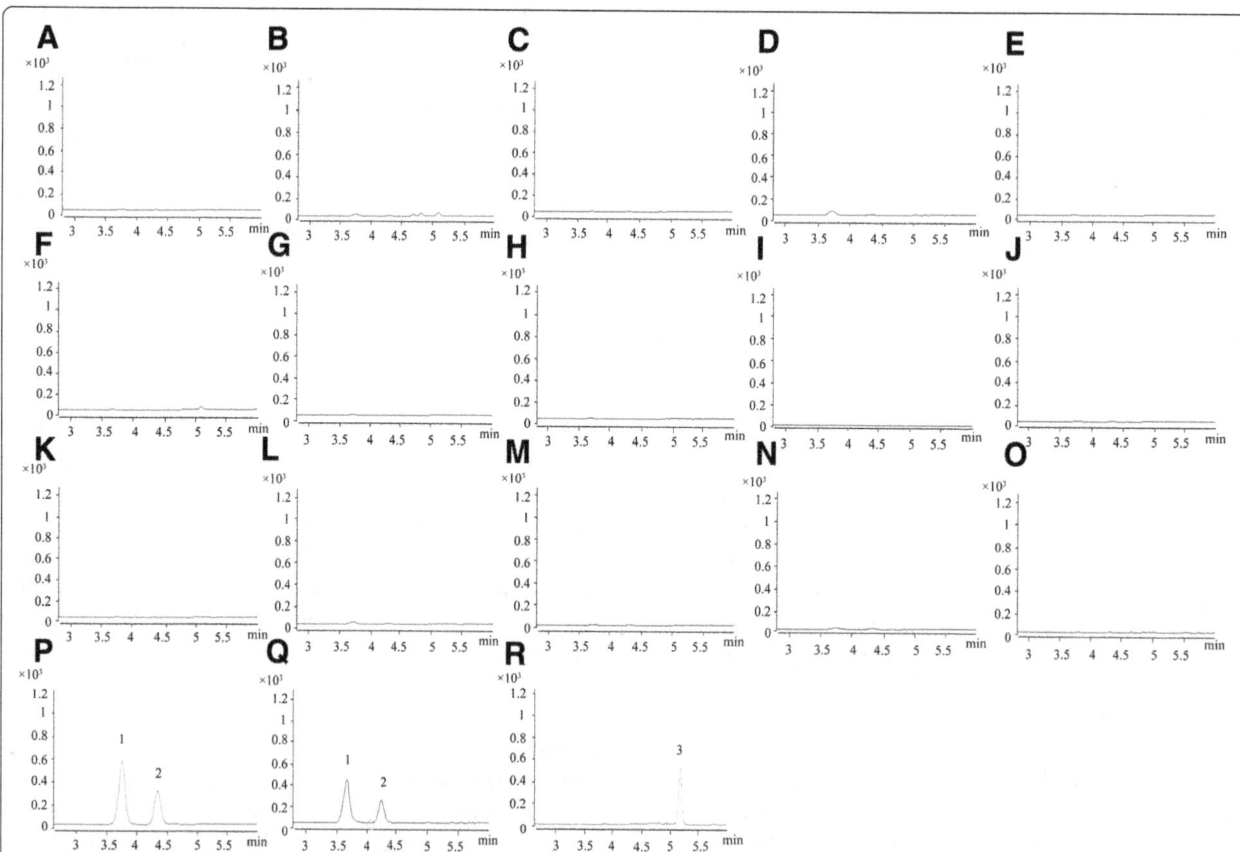

Fig. 2 Representative chromatograms of analytes from rat plasma and tissue. Blank plasma and tissue sample: (**a**) plasma, (**b**) liver, (**c**) stomach, (**d**) kidney, (**e**) uterus, (**f**) heart, (**g**) small intestine, (**h**) large intestine, (**i**) spleen, (**j**) lung, (**k**) thymus, (**l**) hypothalamus, (**m**) ovary, (**n**) testis, and (**o**) marrow. (**p**) actual sample plasma at 2 h after orally administration of 100 mg/kg MOIG, (**q**) hypothalamus sample obtained at 2 h after oral administration of 100 mg/kg MOIG, and (**r**) was IS (10 ng/mL). Peak 1 was MON and peak 2 was DA, and peak 3 was acetaminophen (IS)

from − 7.72% to 0.46% for DA, while the intra-day and inter-day precision were within 9.26% for MON, and 5.75% for DA, demonstrating that the assay precision and accuracy of the analysis were within the acceptable range.

Extraction recovery and matrix effect

As presented in Additional file 3: Table S3, the matrix effect of MON, DA and IS was 85.87–109.26%, illustrating no significant ion inhibition or enhancement in this method. The extraction recoveries ranged between 62.11–107.42% for MON, DA and IS, which were also acceptable.

Carry-over and dilution

No residue was detected in this infinity UHPLC-MS/MS method. The results of the integrity dilution experiment are shown in Additional file 4: Table S4, indicating that the precision was under 10% and the accuracy was within ±15%, which were also acceptable.

Stability

The results of the stability test are shown in Additional file 5: Table S5, indicating that MON and DA were stable in the plasma at indoor temperature for 6 h, at 4 °C in the auto-sampler for 24 h, after three free-thaw cycles, they were kept at − 80 °C for 30 days.

Pharmacokinetic study

The mean plasma concentration-time curves are displayed in Fig. 3. The primary pharmacokinetic parameters are enumerated in Tables 1 and 2. The time from intravenous administration at a dose of 25 mg/kg MOIG to reaching the maximum concentration (T_{max}) for both MON and DA was 0.03 h in both male and female rats; the maximum plasma concentration (C_{max}) of MON and DA was 39,748 ± 3398 μg/mL and 19,126 ± 1461 μg/mL in male rats, and 25,719 ± 12,174 μg/mL and 12,340 ± 5992 μg/mL in female rats, respectively. MON and DA were shown to have a low apparent volume of distribution (V_d from 0.003 ± 0.002 L/g

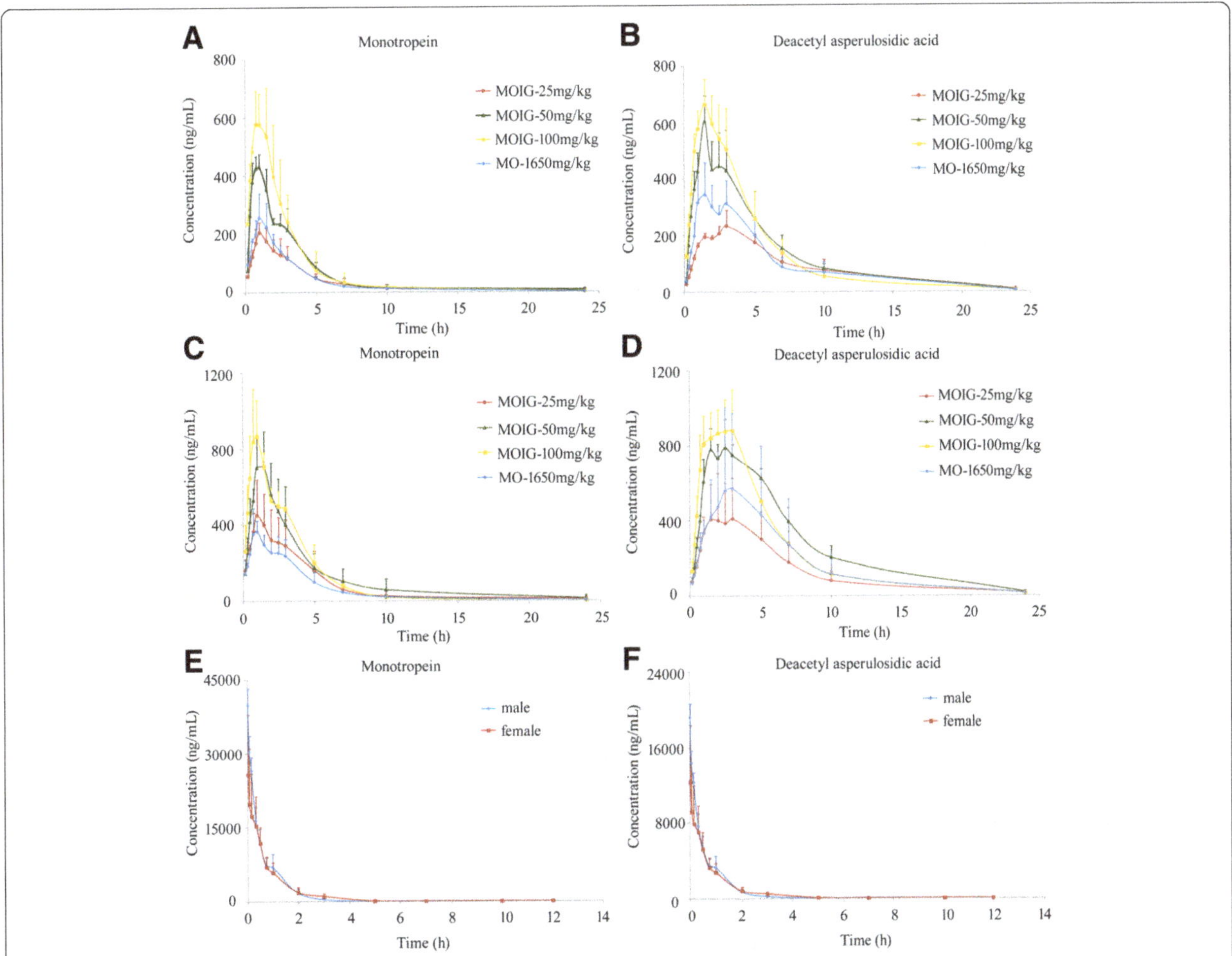

Fig. 3 The mean plasma concentration-time profiles of MON and DA after oral administration of the MOIG at a dose of 25, 50 and 100 mg/kg and the MO extract of 1650 mg/kg in male rats (**a** and **b**), female rats (**c** and **d**) or intravenous administration of 25 mg/kg MOIG (**e** and **f**) in rats ($n = 3$, mean ± SD)

Table 1 The main pharmacokinetic parameters after oral administration of 25, 50, and 100 mg/kg for MOIG, and 1650 mg/kg for MO or intravenous administration of 25 mg/kg MOIG in male rats ($n = 3$, mean ± SD)

Parameters	Component	po-MOIG-25	po-MOIG-50	po-MOIG-100	po-MO-1650	iv-MOIG-25
$AUC_{0\text{-}t}$ (μg·h/L)	MON	832 ± 322	1505 ± 189	1777 ± 537	875 ± 182	21,501 ± 4877
	DA	2010 ± 545	3262 ± 423	3366 ± 753	2220 ± 820	10,239 ± 2044
$AUC_{0\text{-}\infty}$ (μg·h/L)	MON	872 ± 334	1585 ± 279	1812 ± 550	877 ± 182	21,500 ± 4859
	DA	2069 ± 557	3301 ± 411	3397 ± 748	2286 ± 773	10,239 ± 2044
$AUMC_{0\text{-}\infty}$ (μg·h/L)	MON	5121 ± 2698	8645 ± 5804	5011 ± 2132	3064 ± 882	15,255 ± 5098
	DA	14,739 ± 5191	17,844 ± 2090	15,476 ± 3663	12,867 ± 5938	8079 ± 2340
MRT (h)	MON	5.71 ± 1.96	5.17 ± 2.58	2.68 ± 0.40	3.47 ± 0.43	0.70 ± 0.09
	DA	7.03 ± 0.68	5.41 ± 0.24	4.58 ± 0.15	5.43 ± 0.94	0.78 ± 0.09
$t_{1/2}$ (h)	MON	4.60 ± 1.41	7.11 ± 2.18	2.76 ± 1.84	3.00 ± 0.45	1.85 ± 1.67
	DA	4.80 ± 0.62	3.80 ± 1.01	3.76 ± 0.64	3.65 ± 1.16	2.90 ± 0.65
T_{max} (h)	MON	1.00 ± 0.00	0.92 ± 0.14	0.92 ± 0.52	1.17 ± 0.29	0.03 ± 0.00
	DA	2.33 ± 0.76	2.00 ± 0.87	1.5 ± 0.00	2.17 ± 0.76	0.03 ± 0.00
V_d (L/g)	MON	0.20 ± 0.04	0.32 ± 0.04	0.22 ± 0.13	8.51 ± 2.61	0.004 ± 0.004
	DA	0.09 ± 0.04	0.08 ± 0.03	0.17 ± 0.06	3.90 ± 0.90	0.011 ± 0.004
CL (L/g·h)	MON	0.031 ± 0.010	0.032 ± 0.006	0.059 ± 0.020	1.932 ± 0.361	0.001 ± 0.000
	DA	0.013 ± 0.004	0.015 ± 0.002	0.030 ± 0.006	0.791 ± 0.310	0.003 ± 0.001
C_{max} (μg/L)	MON	203 ± 34	451 ± 35	605 ± 114	265 ± 82	39,748 ± 3398
	DA	236 ± 54	624 ± 63	664 ± 89	379 ± 91	19,126 ± 1461
F (%)	MON	4.06 ± 1.55	3.69 ± 0.65	2.11 ± 0.64	2.04 ± 0.42	–
	DA	20.21 ± 5.44	16.12 ± 2.01	8.29 ± 1.83	11.16 ± 3.77	–

to 0.011 ± 0.004 L/g), with a half-life time ($t_{1/2}$) from 1.76 ± 1.32 h to 2.20 ± 1.86 h and a clearance from 0.001 ± 0.000 to 0.003 ± 0.001 L/(g·h). After oral administration of 3-dose levels of MOIGs, C_{max} versus the MON and DA dose distribution was linear with a correlation coefficient being more than 0.90. The increase in C_{max} of MON and DA was positively correlated with the increase in MOIG dosage. The T_{max} of MON and DA were observed about 1 h and 2 h after oral administration respectively, demonstrating that the blood circulatory system could absorb MON and DA. The value of T_{max} and $t_{1/2}$ demonstrated that MON and DA were relatively slowly dispersed. Apparent volume of distribution (V_d) indicated that MON and DA were taken up in the tissue after oral administration, with an absolute bioavailability value of 2.04–3.69% and 8.29–16.12% for MON in male and female rats, and 3.90–10.66% and 16.17–37.23% for DA in male and female rats at an oral dose of 25, 50 and 100 mg/kg MOIG, respectively. These results indicate that the bioavailability of these drugs was dose dependent and showed a significant gender difference.

Tissue distribution study

Tissue distribution of MON and DA was investigated in male and female rats at 0.5, 1, 2, 4, 8, 12 and 24 h after oral administration at a dose of 100 mg/kg MOIG. The level of MON and DA in tissues or organs including the small intestine, large intestine, stomach, spleen, liver, lung, kidney, heart, marrow, thymus, hypothalamus, testis, ovary and uterus was determined. As shown in Tables 3 and 4, MON and DA were widely distributed in all tissues examined after oral administration. MON and DA extensively distributed into the extra-vascular system of the animals. MON and DA levels are significantly reduced to an undetectable level in 12 h or 24 h after oral administration. In male rats, the highest concentration of MON and DA was observed in the intestine and stomach, followed by the spleen, heart, kidney, and testis at 1, 2, and 24 h after oral administration, while the highest concentration of MON and DA in female rats was found in hypothalamus, ovary, uterus, marrow, and liver at 0.5 and 1 h after oral administration. Apart from the intestine and stomach, the spleen and heart had a higher concentration of MON and DA in the male rats. The concentration of MON and DA in the liver, marrow and hypothalamus was higher in female rats than that in male rats.

Discussion

It was found in the present study that the same dosage of MON and DA produced significantly different pharmacokinetic parameters in the treatment of po-MOIG-50 and po-MO-1650. Their comparisons were shown in Fig. 4. The $AUC_{0\text{-}t}$, $AUC_{0\text{-}\infty}$, C_{max} and absolute bioavailability of MON and DA in the treatment of po-MO-1650 were lower

Table 2 The main pharmacokinetic parameters after oral administration of 25, 50, and 100 mg/kg for MOIG, and 1650 mg/kg for MO or intravenous administration of 25 mg/kg MOIG in female rats ($n = 3$, mean ± SD)

Parameters	Component	po-MOIG-25	po-MOIG-50	po-MOIG-100	po-MO-1650	iv-MOIG-25
AUC_{0-t} (μg·h/L)	MON	1988 ± 870	3083 ± 1184	2963 ± 397	1504 ± 244	19,098 ± 4740
	DA	3133 ± 1580	6572 ± 884	5727 ± 992	4254 ± 3301	8910 ± 2343
$AUC_{0-\infty}$ (μg·h/L)	MON	2040 ± 815	3178 ± 1290	2981 ± 400	1507 ± 243	19,129 ± 4743
	DA	3221 ± 1536	6661 ± 935	5785 ± 1024	4308 ± 3367	8945 ± 2349
$AUMC_{0-\infty}$ (μg·h/L)	MON	10,005 ± 3510	16,892 ± 14,358	8895 ± 1596	5589 ± 407	17,847 ± 2842
	DA	20,444 ± 6912	41,101 ± 9585	29,163 ± 7495	25,789 ± 23,049	9214 ± 715
MRT (h)	MON	5.28 ± 2.38	4.78 ± 2.64	2.99 ± 0.43	3.75 ± 0.34	0.98 ± 0.31
	DA	6.77 ± 1.35	6.12 ± 0.60	4.99 ± 0.44	5.66 ± 0.71	1.08 ± 0.31
$t_{1/2}$ (h)	MON	3.61 ± 1.03	4.01 ± 2.35	2.08 ± 0.50	2.51 ± 0.34	1.76 ± 1.32
	DA	4.43 ± 1.12	3.66 ± 0.35	3.64 ± 0.43	3.38 ± 0.44	2.20 ± 1.86
T_{max} (h)	MON	0.94 ± 0.00	1.33 ± 0.29	0.92 ± 0.14	0.92 ± 0.14	0.03 ± 0.00
	DA	2.17 ± 0.76	1.83 ± 0.58	2.33 ± 0.58	2.08 ± 1.18	0.03 ± 0.00
V_d (L/g)	MON	0.08 ± 0.05	0.09 ± 0.04	0.10 ± 0.04	4.07 ± 1.16	0.003 ± 0.002
	DA	0.07 ± 0.06	0.04 ± 0.01	0.09 ± 0.01	2.50 ± 1.25	0.009 ± 0.006
CL (L/g·h)	MON	0.014 ± 0.005	0.018 ± 0.009	0.034 ± 0.05	1.114 ± 0.183	0.001 ± 0.000
	DA	0.010 ± 0.006	0.008 ± 0.001	0.018 ± 0.003	0.532 ± 0.287	0.003 ± 0.001
C_{max} (μg/L)	MON	475 ± 160	761 ± 184	899 ± 197	405 ± 102	25,719 ± 12,174
	DA	445 ± 218	863 ± 112	966 ± 171	584 ± 419	12,340 ± 5992
F (%)	MON	10.66 ± 4.26	8.31 ± 3.37	3.90 ± 0.52	3.94 ± 0.64	–
	DA	36.01 ± 17.17	37.23 ± 5.23	16.17 ± 2.86	24.08 ± 18.82	–

than those in the treatment of po-MOIG-50; the V_d and CL of MON and DA in the treatment of po-MO-1650 were by far higher than those in the treatment of po-MOIG-50. These results suggest that MON and DA were eliminated more quickly and distributed in the tissue under the condition of coexistence of multicomponents in MO-1650.

It was reported that gender was a potential factor affecting drug pharmacokinetics [18], including the absorption process, distribution and bioavailability. The present study showed that the pharmacokinetic parameters for male and female rats were significantly different. The AUC_{0-t}, C_{max} and bioavailability of MON and DA in female rats were higher than those in male rats, but V_d and CL of MON and DA in female rats were lower than those in male rats, indicating that MON and DA were cleared more slowly in female rats than those in male rats.

MON and DA are isomers. Some studies [18, 19] demonstrated that MON and DA were relatively stable in the MO root under normal conditions, while MON may convert to DA in acidic conditions. This may be the reason for the lower bioavailability of MON than DA. In addition, the concentration-time curve of DA showed an obvious double-peak phenomenon. This might be caused by different absorption capacities in different regions of the gut or enterohepatic circulation [20], the conversion of MON or its derivatives into DA through the hydration in gastric acid conditions [17, 18], the pharmacological effect of the MON and DA [21], and gastric emptying-limited absorption [22].

However, we found that MON and DA also distributed in the hypothalamus, implying that they could pass through the blood-brain barrier. The samples collected at 12 h after administration indicated that MON and DA were gradually cleared and no accumulation was observed in the tissues. The compounds absorbed through the blood were transported to the target tissue, and then the unbound portion of the drug exerted the pharmacological effect. MON and DA distributed in the heart, liver, spleen, lung, kidney, especially in the thymus and bone marrow. Thence, we surmised that MON and DA may be able to exert their pharmacological effects in these target organs. MO strengths kidney-*yang* and improves spermatogenesis and the reproductive capacity [23, 24], which is consistent with our finding that MON and DA distributed in the testes at a high concentration. MO and MON showed an obvious anti-osteoporosis effect [10, 11], which is consistent with our finding that MON and DA were also observed in the ovary, uterus and bone marrow at a high concentration. The high concentration of MON and DA in the intestine may be related to their therapeutic effect against colitis [12]. The highest

Table 3 The concentrations (ng/mL) of MON and DA in various tissues after oral administration of 100 mg/kg MOIG in male rats (mean ± SD, $n = 3$)

Tissue/organs	Component	0.5 h	1 h	2 h	4 h	8 h	12 h	24 h
Small intestine	MON	162.8 ± 134.4	19,075.1 ± 16,724.9	3223.4 ± 3453.3	69.2 ± 114.2	24.6 ± 34.1	45.6 ± 78.9	0.1 ± 0.1
	DA	132.2 ± 101.9	13,371.3 ± 11,978.3	2053.3 ± 2478.3	495.0 ± 838.1	110.7 ± 152.2	124.9 ± 197.2	4.3 ± 6.2
Large intestine	MON	706.8 ± 659.0	924.9 ± 972.6	576.9 ± 380.8	66.1 ± 79.2	58.3 ± 29.9	18.6 ± 4.0	1.7 ± 3.0
	DA	2564.7 ± 3177.5	1928.8 ± 1640.6	3135.9 ± 2828.6	1310.0 ± 2008.0	994.9 ± 873.6	334.6 ± 69.8	26.0 ± 23.5
Stomach	MON	2888.7 ± 235.2	1052.1 ± 402.1	364.5 ± 141.9	11.7 ± 11.8	91.0 ± 21.5	12.1 ± 20.9	1.0 ± 1.7
	DA	2451.1 ± 638.1	1124.3 ± 210.2	435.1 ± 96.7	39.5 ± 21.6	84.1 ± 34.5	20.9 ± 34.5	3.2 ± 5.5
Spleen	MON	14.6 ± 9.8	75.2 ± 71.0	5434.0 ± 9376.5	66.6 ± 113.9	4.6 ± 7.9	0.2 ± 0.3	49.8 ± 86.2
	DA	14.1 ± 8.7	58.9 ± 49.4	3563.4 ± 6127.5	9.5 ± 1.9	6.6 ± 6.1	3.2 ± 4.6	29.6 ± 51.2
Testis	MON	18.4 ± 3.8	16.3 ± 15.3	56.6 ± 11.3	188.4 ± 304.1	304.2 ± 513.5	0.0 ± 0.0	0.0 ± 0.0
	DA	17.1 ± 4.9	79.1 ± 67.0	69.1 ± 11.2	24.8 ± 5.6	221.0 ± 358.6	0.0 ± 0.0	0.8 ± 1.3
Heart	MON	24.3 ± 10.6	545.5 ± 908.9	8.9 ± 1.9	0.0 ± 0.0	0.2 ± 0.3	0.0 ± 0.0	269.2 ± 466.2
	DA	22.7 ± 7.4	533.2 ± 856.8	28.9 ± 0.8	10.0 ± 1.9	2.2 ± 1.9	0.0 ± 0.0	214.3 ± 371.2
Kidney	MON	48.6 ± 19.5	147.8 ± 109.9	30.7 ± 4.3	17.0 ± 4.3	3.5 ± 1.7	4.2 ± 7.2	0.0 ± 0.0
	DA	91.7 ± 15.9	303.2 ± 162.0	220.2 ± 19.4	202.2 ± 40.2	66.1 ± 6.5	31.5 ± 18.8	2.5 ± 4.4
Marrow	MON	82.8 ± 46.8	24.2 ± 23.6	10.1 ± 2.9	5.8 ± 6.6	1.2 ± 2.0	0.0 ± 0.0	0.0 ± 0.0
	DA	102.7 ± 90.0	37.8 ± 21.0	24.8 ± 5.1	11.4 ± 3.3	5.6 ± 7.0	0.0 ± 0.0	0.0 ± 0.0
Liver	MON	15.6 ± 7.0	26.5 ± 7.9	20.3 ± 5.2	10.3 ± 3.9	12.6 ± 9.3	20.4 ± 35.3	0.0 ± 0.0
	DA	17.5 ± 2.4	46.9 ± 15.9	52.0 ± 7.6	35.4 ± 7.7	20.9 ± 5.4	22.9 ± 31.9	0.0 ± 0.0
Lung	MON	58.9 ± 29.3	28.7 ± 23.1	34.7 ± 13.9	9.5 ± 6.3	2.0 ± 0.3	64.3 ± 96.8	0.0 ± 0.0
	DA	47.5 ± 23.8	47.1 ± 8.6	48.5 ± 10.5	23.9 ± 2.5	6.4 ± 0.7	72.4 ± 116.7	3.9 ± 6.7
Thymus	MON	16.8 ± 11.5	11.6 ± 3.8	13.0 ± 2.8	13.0 ± 11.1	6.4 ± 1.3	0.0 ± 0.0	0.0 ± 0.0
	DA	22.7 ± 14.6	23.0 ± 3.5	29.7 ± 5.0	10.1 ± 1.9	4.5 ± 3.2	0.8 ± 1.4	1.5 ± 2.0
Hypothalamus	MON	152.5 ± 76.3	110.3 ± 58.0	122.7 ± 137.7	27.7 ± 39.7	16.4 ± 14.2	0.0 ± 0.0	0.0 ± 0.0
	DA	101.0 ± 19.9	70.9 ± 27.6	74.7 ± 88.3	32.5 ± 29.7	17.1 ± 14.9	4.8 ± 8.3	2.6 ± 4.6

concentration of MON and DA in the hypothalamus was observed at 0.5 h, indicating that MON and DA could directly cross the blood-brain barrier and exert their potential pharmacological action on the hypothalamus-gonad system. In addition, the results of tissue distribution of MON and DA maybe implied some new therapeutic areas of MO. The distribution of MON and DA from MO in the stomach, intestine and lung, combined with its anti-inflammatory effects, maybe hint that MO can be used to prevent and treat inflammatory disease in these organs, such as gastritis, pneumonia and colon cancer.

Regarding the toxicity of the MO, there is no literature to report the adverse effect of MO at a normal dose in clinics. The acute toxicity test indicated that MO at a cumulative dose of 250 g/kg/day did not lead to death of mice in 3 days [25]. Some investigation showed that MO extracts had no mutagenic or genotoxic effect on *Escherichia coli* PQ37DNA [26]. Our experiments indicated that MOIG at dose of 22.5 g/kg did not cause any death of mice. These evidence, together with their significant pharmacological properties, implied that iridoid glycosides, such as monotropein and deacetyl asperulosidic acid from Morinda officinalis root in rats, had potential for the use in medication, especially for inflammatory disease.

Conclusion

The two major IGs (MON and DA) from the MO root were simultaneously determined by a simple, rapid and sensitive UHPLC-MS/MS method. This method was also used in the study of pharmacokinetics and tissue distribution after oral administration of 25, 50, and 100 mg/kg MOIGs and 1650 mg/kg MO extract. This is the first report on the pharmacokinetic and tissue distribution of MON and DA after oral administration of the MO extract. We also found that MON and DA exhibited a significant gender difference in terms of the pharmacokinetic parameters. In addition, the absolute bioavailability of MON and DA also showed a significant gender difference. The results of tissue distribution in male and female rats indicated that MON and DA from the MO root mainly distributed in the intestine and stomach after oral administration, followed by the

Table 4 The concentrations (ng/mL) of MON and DA in various tissues after oral administration of 100 mg/kg MOIG in female rats (mean ± SD, *n* = 3)

Tissue/organs	Component	0.5 h	1 h	2 h	4 h	8 h	12 h	24 h
Small intestine	MON	244.3 ± 392.8	19,223.7 ± 9918.4	11,552.4 ± 18,012.3	5751.1 ± 4091.9	26.1 ± 20.4	8.3 ± 14.4	1.9 ± 3.2
	DA	153.0 ± 232.2	11,548.8 ± 3298.3	7897.3 ± 11,589.7	6001.6 ± 2129.6	28.3 ± 10.9	198.7 ± 310.3	3.0 ± 5.2
Large intestine	MON	966.5 ± 1501.4	1089.2 ± 411.5	2949.1 ± 4063.5	215.6 ± 137.4	27.9 ± 5.8	17.4 ± 22.5	0.0 ± 0.0
	DA	1408.8 ± 2274.2	2026.4 ± 1904.6	5383.1 ± 4417.7	5200.8 ± 4470.2	246.3 ± 189.6	374.1 ± 418.7	0.4 ± 0.3
Stomach	MON	1913.2 ± 1817.5	3098.1 ± 3293.7	1226.6 ± 1009.2	39.1 ± 22.2	81.3 ± 25.5	0.0 ± 0.00	0.0 ± 0.0
	DA	1526.7 ± 1436.1	3015.9 ± 3232.2	1328.7 ± 1031.1	83.0 ± 33.6	73.6 ± 22.8	1.0 ± 0.9	0.0 ± 0.0
Spleed	MON	25.0 ± 16.2	102.8 ± 120.3	28.5 ± 21.9	7.7 ± 7.1	14.9 ± 22.5	0.0 ± 0.0	0.0 ± 0.0
	DA	29.4 ± 15.7	83.9 ± 82.6	43.6 ± 31.6	19.9 ± 11.5	16.5 ± 17.7	0.0 ± 0.0	0.0 ± 0.0
Ovary	MON	374.7 ± 318.2	2112.7 ± 2497.3	504.0 ± 470.3	138.4 ± 105.5	45.5 ± 15.6	6.5 ± 11.3	1.7 ± 2.9
	DA	241.9 ± 185.0	854.1 ± 859.3	382.3 ± 298.2	110.4 ± 101.8	33.8 ± 9.5	5.7 ± 9.8	0.7 ± 1.3
Uterus	MON	331.7 ± 229.3	2214.1 ± 2264.0	601.3 ± 664.6	269.9 ± 217.3	97.2 ± 21.0	0.0 ± 0.0	3.0 ± 5.0
	DA	194.0 ± 122.7	1069.7 ± 908.8	426.3 ± 422.7	256.6 ± 340.3	68.4 ± 14.9	1.8 ± 2.1	3.6 ± 3.5
Heart	MON	44.3 ± 18.2	79.0 ± 91.0	21.5 ± 3.6	5.8 ± 5.7	3.7 ± 6.5	0.0 ± 0.0	0.0 ± 0.0
	DA	45.8 ± 19.1	86.1 ± 81.8	42.1 ± 7.7	17.6 ± 4.9	6.3 ± 5.6	0.0 ± 0.0	0.0 ± 0.0
Kidney	MON	146.6 ± 133.3	139.8 ± 98.6	68.3 ± 25.4	48.8 ± 27.5	14.1 ± 10.3	0.0 ± 0.0	8.1 ± 14.0
	DA	1832.9 ± 2990.7	218.6 ± 114.6	264.8 ± 33.7	244.0 ± 25.8	109.0 ± 22.5	44.6 ± 2.5	0.9 ± 1.4
Marrow	MON	583.1 ± 978.7	257.0 ± 226.1	48.4 ± 60.3	10.7 ± 14.8	0.1 ± 0.2	0.0 ± 0.0	0.0 ± 0.0
	DA	446.2 ± 744.7	209.9 ± 183.6	66.1 ± 51.3	27.6 ± 29.1	3.8 ± 1.9	0.0 ± 0.0	0.0 ± 0.0
Liver	MON	729.3 ± 993.8	169.0 ± 129.8	66.4 ± 23.4	13.9 ± 4.6	33.0 ± 36.6	0.0 ± 0.0	0.0 ± 0.0
	DA	536.2 ± 725.7	142.0 ± 83.4	87.2 ± 13.9	42.2 ± 12.1	36.3 ± 14.4	3.1 ± 3.0	0.0 ± 0.0
Lung	MON	72.2 ± 53.3	398.3 ± 491.2	50.6 ± 33.7	244.8 ± 407.7	26.7 ± 25.6	47.6 ± 82.5	0.0 ± 0.0
	DA	56.5 ± 29.8	222.3 ± 257.4	72.1 ± 28.2	180.7 ± 267.3	23.8 ± 16.9	30.2 ± 52.3	0.0 ± 0.0
Thymus	MON	22.3 ± 9.2	140.0 ± 144.2	32.6 ± 36.1	1.8 ± 1.1	22.8 ± 6.3	0.0 ± 0.00	0.0 ± 0.0
	DA	26.50 ± 7.7	136.05 ± 128.2	57.3 ± 45.6	14.1 ± 3.4	30.6 ± 8.6	0.0 ± 0.0	0.0 ± 0.0
Hypothalamus	MON	2209.3 ± 3684.2	504.1 ± 333.9	226.2 ± 264.4	41.1 ± 43.2	72.3 ± 95.2	0.0 ± 0.0	9.7 ± 16.9
	DA	1754.0 ± 2942.7	287.1 ± 176.9	145.8 ± 144.6	47.2 ± 9.2	67.7 ± 77.7	0.0 ± 0.0	21.0 ± 36.4

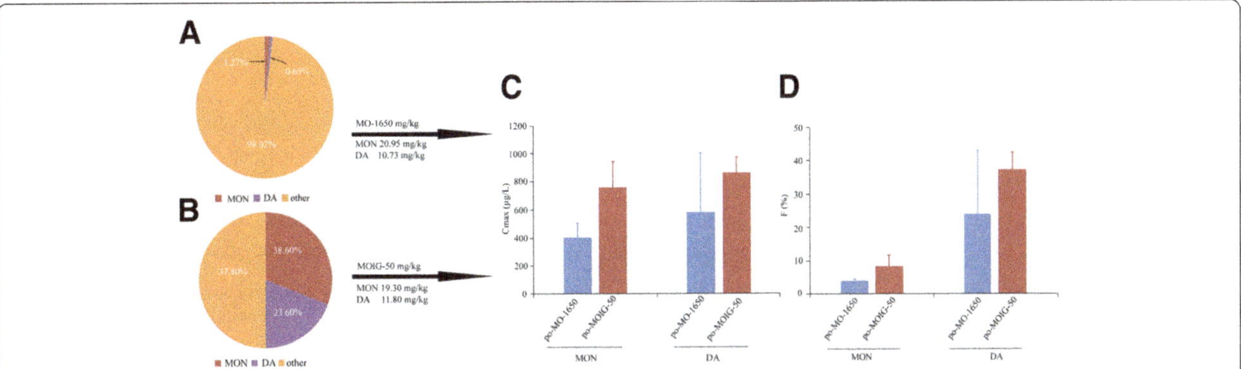

Fig. 4 The pie diagram of actual values of MON and DA in the MO (**a**) and MOIG (**b**). After oral administration of the 50 mg/kg MOIG and 1650 mg/kg MO extract, comparing the C_{max} (**c**) and absolute bioavailability (**d**) of MON and DA in female rats plasma

spleen, hypothalamus, and gonad. These findings may shed new lights on the biological behavior of MOIGs in vivo, help explain some of their pharmacological actions, and provide experimental clues for rational clinical use of these IGs extracted from the MO root.

Additional files

Additional file 1: Table S1. Standard curves, linear ranges, correlation coefficients and lower limit of quantification of MON and DA in biological samples.

Additional file 2: Table S2. Intra-day and inter-day accuracy and precision of analytes in rats blank samples. (DOC 19 kb)

Additional file 3: Table S3. Extraction recovery and matrix effect of MON, DA and IS in rat plasma and tissue homogenates ($n = 6$, mean ± SD).

Additional file 4: Table S4. Dilution integrity experiments of MON and DA ($n = 5$, mean ± SD).

Additional file 5: Table S5. Stability of MON and DA in blank plasma samples ($n = 5$).

Abbreviations

ACE: Acetaminophen; AJS: Agilent jet stream technology; $AUC_{0-\infty}$: Area under the plasma concentration-time curve from zero to time infinity; AUC_{0-t}: Area under the plasma concentration-time curve; CL: Body clearance; C_{max}: Peak concentration; DA: Deacetyl asperulosidic acid; DSS: Dextran sulfate sodium; EMA: European Medicines Agency; ESI: Electrospray source interface; FDA: Food and Drug Administration; F_{oral}: Absolute oral bioavailability; IGs: Iridoid glycosides; IL-1β: Interleukin-1-beta; IS: Internal standard; LLOQ: Lower limit of quantification; ME: Matrix effect; MO: *Morinda officinalis*; MOIGs: *Morinda officinalis* iridoid glycosides; MON: Monotropein; MRM: Multiple reaction monitoring; MRT: Mean residence time; QC: Quality control; $t_{1/2}$: Half-life; T_{max}: Peak time; UHPLC-MS: Ultra high performance liquid chromatography-tandem mass spectrometry; ULOQ: Upper limit of quantification; V_d: Apparent volume of body distribution

Acknowledgements

We would like to thank the Experimental Animal Center of the Second Military Medical University for providing experimental sites.

Funding

This study was supported by the National Natural Science Foundation of China (Grant No. U1505226 and U1603283) and Shanghai Committee of Science and Technology (Grant No.14401902700).

Authors' contributions

SY, ZQY, QYP, and XHL contributed to the study design. HT, HHY, and ZL contributed the reagents, materials and analysis tools. SY, ZQ, HYQ, and ZJH performed the experiments. WYB, SHT, and LB analyzed and interpreted the data. SY, ZQY and QYP wrote and revised the manuscript. All authors read and approved the final manuscript.

Competing interest

The authors declare that they have no competing interests.

Author details

[1]School of Pharmacy, Fujian University of Traditional Chinese Medicine, No. 1 Qiuyang Road, Shangjie Town, Minhou County, Fuzhou 350122, People's Republic of China. [2]School of Pharmacy, Zhejiang University of Traditional Chinese Medicine, Gaoke Road, Fuyang District, Hangzhou 310053, People's Republic of China. [3]School of Pharmacy, Second Military Medical University, No. 325 Guohe Road, Yangpu District, Shanghai 200433, People's Republic of China. [4]Department of Pharmacy, Eastern Hepatobiliary Surgery Hospital, Second Military Medical University, No. 225 Changhai Road, Yangpu District, Shanghai 200438, People's Republic of China. [5]Department of Biotechnology and Laboratory Science in Medicine, National Yang-Ming University, No. 155, Section 2, Li Nong Street, Beitou District, Taipei 112-21, People's Republic of China. [6]Fuzhou General Hospital of Nanjing Military Region, No. 156, West Second Ring North Road, Gulou District, Fuzhou 350025, People's Republic of China.

References

1. Zhang JH, Xin HL, Xu YM, Shen Y, He YQ, Hsien Y, Ling B, Song HT, Juan L, Yang HY, Qin LP, Zhang QY, Du J. Morinda officinalis how. -Acomprehensive review of traditional uses, phytochemistry and pharmacology. J Ethnopharmacol. 2018;213:230–55.
2. Wang YF, Li YH, Xing SQ, Li Y, Yi LZT, Shang XD, Zhao DF, Bai LQ. Review of experiment research progress in treating deficiency of kidney-yang syndrome by Morinda officinalis how. And its effective components. China J Tradit Chin Med Pharm. 2016;31:5165–7.
3. Ye WH, Gong MJ, Zou ZJ. Metabonomic study of anti-inflammatory effect of Morinda officinalis How on acute inflammation induced by carrageenan. Pharm Clin Chin Mater Med. 2013;3:22–5.
4. Chen DL, Yang X, Yang J, Lai GX, Yong TQ, Tang XC, Shuai O, Zhou GL, Xie YZ, Wu QP. Prebiotic effect of fructooligosaccharides from Morinda officinalis on Alzheimer's disease in rodent models by targeting the microbiota-gut-brain axis. Front Aging Neurosci. 2017;9:403–30.
5. Cheng D, Murtaza G, Ma SY, Li LL, Li XJ, Tian FZ, Zheng JC. LuY. In silico prediction of the anti-depression mechanism of a herbal formula (Tiansi liquid) containing Morinda officinalis and Cuscuta chinensis. Molecules. 2017;22:1614–29.
6. Lee YK, Bang HJ, Oh JB, Whang WK. Bioassay-guided isolated compounds from Morinda officinalis inhibit Alzheimer's disease pathologies. Molecules. 2017;22:1638–49.
7. Chen YB, Xue Z. Study on chemical constituents of Morinda officinalis how. Bull Chin Mat Med. 1987;12:27–9.
8. Choi J, Lee KT, Choi MY, Nam JH, Jung HJ, Park SK, Park HJ. Antinociceptive anti-inflammatory effect of monotropein isolated from the root of Morinda officinalis. Biol Pharm Bull. 2005;28:1915–8.
9. Wang YL, Cui HM, Huang SJ, Li Q, Lei HM. Determination ofmajor iridoid glycosides in Morinda officinalis from different origins and batches by HPLC. J Chin Med Mat. 2011;34:1187–90.
10. Zhang ZG, Zhang QY, Yang H, Liu W, Zhang ND, Qin LP, Xin HL. Monotropeinisolated from the roots of Morinda officinalis increases osteoblastic bone formation and prevents bone loss in ovariectomized mice. Fitoterapia. 2016;110:166–72.
11. Wang F, Wu LH, Li LF, Chen SY. Monotropein exerts protective effects against IL-1β-induced apoptosis and catabolic responses on osteoarthritis chondrocytes. Int Immunopharmacol. 2014;23:575–80.
12. Shin JS, Yun KJ, Chung KS, Seo KH, Park HJ, Cho YW, Baek NI, Jang D, Lee KT. Monotropein isolated from the roots of Morinda officinalis ameliorates proinflammatory mediators in RAW 264.7 macrophages and dextran sulfate sodium (DSS)-induced colitis via NF-κB inactivation. Food Chem Toxicol. 2013;53:263–71.
13. Zhang JH, Xu YM, He YQ, Song HT, Du J, Zhang QY. Study on determination and extraction of iridoid glycosides from Morinda officinalis. J Pharm Pract. 2017;35:328–33.
14. Li C, Dong J, Tian JC, Deng ZP, Song XJ. LC/MS/MS determination and pharmacokinetic study of iridoid glycosides monotropein and deacetyl asperulosidic acid isomers in rat plasma after oral administration of Morinda officinalis extract. Biomed Chromatogr. 2016;30:163–68.
15. Ganzera M, Sturm S. Recent advances on HPLC/MS in medicinal plant analysis-an update covering 2011-2016. J Pharm Biomed Anal. 2018;147:211–33.
16. U.S. Food and Drug Administration, Guidance for Industry, Bioanalytical Method Validation, 2013. https://www.yumpu.com/en/document/view/21736056/bioanalytical-method-validation-guidance-for-industry-draft-guidance-2013.
17. European Medicines Agency, Guideline on Bioanalytical Method Validation, 2012. https://www.ema.europa.eu/documents/scientific-guideline/guideline-bioanalytical-method-validation_en.pdf.
18. Franconi F, Campesi I. Sex impact on biomarkers, pharmacokinetics and pharmacodynamics. Curr Med Chem. 2017;24:2561–75.
19. Wang YL, Huang SJ, Chi DJ, Li Q, Lei HM, Cui HM. Study on stability of main iridoid glucosides from Morinda officinalis radix. China J Exper Tradit Med Form. 2011;17:65–8.

20. Parquet M, Metman EH, Raizman A, Rambaud JC, Berthaux N, Infante R. Bioavailability, gastrointestinal transit, solubilization and faecal excretion of ursodeoxycholic acid in man. Eur J Clin Investig. 1985;15:171–8.
21. Zhou H. Pharmacokinetic strategies in deciphering atypical drug absorption profiles. J Clin Pharmacol. 2003;43:211–27.
22. Ogungbenro K, Pertinez H, Aarons L. Empirical and semi-mechanistic modelling of double-peaked pharmacokinetic profile phenomenon due to gastric emptying. AAPS J. 2015;17:227–36.
23. Chen TJ, Wang W. Morinda officinalis extract repairs cytoxan-impaired spermatogenesis of male rats. Zhonghua Nan Ke Xue. 2015;21:436–42.
24. Song B, Wang FJ, Wang W. Effect of aqueous extract from *Morinda officinalis* F. C. How on microwave-induced hypothalamic-pituitary-testis axis impairment in male Sprague-dawley rats. Evid Based Complement Alternat Med. 2015;2015:1–9.
25. Zhang ZQ, Yuan L, Zhao N, Xu YK, Yang M, Luo ZP. Antidepressant effect of the ethanolic extracts of the roots of Morinda officinalis in rats and mice. Chin Pharm J. 2000;35:739–41.
26. Sun YL. Study on the genotoxicity of Panax, Atractylodes, and Morinda. Master Thesis of Sichuan University 2003. Sichuan Province, China.

10

Acid-base fractions separated from *Streblus asper* leaf ethanolic extract exhibited antibacterial, antioxidant, anti-acetylcholinesterase, and neuroprotective activities

Anchalee Prasansuklab[1], Atsadang Theerasri[1], Matthew Payne[2], Alison T. Ung[2*] and Tewin Tencomnao[3*]

Abstract

Background: *Streblus asper* is a well-known plant native to Southeast Asia. Different parts of the plant have been traditionally used for various medicinal purposes. However, there is very little scientific evidence reporting its therapeutic benefits for potential treatment of Alzheimer's disease (AD). The study aimed to evaluate antibacterial, antioxidant, acetylcholinesterase (AChE) inhibition, and neuroprotective properties of *S. asper* leaf extracts with the primary objective of enhancing therapeutic applications and facilitating activity-guided isolation of the active chemical constituents.

Methods: The leaves of *S. asper* were extracted in ethanol and subsequently fractionated into neutral, acid and base fractions. The phytochemical constituents of each fraction were analyzed using GC-MS. The antibacterial activity was evaluated using a broth microdilution method. The antioxidant activity was determined using DPPH and ABTS radical scavenging assays. The neuroprotective activity against glutamate-induced toxicity was tested on hippocampal neuronal HT22 cell line by evaluating the cell viability using MTT assay. The AChE inhibitory activity was screened by thin-layer chromatography (TLC) bioautographic method.

Results: The partition of the *S. asper* ethanolic leaf extract yielded the highest mass of phytochemical constitutions in the neutral fraction and the lowest in the basic fraction. Amongst the three fractions, the acidic fraction showed the strongest antibacterial activity against gram-positive bacteria. The antioxidant activities of three fractions were found in the order of acidic > basic > neutral, whereas the decreasing order of neuroprotective activity was neutral > basic > acidic. TLC bioautography revealed one component in the neutral fraction exhibited anti-AChE activity. While in the acid fraction, two components showed inhibitory activity against AChE. GC-MS analysis of three fractions showed the presence of major phytochemical constituents including terpenoids, steroids, phenolics, fatty acids, and lipidic plant hormone.

(Continued on next page)

* Correspondence: Alison.Ung@uts.edu.au; tewin.t@chula.ac.th
[2]School of Mathematical and Physical Sciences, Faculty of Science, The University of Technology Sydney, Sydney, NSW 2007, Australia
[3]Age-Related Inflammation and Degeneration Research Unit, Department of Clinical Chemistry, Faculty of Allied Health Sciences, Chulalongkorn University, Bangkok 10330, Thailand
Full list of author information is available at the end of the article

(Continued from previous page)
Conclusions: Our findings have demonstrated the therapeutic potential of three fractions extracted from *S. asper* leaves as a promising natural source for neuroprotective agents with additional actions of antibacterials and antioxidants, along with AChE inhibitors that will benefit in the development of new natural compounds in therapies against AD.

Keywords: Acid-base extraction, *Streblus asper*, Glutamate toxicity, HT22 cells, Neuroprotection, Alzheimer's disease, Neurodegenerative diseases

Background

Herbal medicines are gaining significant attention globally in primary health care due to its various advantages over prescribed synthetic drugs, especially in long-term usage [1–3]. Synthetic FDA approved drugs, during long-term usage, may have adverse side effects [4, 5], and are not cost-effective or readily affordable in under developed and developing countries [6–10]. The use of medicinal plants or plant-derived substances in the prevention and treatment of various diseases including Alzheimer's disease (AD) has been proven to be effective and is on the rise [11–15]. Two examples of plant-derived FDA approved drugs used for the treatment of AD are rivastigmine and galantamine, which were isolated from *Physostigma venenosum* and *Galanthus caucasicus*, respectively [16, 17]. Other promising natural products such as Huperzine A (derived from *Huperzia serrata*), curcumin (derived from *Curcuma longa*), and resveratrol (derived from *Vitis vinifera*) also possess excellent anti-AD activity and they are in Phase II or III clinical trials [18, 19]. Moreover, a number of medicinal plants with antioxidant, anti-inflammatory, and anti-apoptotic effects are currently being researched as an excellent source of neuroprotective agents and/or anti-AD drugs [16, 17, 20–23].

AD is one of the most common neurodegenerative diseases, characterized by the progressive loss of neuronal cells in the central nervous system which eventually contributes to memory impairment. Moreover, as the result of abnormal functioning in several areas of the patient's brain in the late stage of disease, AD can be fatal and it is officially ranked as the sixth-leading cause of death in the United States (U.S.) in 2018 [24]. AD is suffered by 35–40 million patients worldwide and there is currently no proven complete cure [25]. Although the exact pathogenic mechanisms underlying AD remains unknown, the neurotransmitter acetylcholine and glutamate are potentially considered as therapeutic targets and have been focused since both neurotransmission systems were found aberrant in the brains of individuals with AD [26]. Drugs commonly used to treat AD include acetylcholinesterase (AChE) inhibitors (e.g., galantamine and donepezil) and *N*-methyl-D-aspartate (NMDA)-type glutamate receptor antagonists (e.g., memantine). Nevertheless, these drugs provide only symptomatic relief but not a cure. The debate over the therapeutic benefits versus the side effects and the financial cost of these drugs has continued for decades [27–29]. The discovery of therapeutic, cost effective AD drugs devoid of adverse side effects is a very active area of research [30].

Besides disturbances of neurotransmitters, oxidative stress and exacerbation of inflammatory responses have been associated with AD as significant contributors to neuronal damage and neurodegeneration [31–33]. Interestingly, bacterial infection is now considered as a risk or causative factor of AD by triggering chronic inflammation in the brain that may subsequently promote the initiation and progression of the disease [34–36]. Additionally, the presence of bacteria in the brain may play a role in the accumulation and deposition of amyloid beta (Aβ) peptides, the major pathological hallmark of AD, which these peptides may be recruited to the site of infection due to their functions in innate immunity as antimicrobials [37, 38]. A dramatic reduction of cerebral Aβ levels was observed when transgenic mouse model of AD was in the absence of gut microbiota [39] or in the prolonged shift of gut microbial composition induced by broad-spectrum combinatorial antibiotic treatment [40]. Recent evidence using next generation sequencing (NGS) analysis that observed an increase of bacterial populations in post-mortem brains from patients with AD, also supports the involvement of bacterial infection in AD [41]. Hence, controlling AD-associated infections by using compounds with bactericidal or antibacterial activities was highlighted as an alternative strategy for disease prevention and treatment [34, 35, 42, 43].

Medicinal plants can be of important natural resources for novel agents that may constitute an alternative to the present drugs used in the treatment of several illnesses including AD [11]. *Streblus asper* Lour. is a well-known medicinal plant that belongs to family Moraceae and distributes mainly over the region of Southeast Asia. Different parts of the plant have been traditionally used for various medicinal purposes such as treatment of fever, toothache, filariasis, leprosy, snakebite, diarrhoea, piles, epilepsy, epistaxis, heart disease, urinary tract complaints, stomachache, obesity, skin diseases, wounds, and cancer [44, 45]. It has also been used as an ingredient in a traditional Thai formula for longevity [46]. Studies on the crude plant extract as well as the isolated compounds have demonstrated that *S. asper* exhibits various pharmacological properties including antioxidant, anticancer [47], antimicrobial [48], antimalarial [49], anti-filarial [50], anti-inflammation [51], and anti-hepatitis B activities [52]. Moreover, the neuroprotective properties of *S. asper* leaf extracts in both in vivo and in vitro models of neurodegenerative diseases were recently reported [53, 54]. However, the active phytochemical ingredients responsible for neuroprotection have not been clearly identified. The main objective of our research is to enhance the utilization of this plant extract with the best efficacy for therapeutic applications and facilitate the clarification of its active components. This was achieved by first carrying out the fractionation of the crude ethanolic extract of *S. asper* leaves using liquid-liquid extraction based on pH properties of its phytochemical constituents. The resulting fractions of organic neutral, acidic, and basic components were investigated and compared to each other for their pharmacological potentials including antibacterial, antioxidant, anti-AChE, and neuroprotective activities.

Methods

Chemicals and reagents

Acetylcholinesterase from electric eel (EC 3.1.1.7, type V-S), bovine serum albumin (BSA), 1-naphthyl acetate, Fast Blue B salt, galantamine, Tris-HCl, dimethyl sulfoxide (DMSO), Dulbecco's modified Eagle's medium (DMEM), fetal bovine serum (FBS), 2,2′-Azino-bis(3-ethylbenzothiazoline-6-sulfonic acid) diammonium salt (ABTS), and 2,2-Diphenyl-1-picrylhydrazyl (DPPH) were purchased from Sigma-Aldrich (St. Louis, MO, USA). Phosphate buffer saline (PBS) and Penicillin/Streptomycin solution were purchased from Hyclone (Logan, Utah, USA). Trypsin-EDTA was purchased from Gibco (Waltham, MA, USA). 3-(4,5-dimetylthiazol-2-yl)-2,5-diphenyltetrazoliumbromide (MTT) was purchased from Bio Basic (Markham, Ontario, Canada). L-ascorbic acid was purchased from Calbiochem (San Diego, CA, USA). Mueller-Hinton broth was purchased from Himedia laboratories (Mumbai, MH, India). Other reagents used in extraction process were of analytical grade.

Plant collection and identification

Leaves of *S. asper* were collected from the Princess Maha Chakri Sirindhorn Herbal Garden (Rayong Province, Thailand). The plant was authenticated by Professor Dr. Thaweesakdi Boonkerd and deposited in the herbarium of Kasin Suvatabhandhu (Department of Botany, Faculty of Science, Chulalongkorn University, Thailand) under voucher number A013419 (BCU).

Preparation of crude extract

After collection, the ethanolic extract of *S. asper* leaves was prepared as previously described [54]. In brief, the dry powered plant material (0.73 kg) was soaked in 100% ethanol (7.3 L) with a 1:10 sample-solvent ratio for 48 h at room temperature (RT) in the dark with continuous shaking. The resulting liquid extract was filtered and concentrated using rotary evaporator to give 29.44 g of crude extract. Part of this concentrated extract was dissolved in DMSO, passed through a 0.2-μm filter, and stored at − 20 °C as a stock solution for evaluating biological activities.

Preparation of acid-base fractions

For efficient acid-base extraction, crude ethanolic extract of *S. asper* leaves (29.44 g) was firstly dissolved in ethyl acetate (EtOAc) (700 mL) and partitioned with distilled water (700 mL). The resulting organic solution was concentrated, re-dissolved in dioxane (200 mL) and slowly added dropwise of distilled water (80 mL) while stirring continuously to induce the precipitation of chlorophyll [55]. Then, the precipitates were removed by three rounds of centrifugation (4400 rpm for 20 min) with each round being followed by filtration through filter papers. The chlorophyll-removed extracts were combined, and solvents were removed to give a thick paste. The paste was used for fractionation into neutral, acidic, and basic fractions based on the method of alkaloid extraction previously used by Mungkornasawakul et al. [56], with some modifications. The procedure of acid-base extraction was summarized in Fig. 1. The crude paste was dissolved in EtOAc (150 mL) and extracted with 5% hydrochloric acid (HCl) (700 mL). The ethyl acetate (Organic phase-1) layer was separated from the 5% HCl (Aqueous phase-1) layer and set aside for basic extraction. The 5% HCl solution was made basic (pH 10) with 10 M sodium hydroxide (NaOH) and the resulting solution was further extracted with EtOAc (200 mL × 2). The ethyl acetate extracts were washed with saturated NaCl solution and dried over anhydrous potassium carbonate (K_2CO_3). The solvent was removed to afford the basic fraction.

Simultaneously, ethyl acetate (Organic phase-1) layer was extracted with an equal volume of 0.5 M NaOH solution. The top organic layer (Organic phase-2) was separated from the aqueous NaOH layer (Aqueous phase-2), then washed with a saturated solution NaCl and dried over anhydrous sodium sulfate (Na_2SO_4) and the solvent was removed under reduced pressure to afford the neutral fraction. Finally, the remaining the aqueous NaOH layer (Aqueous phase-2) was then acidified to pH 1 with 5% HCl and extracted with EtOAc (200 mL × 2). The combined ethyl acetate extracts were washed with a saturated solution NaCl and dried over

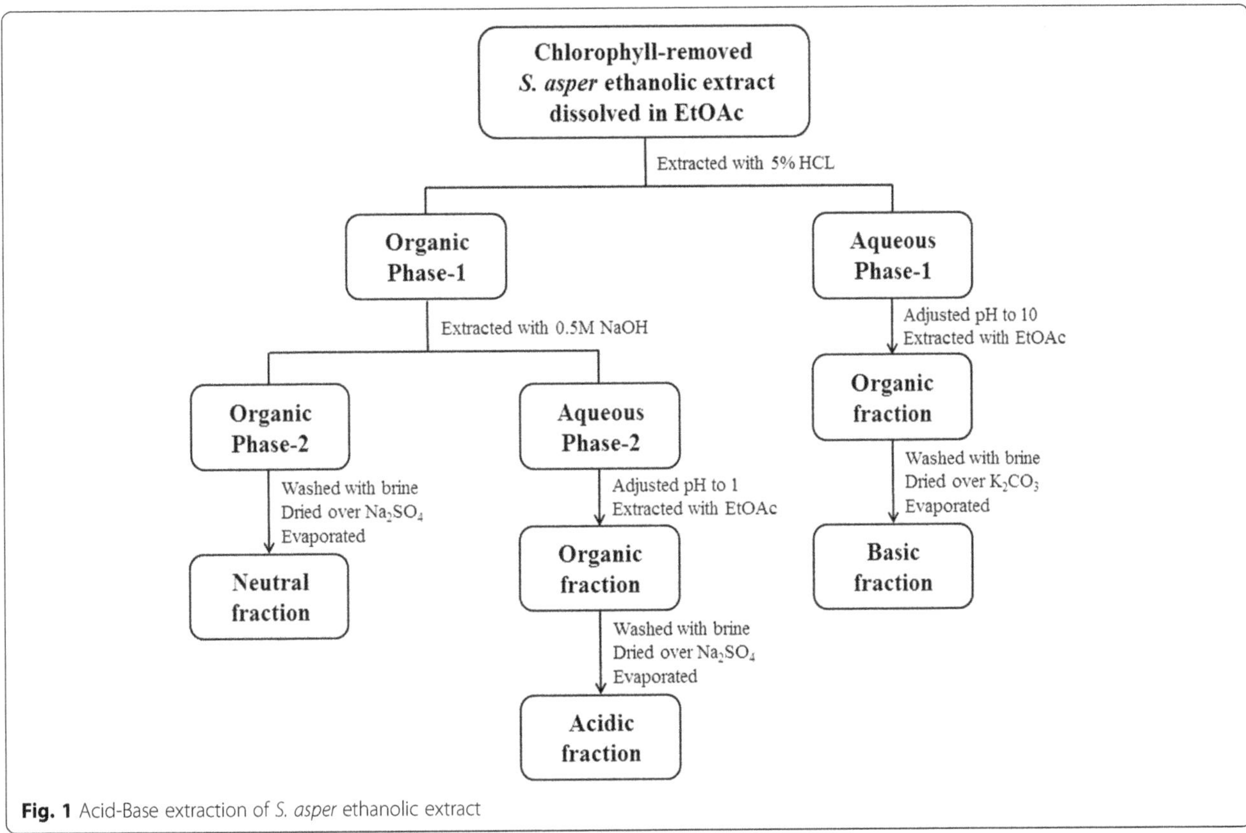

Fig. 1 Acid-Base extraction of *S. asper* ethanolic extract

anhydrous Na_2SO_4, and the solvent was removed under reduced pressure to afford the acidic fraction. Parts of three fractions obtained after acid-base extraction were dissolved in DMSO, filtered through a 0.2-μm filter, and stored at − 20 °C as a stock solution for evaluating biological activities.

GC-MS analysis

Analysis of volatile chemical constituents was performed using Agilent 6890 gas chromatograph fitted with an Agilent HP-5 MS fused-silica capillary column (5% polysilphenylene, 95% polydimethylsiloxane column, 30 m × 0.25 mm, i.d. 0.25 μm film thickness), coupled to an Agilent 5973 N mass selective detector with electron-ionization (EI) source (Agilent Technologies, Palo Alto, CA, USA). The samples were dissolved in ethyl acetate and injected automatically in the split mode with a split ratio of 1:25 and injection volume of 1 μL. Helium was used as the carrier gas at a constant flow rate of 1.2 mL/min. The total run time was 10.8 min. The column oven temperature was programmed initially at 50 °C for 2 min. Then, it was raised to 290 °C with a rate of 50 °C/min and held at 290 °C for 4 min. The mass spectrometer was operated with ionization energy of 70 eV, ion source temperature of 230 °C, detector temperature of 150 °C, and in the scan mode over the mass range of m/z 40–450. The compounds were identified by matching their recorded retention times and mass spectral patterns with the NIST mass spectral library (NIST08.L).

Determination of antibacterial activity

The antibacterial activity was determined by broth microdilution according to CLSI guidelines. The test medium was cation-adjusted Mueller-Hinton broth (CAMHB). Test Medium was used for *S. aureus* ATCC25923, *B. subtilis* SU5, *E. coli* MG1655 and *P. aeruginosa* PA14. Serially diluted concentrations of samples or standard antibiotic ampicillin (a positive inhibition control) were tested using a 96 well plate, which was inoculated with a bacterium cell concentration of approximately 5×10^5 CFU. The CAMHB medium plus sample without inoculum was used as a negative control. After 20 h of incubation at 37 °C statically, the minimum inhibitory concentration (MIC) was defined as the lowest concentration of compound that showed 95% cell growth inhibition, determined by measuring absorbance at 595 nm. The experiment was performed in biological triplicates.

Determination of antioxidant activity

The antioxidant activity was evaluated in vitro using the DPPH and ABTS radical scavenging assays modified for a 96-well microtiter plate format as described previously [54]. Briefly, various concentrations of samples or ascorbic acid (a positive control) in absolute ethanol and the DPPH• or ABTS• + working solution were mixed in a ratio of 9:1 (*v*/v) in a 96 well-plate. The working solution plus absolute ethanol was used as a negative control. The reaction mixture was incubated in the dark at RT for 15 min or 30 min and the absorbance was recorded using a microplate reader (BioTek Instruments, Winooski, VT, USA) at 517 nm or 734 nm for DPPH or ABTS assay, respectively. Radical scavenging activity was calculated as the percent inhibition of free radicals using the following equation: % Inhibition = 100 - [(Abs of the sample - Abs of blank) × 100/ Abs of control]. The antioxidant capacity of each sample was also compared with those of ascorbic acid (vitamin C) and was expressed as vitamin C equivalent antioxidant capacity (VCEAC) in mg per g of dry weight sample.

Determination of anti-acetylcholinesterase activity

The AChE inhibitory activity was screened by using thin-layer chromatography (TLC)-direct bioautographic assay adapted from Marston's method [57]. This assay is based on the activity of AChE in converting the substrate 1-naphthyl acetate to 1-naphthol, which in turn reacts with the chromogenic agent Fast Blue B salt to produce a purple-coloured diazonium dye. The working solution of AChE was prepared by dissolving 1.21 mg of lyophilized powder of AChE from electric eel in 135 mL of 0.05 M Tris-HCl buffer at pH 7.8 with 150 mg of bovine serum albumin. The silica gel F_{254} TLC plates (Merck, Darmstadt, Germany) were prewashed with acetone and thoroughly dried before use. Briefly, 1 mg of each sample was dissolved in ethyl acetate (1000 ppm), 6.7 μL (6.7 μg) of the solution was spotted on a pre-washed TLC plate and developed with the solvent system of hexane: ethyl acetate (7:3, *v*/v). Then, 3.3 μL (0.3 μg) of galantamine solution (0.1 mg/mL, 100 ppm) was also applied on the plate as a positive control. After completely air-dried, the TLC plates were then saturated by spraying with the enzyme stock solution (6.71 U/mL) and incubated in a humidified chamber for 20 min at 37 °C. Afterwards, the enzyme activity was detected by spraying with the mixture solution containing a part of 13.8 mM of 1-naphthyl acetate in ethanol plus four parts of 5.27 mM of Fast Blue B salt in distilled water, onto the moist TLC plates. The presence of potential compounds with anti-AChE activity was determined as the appearance of white (clear) spot on the purple-coloured background.

Cell culture and treatments

Immortalized mouse hippocampal HT22 cell line, a kind gift from Prof. David Schubert at the Salk Institute (San Diego, CA, USA), was grown in DMEM supplemented with 10% FBS and 1% Penicillin/Streptomycin solution. The cells were maintained at 37 °C in a 5% CO_2 humidified incubator and sub-cultured when they reach about 80–90% confluency. For cell viability assay, HT22 cells were seeded onto a 96-well microtiter plate at a density of 6×10^3 cells per well and allowed to attach. Twenty-four hours later, the cells were incubated for additional 18 h with the medium in the absence or presence of 5 mM glutamate or in the presence of 5 mM glutamate plus various concentrations of tested extracts.

Determination of cell viability

The cell viability of HT22 cells was measured by the MTT colourimetric assay to determine the neuroprotective property of tested extracts against glutamate cytotoxicity. In the assay, untreated HT22 cells served as a negative control, while cells treated with 100% DMSO served as a positive control. MTT was prepared as a stock solution of 5 mg/ml in PBS, pH 7.2, sterilized through a 0.2-μm filter, and stored at − 20 °C. At the end of incubation time, 20 μL of MTT solution was added to each well, followed by incubation at 37 °C for 4 h. The medium containing MTT solution was then removed and 100 μL of DMSO was replaced in each well to dissolve the purple formazan crystals produced from viable cells. The absorbance was read by a microplate reader (BioTek Instruments, Winooski, VT, USA) at 550 nm. The percentage of cell viability was calculated by the following formula: Cell viability (%) = [Abs of treated cells/ Abs of untreated cells (control)] × 100.

Statistical evaluation

For antioxidant and cell viability assays, the experiments were performed at least in triplicate and the data are represented as means ± standard deviation (SD) or means ± standard error of the mean (SEM) as indicated in figures. The statistical analyses were performed using SPSS software version 17.0 (SPSS Inc., Chicago, IL, USA). Pearson's correlation test was conducted to evaluate the relationship between two antioxidant assays. One-way analysis of variance (ANOVA), followed by the post hoc Tukey HSD multiple comparison tests was employed to determine the differences among group means. P values < 0.05 were considered statistically significant.

Results

Extraction yields and the chemical composition of the *S. asper* fractions obtained by acid-base extraction

Acid-base extraction of 29.44 g of the *S. asper* ethanolic leaf extract yielded 0.158 g (0.54%, *w*/w) of basic fraction, 0.476 g (1.62%, w/w) of acidic fraction, and 1.128 g (3.83%, w/w) of neutral fraction. Figure 2 shows the color of crude leaf extract and the fractions obtained. The brownish and yellowish colors observed in the

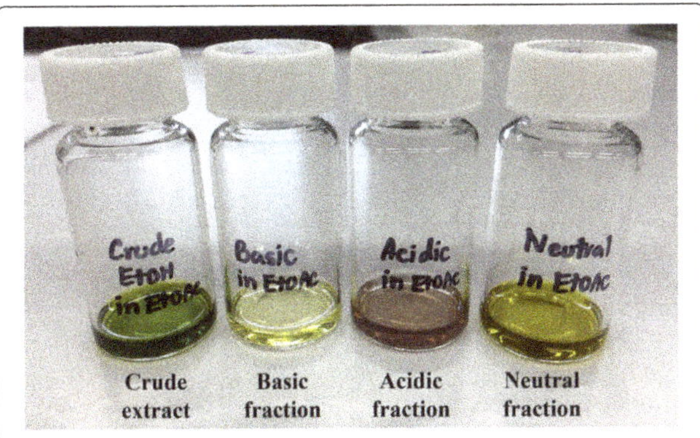

Fig. 2 Crude ethanolic extract of *S. asper* leaves and its acid-base fractions

acid-base fractions suggested that most of the chlorophyll (green pigment) in the leaves was successfully removed from crude leaf extract. Each fraction was further analyzed by GC-MS and tentative compounds were identified by comparing their GC retention indices and mass spectral patterns with the database at the match quality value above 80%. A total of 11 tentative volatile compounds were proposed including terpenoids, steroids, phenolics, fatty acids, nitrogen-sulfur containing compounds, as well as lipidic plant hormone were listed in Table 1.

Antibacterial activity of the *S. asper* fractions

The antibacterial activity of the crude *S. asper* ethanolic extract and its acid-base fractions are presented in Table 2. Amongst the three fractions examined, the acidic fraction exhibited the strongest antibacterial activity against two gram-positive bacteria *S. aureus* and *B. subtilis*, with a MIC value of 125 μg/mL. However, at the highest tested concentration of 1000 μg/mL, none of the three fractions showed inhibition of bacterial growth at ≥95% against the two gram-negative bacteria *E. coli* and *P. aeruginosa*.

Antioxidant capacity of the *S. asper* fractions

The DPPH radical scavenging activities at 1 mg/mL concentration of the crude *S. asper* ethanolic extract and its acid-base fractions varied ranging from 8.94 to 17.16% (10.00 to 18.88 mg VCEAC/g dry weight), whereas their scavenging activities on ABTS radical were found much higher than those on DPPH radical in the range of 34.29 to 48.45% (29.02 to 39.45 mg VCEAC/g dry weight) (Table 3). All the crude extract and its acid-base fractions exhibited concentration-dependent scavenging effects towards the DPPH (Fig. 3a) and ABTS radicals (Fig. 3b). Amongst all the extract and three fractions examined, the acidic fraction possessed the strongest antioxidant capacity, while the neutral fraction showed relatively weak antioxidant property based on the results from both DPPH and ABTS assays. The descending order of antioxidant potential among three isolated fractions was as acidic > basic > neutral. Pearson's correlation revealed a significant positive moderate relationship ($r = 0.7275$, $p = 0.0014$) between the DPPH and ABTS antioxidant activities of all tested samples (Fig. 3c).

Neuroprotective activity of the *S. asper* fractions

The neuroprotective properties of the crude *S. asper* ethanolic extract and its acid-base fractions were evaluated against glutamate toxicity in hippocampal neuronal HT22 cells. The crude extract, neutral and acidic fractions did not exhibit a noticeable cytotoxic effect on HT22 cells whose cell viabilities were above 90% following exposure to varying concentrations ranging from 1 to 50 μg/mL (Fig. 4a). The basic fraction became toxic to the cells when the concentration was increased above 25 μg/mL. Treatment of HT22 cells with 5 mM glutamate significantly reduced cell viability by approximately 80%. However, co-treatment with crude extract, either neutral fraction or basic fraction significantly increased the viability of glutamate-treated HT22 cells in a dose-dependent manner, as determined using MTT assay (Fig. 4b) and examined morphologically under a phase contrast microscope (Fig. 4c). The cytotoxic effect of glutamate could be considerably restored (comparable to about 80% of the control level) in the presence of the crude extract, neutral fraction, and the basic fraction at the minimum concentration of 25, 5, and 10 μg/mL, respectively. The acidic fraction did not show any protective effects against glutamate-induced cytotoxicity.

Anti-acetylcholinesterase activity of the *S. asper* fractions

TLC chromatogram of the neutral fraction isolated at least 9 visible spots of constituents under visible light (Fig. 5a) and confirmed by visualizing under short-wavelength UV radiation (254 nm), in which three of them were also observed by $KMnO_4$ staining (Fig. 5b). However, in the acidic fraction, there was only one spot visible under visible light (Fig. 5a), while three more spots could be only viewed under UV light, in which one of them was also observed by $KMnO_4$ staining (Fig. 5b). Using a similar solvent system to that employed in the experiment mentioned above, the AChE inhibitory properties of the neutral and acidic fractions were further evaluated on TLC plates by the bioautographic method and are shown in Fig. 5c. In this assay, the white spot of inhibition on a dark purple background of the plate represented the chemical components with AChE inhibitory activity. A total of three chemical constituents corresponding to AChE inhibitory activity in the neutral and acidic fractions were found. TLC bioautogram of the neutral fraction showed one spot of inhibition with

Table 1 GC-MS analysis of the volatile components presented in the *S. asper* fractions

Fraction	Retention time (min)	Relative area (%)	Tentative identification	Match quality (%)
Neutral	6.111	2.6	Dihydroactinidiolide	94
	6.548	5.5	Cadalene	80
	6.696	11.7	n.i.	–
	7.124	7.0	Benzothiazole, 2-(2-hydroxyethylthio)-	99
	7.466	5.9	n.i.	–
	8.370	9.4	Cholest-14-en-3-ol, 4-methyl-, (3.beta.,4.alpha.,5.alpha.)-	93
	8.417	10.8	n.i.	–
	8.612	7.4	2,4-Bis(1-phenylethyl)phenol	86
	10.072	7.3	n.i.	–
Acidic	5.531	0.6	4-Hydroxybenzaldehyde	91
	5.683	0.2	Vanillin	96
	6.477	0.3	(+/–)-Jasmonic acid	95
	6.543	3.6	Cadalene	83
	6.686	3.1	n.i.	–
	7.010	2.2	Palmitic acid	99
	7.114	6.9	Benzothiazole, 2-(2-hydroxyethylthio)-	98
	7.457	12.6	Linolenic acid	99
	7.485	8.5	n.i.	–
	8.355	6.8	Cholest-14-en-3-ol, 4-methyl-, (3.beta.,4.alpha.,5.alpha.)-	91
	8.398	7.2	n.i.	–
	8.593	5.8	2,4-Bis(1-phenylethyl)phenol	93
Basic	5.421	1.6	n.i.	–
	6.543	2.2	Phenol, 2-(1-phenylethyl)-	91
	6.686	30.1	n.i.	–
	6.762	4.9	n.i.	–
	7.109	6.0	Benzothiazole, 2-(2-hydroxyethylthio)-	99
	7.295	8.2	n.i.	–
	7.471	12.4	n.i.	–
	8.350	4.2	n.i.	–
	8.398	4.6	n.i.	–
	8.588	3.3	Phenol, 2,4-bis(1-phenylethyl)-	91

n.i. Not identified

Table 2 Antibacterial activities of crude ethanolic extract of *S. asper* leaves and its fractions against a range of microorganisms determined by the broth microdilution method

Microorganisms	Minimum inhibitory concentration (MIC) in μg/mL			
	Crude extract	Neutral fraction	Acidic fraction	Basic fraction
Gram-positive bacteria				
Staphylococcus aureus (ATCC25923)	1000	1000	125	1000
Bacillus subtilis (SU5)	1000	250	125	500
Gram-negative bacteria				
Escherichia coli (MG1655)	> 1000	> 1000	> 1000	> 1000
Pseudomonas aeruginosa (PA14)	> 1000	> 1000	> 1000	> 1000

MIC values are the lowest concentrations at which at least 95% bacterial growth reduction
The tested concentration of samples ranged from 125 to 1000 μg/mL

Table 3 Antioxidant capacities of the crude ethanolic extract of *S. asper* leaves and its fractions determined by the DPPH and ABTS scavenging assays

Sample	DPPH scavenging assay		ABTS scavenging assay	
	%Radical Scavenging activity (of 1 mg/mL sample)	mg VCEAC/g dry weight sample	%Radical Scavenging activity (of 1 mg/mL sample)	mg VCEAC/g dry weight sample
Crude extract	16.58 ± 1.33^{a}	18.37 ± 1.25^{a}	37.69 ± 1.81^{a}	31.52 ± 1.63^{a}
Neutral fraction	8.94 ± 0.78^{b}	10.63 ± 1.38^{b}	34.29 ± 1.56^{b}	29.02 ± 1.43^{b}
Acidic fraction	17.16 ± 1.74^{a}	18.88 ± 1.39^{a}	48.45 ± 1.55^{c}	39.45 ± 1.43^{c}
Basic fraction	8.94 ± 1.62^{b}	10.00 ± 0.77^{b}	39.23 ± 0.66^{a}	32.66 ± 0.84^{a}

Results are expressed as mean ± SD of at least three replicates
Different superscript letters in the same column indicate a significant difference between the means by one-way ANOVA ($p < 0.05$) and the same letter indicates that there is no statistical difference

R_f value of 0.44 and positive staining for $KMnO_4$ (Fig. 5b and c). TLC bioautogram of the acidic fraction showed two spots of inhibition with R_f values of 0.15 and 0.55. The spot with R_f 0.15 was also positively stained with $KMnO_4$ (Fig. 5b and c).

Discussion

The current available medications can only reduce the severity of AD in certain patient groups, since there has been no complete cure known for it. Importantly, AD can be fatal and is now recognized as one of the major global health problems [24]. Therefore, its prevalence continues to rise rapidly, along with the burden on public healthcare costs. This has a long-term impact on the socio-economic development of the developing countries. In challenging this difficult situation, a number of researchers have put a considerable effort for decades in search of alternative treatment methods. Research in the

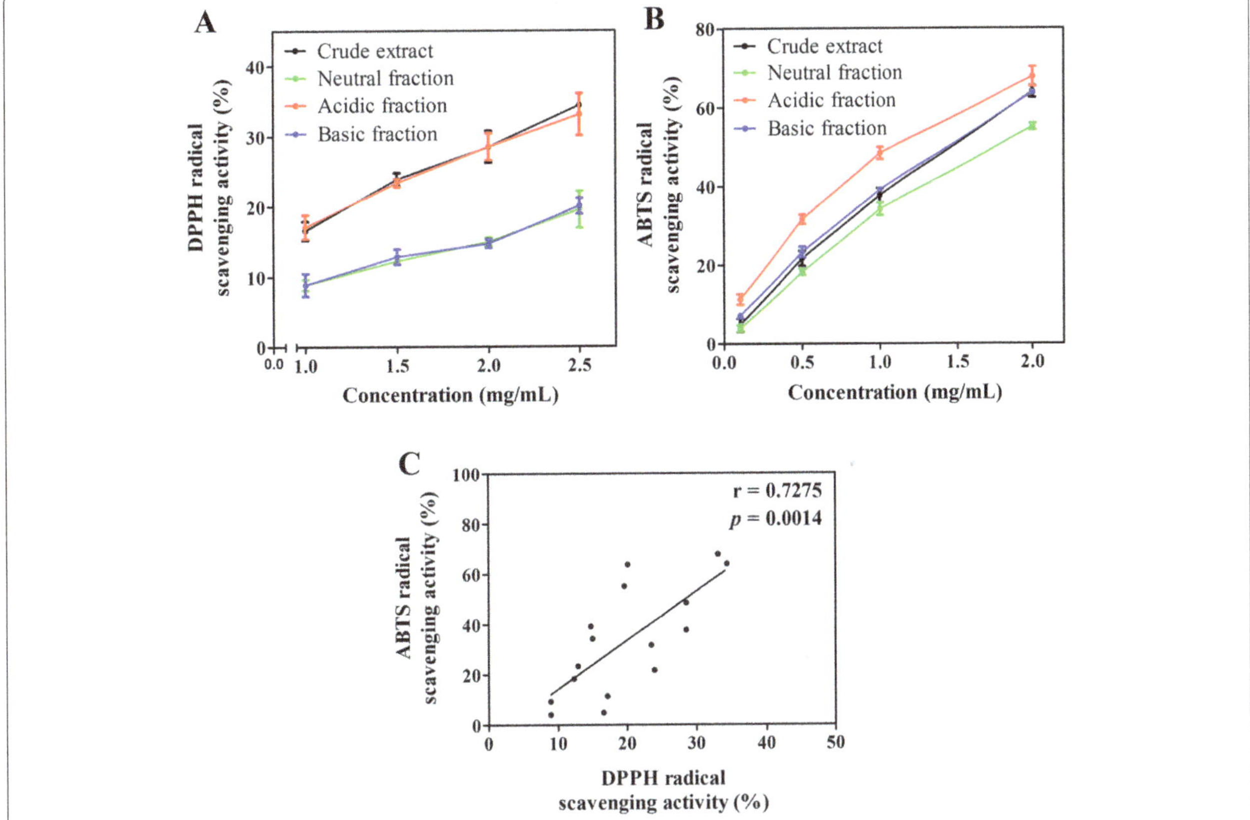

Fig. 3 The dose-response scavenging effects of the crude ethanolic extract of *S. asper* leaves and its fractions on **a** DPPH and **b** ABTS free radicals. Data are expressed as means ± SD of 3–7 replicates. **c** Pearson's correlation analysis between DPPH and ABTS scavenging activities based on mean values of all samples analyzed

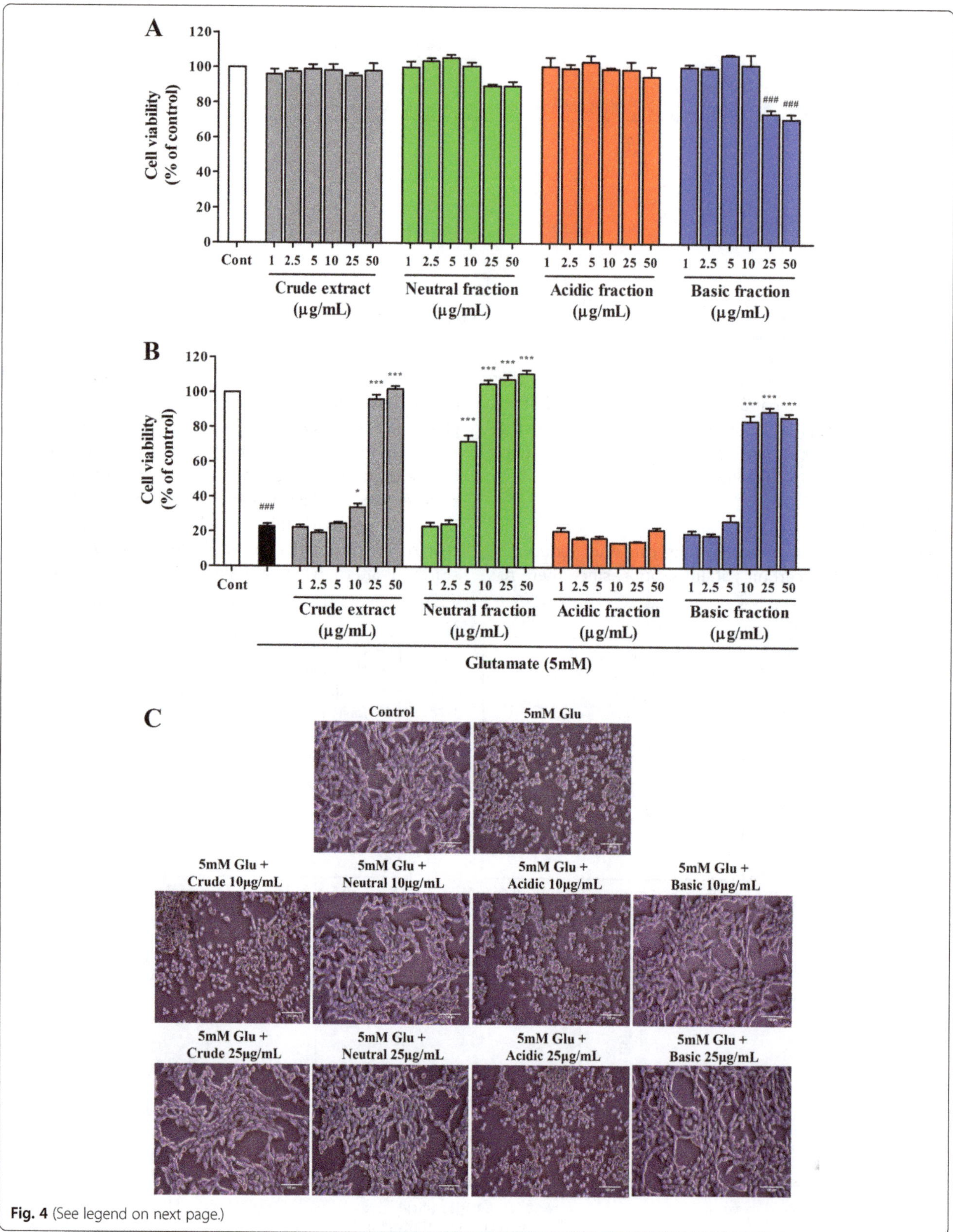

Fig. 4 (See legend on next page.)

(See figure on previous page.)
Fig. 4 Protective effects of the crude ethanolic extract of *S. asper* leaves and its fractions against glutamate-induced neuronal cell death. **a** Relative MTT viability of HT22 cells exposed to various concentrations of extracts. $^{###}P = 8.8 \times 10^{-5}$ for 25 μg/mL and $^{###}P = 7.5 \times 10^{-6}$ for 50 μg/mL of basic fraction vs. control. **b** Relative MTT viability of HT22 cells exposed to glutamate alone or glutamate combined with different concentrations of extracts. $^{###}P = 2.9 \times 10^{-11}$ vs. control; $^{*}P = 3.1 \times 10^{-2}$ and $^{***}P = 2.9 \times 10^{-11}$ vs. glutamate-treated cells. **c** Representative morphological images at 5X magnification (scale bar = 100 μm) of untreated HT22 cells (control), or cells treated with glutamate alone, or with glutamate plus crude extract or fractions at 1 and 10 μg/mL. Data are expressed as means ± SEM of 4 independent experiments with 2–3 replicates each

field of herbal medicines has attracted much attention in recent years, as it is believed to have advantages over modern synthetic medicines with regard to efficacy, safety, and cost for treatment of various medical problems. In Southeast-Asian countries, *S. asper* is a well-known medicinal plant that has been traditionally used for a variety of illness conditions despite limited scientific evidence [44–46]. Interestingly, the ethanolic leaf extracts of this plant have shown pharmacological properties including antibacterial, neuroprotective, and cognitive-improving effects that can be beneficial for the treatment of AD [48, 53, 54]. However, the active constituents responsible for those different activities have not been clearly identified. In this study, the *S. asper* leaf ethanolic extract was fractionated into fractions based on pH properties and further evaluated for their antibacterial, antioxidant, anti-AChE, and neuroprotective activities. These biological activities could enhance the therapeutic applications and facilitating activity-guided isolation of active compounds of the *S. asper* extract in the near future.

S. asper is commonly used to treat skin infections (e.g. boils, leprosy, and wounds) and has beneficial role for oral health and hygiene (e.g. relief of toothache, antigingivatis, and strengthening teeth and gum) [44]. The bacterial species, which are most frequently found associated with AD, are commonly found in oral cavities such as spirochetes [42] and actinobacteria [41], thus it is tempting us to investigate the antibacterial properties of this plant. In this study, the crude ethanolic extract was found to inhibit cell growth of gram-positive bacteria, *S. aureus* and *B. subtilis*. This effect was more profound when the extract was fractionated to the acidic fraction (MIC of 125 μg/mL) with at least eight-fold higher than to ethanol crude extract. Neither the ethanol extract nor acid-base fractions inhibit the growth of gram-negative bacteria, *E. coli* and *P. aeruginosa*. Previous work by Wongkam et al. on the crude 50% ethanolic extract, reported no antibacterial activity when tested on the bacteria strains used in our study. Their study instead showed weak MIC and MBC of 1.93 mg/mL against *Streptococcus mutans, Porphyromonas gingivalis, and Actinobacillus actinomycetemcomitans;* bacteria that are commonly associated with dental caries and gingivitis [48, 58, 59]. The source of plant collection and the percentage of ethanol used for extraction may be the critical factors for the different findings. Although gram-negative bacteria are generally more harmful, some

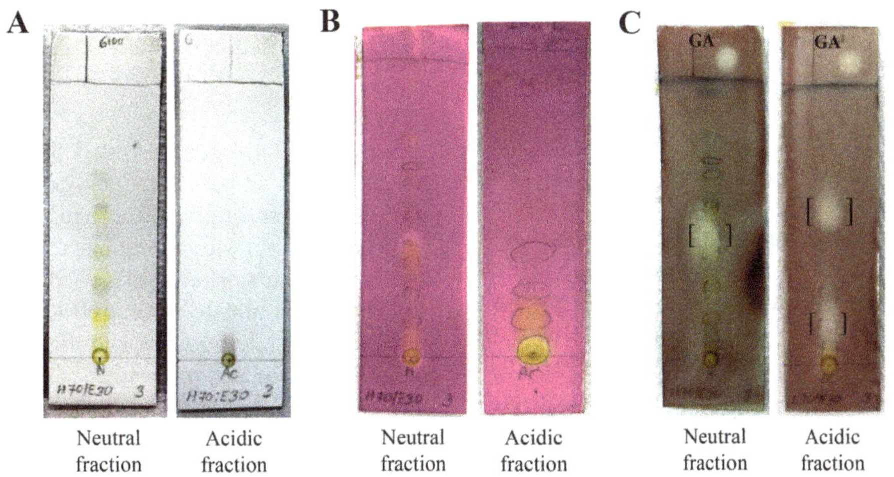

Fig. 5 Anti-AChE activities of neutral and acidic fractions obtained from *S. asper* leaves. TLC chromatograms of neutral and acidic fractions (at 6.7 μg application) in a solvent system of hexane:ethyl acetate (7:3, *v/v*) were observed **a** under visible light, **b** by staining with $KMnO_4$, and **c** by bioautographic method for screening on AChE inhibitory activity, where white spots against the dark background represent the inhibition. Galantamine (GA) was used as a positive control at 0.3 μg. Brackets indicate AChE inhibiting constituents

of the gram-positive bacteria can also be pathogenic in humans. *S. aureus* is one of the most common causes of skin and nosocomial infections as well as other infections at various sites of the body (e.g. bone, joint, lung, and gastrointestinal tract) with symptoms ranging from minor to life-threatening [60]. Here, our study provides supporting evidence for the use of acidic fraction from SA leaves to treat gram-positive bacterial infections particularly caused by *S. aureus*. Moreover, the promising antibacterial activity of the acidic fraction relative to other fractions could be contributed by the action of its major volatile component, linolenic acid (Table 1, [54]). It has been demonstrated that long-chain unsaturated fatty acids including linolenic acid exerted highly potent activity against gram-positive bacteria [61–64].

Free radicals are groups of atoms with an unpaired number of electrons residing in the outermost shell. The majority of free radicals are generated from oxygen molecules and called reactive oxygen species (ROS). Once formed in excess, these highly reactive free radicals can cause damage, in the process called oxidative stress, to important cellular components such as lipids, proteins and nucleic acids, subsequently, alter the structures and functions that are associated with various human diseases including AD [65]. In general, these detrimental effects of free radicals can be counterbalanced by antioxidants, which are naturally derived from plants. *S. asper* can be considered as an alternative source for antioxidants since this plant has been shown promising antioxidant properties in both in vitro and in vivo [54, 66–70]. In line with the previous reports, our present study also revealed the antioxidant properties, like free radical scavenging, in *S. asper* leaf extracts. The ethanol crude extract, neutral, acidic and basic fractions exhibited relatively two- to four-fold higher activities in the ABTS assay than in the DPPH assay and the percentage of scavenging activities determined in both assays were moderately correlated ($r = 0.73$). The slight difference in results could be probably due to the distinct solubility of tested substances in water, as hydrophilic antioxidants were found better reflected by the ABTS than the DPPH assay [71, 72]. Interestingly, after fractionation of crude ethanolic leaf extract, the scavenging activities on DPPH and ABTS radicals were found significantly higher in the acidic fraction when compared to the crude extract and other fractions, while the neutral fraction showed the lowest antioxidant capacity in both assays. These findings suggest that the components with antiradical activity in *S. asper* leaves are majorly in acidic and water-soluble forms. Nevertheless, the DPPH and ABTS radicals used in this study are uncommonly found in the human body, the antioxidant capacity has to be further investigated using ROS, which are produced as by-products during cellular metabolism such as superoxide radicals ($O_2{\bullet}-$), hydrogen peroxide (H_2O_2), or highly reactive hydroxyl radicals ($OH{\bullet}$) for a better idea.

In an effort to develop a more effective treatment for AD, several studies have been searching for new therapeutic targets underlying the disease pathology. Apart from the cholinergic hypothesis that has been proposed in the etiology of AD for several decades [73], growing evidence links oxidative glutamate toxicity (or oxytosis) to AD by supporting that glutamate-induced neuronal cell death via non-receptor-mediated oxidative toxicity pathway involves in the pathogenic mechanism of neurodegeneration [74–76]. Hence, targeting towards the glutamate-mediated oxidative toxicity pathway may offer a new approach for treating AD as well as other neurodegenerative diseases. In accordance with our previous results, the present study demonstrated that crude ethanolic extract from *S. asper* leaves exerted neuroprotective property against glutamate-induced HT22 neuronal cell death [54]. This protective activity was also found higher following fractionation of crude ethanolic leaf extract. The strongest protective activity against glutamate toxicity in HT22 cells was observed in the neutral fraction, wherein the minimum concentration showing recovery of 80% cell viability was five-fold lower than that of the crude extract. Interestingly, TLC bioautography also suggested that neutral fraction contains at least one compound with AChE inhibitory activity with minimum inhibitory concentration requirement of approximately 6.7 μg. Therefore, this finding indicates that neutral fraction can be further developed as a potential multi-target agent for AD treatment. However, due to the weak antiradical activity of neutral fraction, it may exert neuroprotective capacity against glutamate-induced oxidative damage via other antioxidative mechanisms. For instance, induction of nuclear translocation of nuclear factor erythroid 2-related factor 2 (Nrf2) is a protective pathway proposed in our previous work [54].

Conclusions

Our findings have demonstrated the therapeutic potential of three acid-base fractions extracted from the leaf part of *S. asper* as promising natural source for neuroprotective agents with additional actions of antibacterials and antioxidants, along with AChE inhibitors. Further studies should aim to isolate bioactive substances from neutral and acidic fractions and identify the mechanisms underlying their actions, which can be used to develop new natural agents as therapeutic drugs for the treatment of AD.

Abbreviations

ABTS: 2,2′-Azino-bis(3-ethylbenzothiazoline-6-sulfonic acid) diammonium salt; AChE: Acetylcholinesterase; AD: Alzheimer's disease; DPPH: 2,2-Diphenyl-1-picrylhydrazyl; GC-MS: Gas chromatography-mass spectrometry; MIC: Minimum inhibitory concentration; MTT: 3-(4,5-dimetylthiazol-2-yl)-2,5-

diphenyltetrazoliumbromide; NMDA: *N*-methyl-D-aspartate; Nrf2: Nuclear factor erythroid 2-related factor 2; TLC: Thin-layer chromatography; VCEAC: Vitamin C equivalent antioxidant capacity

Acknowledgements
The authors are very grateful to the Princess Maha Chakri Sirindhorn Herbal Garden (Rayong Province, Thailand) for providing plant material, to Prof. David Schubert (The Salk Institute, San Diego, CA, USA) for his generous gift of HT22 cells and to Dr. Prasanth M. Iyer for his kind help in language editing. We are grateful to the Faculty of Science, UTS for providing support to this project.

Funding
This work was financially supported by the 90th anniversary of Chulalongkorn University fund. AP was supported by a Chulalongkorn University Graduate Scholarship to commemorate the 72nd Anniversary of His Majesty King Bhumibol Adulyadej, an Overseas Research Experience Scholarship for Graduate Student by the Graduate School, Chulalongkorn University, and a Grant for Joint Funding, Ratchadaphiseksomphot Endowment Fund. The study conducted by AP for 6 months in School of Mathematical and Physical Sciences, UTS was supported by the University of Technology of Sydney.

Authors' contributions
AU and TT designed the research study, supervised, and corrected the manuscript. AP, AT, and MP performed the experiments. AP analyzed data and wrote the manuscript. All authors approved the final version of the manuscript.

Competing interests
The authors declared that they have no competing interests.

Author details
[1]Program in Clinical Biochemistry and Molecular Medicine, Department of Clinical Chemistry, Faculty of Allied Health Sciences, Chulalongkorn University, Bangkok 10330, Thailand. [2]School of Mathematical and Physical Sciences, Faculty of Science, The University of Technology Sydney, Sydney, NSW 2007, Australia. [3]Age-Related Inflammation and Degeneration Research Unit, Department of Clinical Chemistry, Faculty of Allied Health Sciences, Chulalongkorn University, Bangkok 10330, Thailand.

References

1. Ubel PA, Abernethy AP, Zafar SY. Full disclosure--out-of-pocket costs as side effects. N Engl J Med. 2013;369(16):1484–6.
2. Wang Z, Liu X, Ho RL, Lam CW, Chow MS. Precision or personalized medicine for Cancer chemotherapy: is there a role for herbal medicine. Molecules. 2016;21(7)
3. Augustine NR, Madhavan G, Nass SJ (Eds). Committee on Ensuring Patient Access to Affordable Drug Therapies; Board on Health Care Services; Health and Medicine Division; National Academies of Sciences, Engineering, and Medicine, Making Medicines Affordable A National Imperative. Washington (DC): National Academies Press (US); 2017.
4. Kroger E, Mouls M, Wilchesky M, Berkers M, Carmichael PH, van Marum R, et al. Adverse drug reactions reported with cholinesterase inhibitors: an analysis of 16 years of individual case safety reports from VigiBase. Ann Pharmacother 2015; 49(11):1197–1206.
5. Shehab N, Patel PR, Srinivasan A, Budnitz DS. Emergency department visits for antibiotic-associated adverse events. Clin Infect Dis. 2008;47(6):735–43.
6. Cummings JL, Morstorf T, Zhong K. Alzheimer's disease drug-development pipeline: few candidates, frequent failures. Alzheimers Res Ther. 2014;6(4):37.
7. Hung SY, Fu WM. Drug candidates in clinical trials for Alzheimer's disease. J Biomed Sci. 2017;24(1):47.
8. Ventola CL. The antibiotic resistance crisis: part 1: causes and threats. P T. 2015;40(4):277–83.
9. Ventola CL. The antibiotic resistance crisis: part 2: management strategies and new agents. P T. 2015;40(5):344–52.
10. Rex JH, Talbot GH, Goldberger MJ, Eisenstein BI, Echols RM, Tomayko JF, et al. Progress in the fight against multidrug-resistant Bacteria 2005-2016: modern noninferiority trial designs enable antibiotic development in advance of epidemic bacterial resistance. Clin Infect Dis 2017; 65(1):141–146.
11. Newman DJ, Cragg GM. Natural products as sources of new drugs from 1981 to 2014. J Nat Prod. 2016;79(3):629–61.
12. Owen L, Laird K. Synchronous application of antibiotics and essential oils: dual mechanisms of action as a potential solution to antibiotic resistance. Crit Rev Microbiol. 2018:1–22.
13. Akhondzadeh S, Abbasi SH. Herbal medicine in the treatment of Alzheimer's disease. Am J Alzheimers Dis Other Demen. 2006;21(2):113–8.
14. Tian J, Shi J, Zhang X, Wang Y. Herbal therapy: a new pathway for the treatment of Alzheimer's disease. Alzheimers Res Ther. 2010;2(5):30.
15. Yang WT, Zheng XW, Chen S, Shan CS, Xu QQ, Zhu JZ, et al. Chinese herbal medicine for Alzheimer's disease: clinical evidence and possible mechanism of neurogenesis. Biochem Pharmacol 2017; 141:143–155.
16. Syad AN, Devi K. Botanics: a potential source of new therapies for Alzheimer's disease. Botanics. 2014;4:11–6.
17. Kumar A, Singh A, Aggarwal A. Therapeutic potentials of herbal drugs for Alzheimer's disease - an overview. Indian J Exp Biol. 2017;55:63–73.
18. Zangara A. The psychopharmacology of huperzine a: an alkaloid with cognitive enhancing and neuroprotective properties of interest in the treatment of Alzheimer's disease. Pharmacol Biochem Behav. 2003;75(3):675–86.
19. Mazzanti G, Di Giacomo S. Curcumin and resveratrol in the Management of Cognitive Disorders: what is the clinical evidence? Molecules. 2016;21:9.
20. Suk K. Regulation of neuroinflammation by herbal medicine and its implications for neurodegenerative diseases. A focus on traditional medicines and flavonoids. Neurosignals. 2005;14(1–2):23–33.
21. Hugel HM. Brain food for Alzheimer-free ageing: focus on herbal medicines. Adv Exp Med Biol. 2015;863:95–116.
22. Abushouk AI, Negida A, Ahmed H, Abdel-Daim MM. Neuroprotective mechanisms of plant extracts against MPTP induced neurotoxicity: future applications in Parkinson's disease. Biomed Pharmacother. 2017;85:635–45.
23. Dey A, Bhattacharya R, Mukherjee A, Pandey DK. Natural products against Alzheimer's disease: Pharmaco-therapeutics and biotechnological interventions. Biotechnol Adv. 2017;35(2):178–216.
24. Alzheimer's Association: 2018 Alzheimer's Disease Facts and Figures. https://www.alz.org/media/HomeOffice/Facts%20and%20Figures/facts-and-figures.pdf. Accessed 18 July 2018.
25. Biran Y, Masters CL, Barnham KJ, Bush AI, Adlard PA. Pharmacotherapeutic targets in Alzheimer's disease. J Cell Mol Med. 2009;13(1):61–86.
26. Wenk GL. Neuropathologic changes in Alzheimer's disease: potential targets for treatment. J Clin Psychiatry. 2006;67(Suppl 3):3–7.
27. Lanctot KL, Rajaram RD, Herrmann N. Therapy for Alzheimer's disease: how effective are current treatments? Ther Adv Neurol Disord. 2009;2(3):163–80.
28. Casey DA, Antimisiaris D, O'Brien J. Drugs for Alzheimer's disease: are they effective? P T. 2010;35(4):208.
29. Bond M, Rogers G, Peters J, Anderson R, Hoyle M, Miners A, et al. The effectiveness and cost-effectiveness of donepezil, galantamine, rivastigmine and memantine for the treatment of Alzheimer's disease (review of technology appraisal no. 111): a systematic review and economic model. Health Technol Assess. 2012;16(21):1–470.
30. Cacabelos R. Have there been improvements in Alzheimer's disease drug discovery over the past 5 years? Expert Opin Drug Discov. 2018;13(6):523–38.
31. Agostinho P, Cunha RA, Oliveira C. Neuroinflammation, oxidative stress and the pathogenesis of Alzheimer's disease. Curr Pharm Des. 2010;16(25):2766–78.
32. Zotova E, Nicoll JA, Kalaria R, Holmes C, Boche D. Inflammation in Alzheimer's disease: relevance to pathogenesis and therapy. Alzheimers Res Ther. 2010;2(1):1.

33. Zhao Y, Zhao B. Oxidative stress and the pathogenesis of Alzheimer's disease. Oxidative Med Cell Longev. 2013;2013:316523.
34. Bibi F, Yasir M, Sohrab SS, Azhar EI, Al-Qahtani MH, Abuzenadah AM, et al. Link between chronic bacterial inflammation and Alzheimer disease. CNS Neurol Disord Drug Targets 2014; 13(7):1140–1147.
35. Itzhaki RF, Lathe R, Balin BJ, Ball MJ, Bearer EL, Braak H, et al. Microbes and Alzheimer's disease. J Alzheimers Dis 2016; 51(4):979–984.
36. Miklossy J, McGeer PL. Common mechanisms involved in Alzheimer's disease and type 2 diabetes: a key role of chronic bacterial infection and inflammation. Aging (Albany NY). 2016;8(4):575–88.
37. Soscia SJ, Kirby JE, Washicosky KJ, Tucker SM, Ingelsson M, Hyman B, et al. The Alzheimer's disease-associated amyloid beta-protein is an antimicrobial peptide. PLoS One 2010; 5(3):e9505.
38. Kumar DK, Choi SH, Washicosky KJ, Eimer WA, Tucker S, Ghofrani J, et al. Amyloid-beta peptide protects against microbial infection in mouse and worm models of Alzheimer's disease. Sci Transl Med 2016; 8(340):340ra372.
39. Harach T, Marungruang N, Duthilleul N, Cheatham V, Mc Coy KD, Frisoni G, et al. Reduction of Abeta amyloid pathology in APPPS1 transgenic mice in the absence of gut microbiota. Sci Rep 2017; 7:41802.
40. Minter MR, Hinterleitner R, Meisel M, Zhang C, Leone V, Zhang X, et al. Antibiotic-induced perturbations in microbial diversity during post-natal development alters amyloid pathology in an aged APPSWE/PS1DeltaE9 murine model of Alzheimer's disease. Sci Rep 2017; 7(1):10411.
41. Emery DC, Shoemark DK, Batstone TE, Waterfall CM, Coghill JA, Cerajewska TL, et al. 16S rRNA next generation sequencing analysis shows Bacteria in Alzheimer's post-mortem brain. Front Aging Neurosci 2017; 9:195.
42. Allen HB. Alzheimer's disease: assessing the role of spirochetes, biofilms, the immune system, and amyloid-beta with regard to potential treatment and prevention. J Alzheimers Dis. 2016;53(4):1271–6.
43. Hefendehl JK, LeDue J, Ko RW, Mahler J, Murphy TH, MacVicar BA. Mapping synaptic glutamate transporter dysfunction in vivo to regions surrounding Abeta plaques by iGluSnFR two-photon imaging. Nat Commun. 2016;7:13441.
44. Rastogi S, Kulshreshtha DK, Rawat AK. Streblus asper Lour. (Shakhotaka): a review of its chemical, pharmacological and Ethnomedicinal properties. Evid Based Complement Alternat Med. 2006;3(2):217–22.
45. Verma NK, Singh SP, Singh AP, Singh R, Rai PK, Tripathi AK. A brief study on Strebulus asper L.-a review. RJP. 2015;1(2):65–71.
46. Luanchoy S, Tiangkul S, Wongkrajang Y, Temsiririrkkul R, Peungvicha P, Nakornchai S. Antioxidant activity of a Thai traditional formula for longevity. Mahidol J Pharm Sci. 2014;41:1–5.
47. Ren Y, Chen W-L, Lantvit DD, Sass EJ, Shriwas P, Ninh TN, et al. Cardiac glycoside constituents of Streblus asper with potential antineoplastic activity. J Nat Prod 2016; 80(3):648–658.
48. Wongkham S, Laupattarakasaem P, Pienthaweechai K, Areejitranusorn P, Wongkham C, Techanitiswad T. Antimicrobial activity of Streblus asper leaf extract. Phytother Res. 2001;15(2):119–21.
49. Das MK, Beuria MK. Anti-malarial property of an extract of the plant Streblus asper in murine malaria. Trans R Soc Trop Med Hyg. 1991;85(1):40–1.
50. Chatterjee RK, Fatma N, Murthy PK, Sinha P, Kulshrestha DK, Dhawan BN. Macrofilaricidal activity of the stembark of Streblus asper and its major active constituents. Drug Dev Res. 1992;26(1):67–78.
51. Sripanidkulchai B, Junlatat J, Wara-aswapati N, Hormdee D. Anti-inflammatory effect of Streblus asper leaf extract in rats and its modulation on inflammation-associated genes expression in RAW 264.7 macrophage cells. J Ethnopharmacol. 2009;124(3):566–70.
52. Li J, Huang Y, Guan XL, Li J, Deng SP, Wu Q, et al. Anti-hepatitis B virus constituents from the stem bark of Streblus asper. Phytochemistry 2012; 82:100–109.
53. Singsai K, Akaravichien T, Kukongviriyapan V, Sattayasai J. Protective effects of Streblus asper leaf extract on H2O2-induced ROS in SK-N-SH cells and MPTP-induced Parkinson's disease-like symptoms in C57BL/6 mouse. Evid Based Complement Alternat Med. 2015;2015:970354–9.
54. Prasansuklab A, Meemon K, Sobhon P, Tencomnao T. Ethanolic extract of Streblus asper leaves protects against glutamate-induced toxicity in HT22 hippocampal neuronal cells and extends lifespan of Caenorhabditis elegans. BMC Complement Altern Med. 2017;17(1):551.
55. Iriyama K, Ogura N. Takamiya a. A simple method for extraction and partial purification of chlorophyll from plant material, using dioxane. J Biochem. 1974;76(4):901–4.
56. Mungkornasawakul P, Pyne SG, Jatisatienr A, Supyen D, Lie W, Ung AT, et al. Stemocurtisine, the first pyrido[1,2-a]azapine Stemona alkaloid. J Nat Prod 2003; 66(7):980–982.
57. Marston A, Kissling J, Hostettmann K. A rapid TLC bioautographic method for the detection of acetylcholinesterase and butyrylcholinesterase inhibitors in plants. Phytochem Anal. 2002;13(1):51–4.
58. Taweechaisupapong S, Wongkham S, Chareonsuk S, Suparee S, Srilalai P, Chaiyarak S. Selective activity of Streblus asper on Mutans streptococci. J Ethnopharmacol. 2000;70(1):73–9.
59. Taweechaisupapong S, Singhara S, Choopan T. Effect of Streblus asper leaf extract on selected anaerobic Bacteria. In: ISHS Acta Horticulturae 680: III WOCMAP congress on medicinal and aromatic plants, Vol. 6. Traditional medicine and nutraceuticals; 2005. p. 177–81.
60. Tong SY, Davis JS, Eichenberger E, Holland TL, Fowler VG, Jr. Staphylococcus aureus infections: epidemiology, pathophysiology, clinical manifestations, and management. Clin Microbiol Rev 2015; 28(3):603–661.
61. Zheng CJ, Yoo JS, Lee TG, Cho HY, Kim YH, Kim WG. Fatty acid synthesis is a target for antibacterial activity of unsaturated fatty acids. FEBS Lett. 2005;579(23):5157–62.
62. Asthana RK, Srivastava A, Kayastha AM, Nath G, Singh SP. Antibacterial potential of γ-linolenic acid from Fischerella sp. colonizing neem tree bark. World J Microbiol Biotechnol. 2006;22(5):443–8.
63. Huang CB, George B, Ebersole JL. Antimicrobial activity of n-6, n-7 and n-9 fatty acids and their esters for oral microorganisms. Arch Oral Biol. 2010;55(8):555–60.
64. Desbois AP, Lawlor KC. Antibacterial activity of long-chain polyunsaturated fatty acids against Propionibacterium acnes and Staphylococcus aureus. Mar Drugs. 2013;11(11):4544–57.
65. Smith MA, Rottkamp CA, Nunomura A, Raina AK, Perry G. Oxidative stress in Alzheimer's disease. Biochim Biophys Acta. 2000;1502(1):139–44.
66. Gadidasu K, Reddy ARN, Umate P, Reddy YN. Antioxidant and anti-diabetic activities from leaf extracts of Streblus asper Lour. Biotechnol Ind J. 2009;3(4):231–5.
67. Ibrahim NM, Mat I, Lim V, Ahmad R. Antioxidant activity and phenolic content of Streblus asper leaves from various drying methods. Antioxidants (Basel). 2013;2(3):156–66.
68. Kumar RS, Kar B, Dolai N, Bala A, Haldar PK. Evaluation of antihyperglycemic and antioxidant properties of Streblus asper Lour against streptozotocin–induced diabetes in rats. Asian Pac J Trop Dis. 2012;2(2):139–43.
69. Kumar RB, Kar B, Dolai N, Karmakar I, Haldar S, Bhattacharya S, et al. Antitumor activity and antioxidant role of Streblus asper bark against Ehrlich ascites carcinoma in Swiss albino mice. J Exp Ther Oncol 2013; 10(3):197–202.
70. Kumar RB, Kar B, Dolai N, Karmakar I, Bhattacharya S, Haldar PK. Antitumor activity and antioxidant status of Streblus asper bark against Dalton's ascitic lymphoma in mice. Interdiscip Toxicol. 2015;8(3):125–30.
71. Lachman J, Šulc M, Schilla M. Comparison of the total antioxidant status of bohemian wines during the wine-making process. Food Chem. 2007;103(3):802–7.
72. Floegel A, Kim D-O, Chung S-J, Koo SI, Chun OK. Comparison of ABTS/DPPH assays to measure antioxidant capacity in popular antioxidant-rich US foods. J Food Compost Anal. 2011;24(7):1043–8.
73. Craig LA, Hong NS, McDonald RJ. Revisiting the cholinergic hypothesis in the development of Alzheimer's disease. Neurosci Biobehav Rev. 2011;35(6):1397–409.
74. Tan S, Schubert D, Maher P. Oxytosis: a novel form of programmed cell death. Curr Top Med Chem. 2001;1(6):497–506.
75. Sheldon AL, Robinson MB. The role of glutamate transporters in neurodegenerative diseases and potential opportunities for intervention. Neurochem Int. 2007;51(6–7):333–55.
76. Kritis AA, Stamoula EG, Paniskaki KA, Vavilis TD. Researching glutamate - induced cytotoxicity in different cell lines: a comparative/collective analysis/study. Front Cell Neurosci. 2015;9:91.

11

Dendrobium nobile Lindley and its bibenzyl component moscatilin are able to protect retinal cells from ischemia/hypoxia by downregulating placental growth factor and upregulating Norrie disease protein

Wen-Haur Chao[1†], Ming-Yi Lai[1†], Hwai-Tzong Pan[1], Huei-Wen Shiu[1], Mi-Mi Chen[1] and Hsiao-Ming Chao[1,2,3,4*]

Abstract

Background: Presumably, progression of developmental retinal vascular disorders is mainly driven by persistent ischemia/hypoxia. An investigation into vision-threatening retinal ischemia remains important. Our aim was to evaluate, in relation to retinal ischemia, protective effects and mechanisms of Dendrobium nobile Lindley (DNL) and its bibenzyl component moscatilin. The therapeutic mechanisms included evaluations of levels of placental growth factor (PLGF) and Norrie disease protein (NDP).

Methods: An oxygen glucose deprivation (OGD) model involved cells cultured in DMEM containing 1% O_2, 94% N_2 and 0 g/L glucose. High intraocular pressure (HIOP)-induced retinal ischemia was created by increasing IOP to 120 mmHg for 60 min in Wistar rats. The methods included electroretinogram (ERG), histopathology, MTT assay and biochemistry.

Results: When compared with cells cultured in DMEM containing DMSO (DMSO+DMEM), cells subjected to OGD and pre-administrated with DMSO (DMSO+OGD) showed a significant reduction in the cell viability and NDP expression. Moreover, cells that received OGD and 1 h pre-administration of 0.1 μM moscatilin (Pre-OGD Mos 0.1 μM) showed a significant counteraction of the OGD-induced decreased cell viability. Furthermore, compared with the DMSO+OGD group (44.54 ± 3.15%), there was significant elevated NDP levels in the Pre-OGD Mos 0.1 μM group (108.38 ± 29.33%). Additionally, there were significant ischemic alterations, namely reduced ERG b-wave, less numerous retinal ganglion cells, decreased inner retinal thickness, and reduced/enhanced amacrine's ChAT/Müller's GFAP or vimentin immunolabelings. Moreover, there were significantly increased protein levels of HIF-1α, VEGF, PKM2, RBP2 and, particularly, PLGF (pg/ml; Sham vs. Vehicle: 15.11 ± 1.58 vs. 39.53 ± 5.25). These ischemic effects were significantly altered when 1.0 g/Kg/day DNL (DNL1.0 + I/R or I/R+ DNL1.0) was applied before and/or after ischemia, but not vehicle (Vehicle+I/R). Of novelty and significance, the DNL1.0 action mechanism appears to be similar to that of the anti-PLGF Eylea [PLGF (pg/ml); DNL1.0 vs. Eylea+I/R: 19.93 ± 2.24 vs. 6.44 ± 0.60].

(Continued on next page)

* Correspondence: hsiaoming.chao@gmail.com
†Wen-Haur Chao and Ming-Yi Lai contributed equally to this work.
1Institute of Pharmacology, School of Medicine, National Yang-Ming University, Taipei, Taiwan
2Department of Ophthalmology, Cheng Hsin General Hospital, Taipei, Taiwan
Full list of author information is available at the end of the article

(Continued from previous page)
Conclusions: DNL and moscatilin are able to protect against retinal ischemic/hypoxic changes respectively by downregulating PLGF and upregulating NDP. Progression of developmental retinal vascular disorders such as Norrie disease due to persistent ischemia/hypoxia might be thus prevented.

Keywords: Dendrobium nobile Lindley, Moscatilin, Retinal ischemia, Oxygen glucose deprivation, Placental growth factor, Norrie disease protein

Background

Defects in vasculogenesis (early retinal vessel development) seem to be mediated through the Norrin-dependent Wnt signaling pathway [1–3]. Norrin/Frizzled-4 signaling seems to play a crucial role in vasculogenesis such as in Norrie disease and familial exudative vitreoretinopathy [1–4], which might eventually progress into retinal ischemia and neovascularization (NV; angiogenesis). In addition to Norrie disease and familial exudative vitreoretinopathy, there were other developmental retinal vascular disorders, namely Coats disease and persistent hyperplastic primary vitreous that share similar fundus pictures, namely peripheral retinal avascularization and subretinal exudation [1–5]. As above mentioned, these vitreoretinopathies may also cause retinal ischemia, thus giving rise to a similar threat to the patient's vision, although they are not as common as other retinal ischemic disorders such as central/branch retinal artery occlusion (CRAO/BRAO), central/branch retinal vein occlusion (CRVO/BRVO), glaucoma, diabetic retinopathy (DR) and neovascular age related macular degeneration (nvAMD) [6]. As indicated by Beck et al. (2017) [7], persistent hypoxia has been assumed to be one of the major driving forces involved in progression of these developmental retinal vascular disorders such as Norrie disease [5, 7]. Based on the role of Norrin in vasculogenesis [1–5, 7], we investigated here whether the level of Norrie disease protein (NDP; Norrin) might change in cells subjected to a hypoxia model system (oxygen glucose deprivation, OGD). We also investigated whether moscatilin, the bibenzyl component of Dendrobium nobile Lindley (DNL), might have the capacity to upregulate the expression level of NDP, which could potentially protect retinal cells from ischemia/hypoxia that seems to induce the progression of these developmental retinal vascular disorders.

Retinal ganglion cells (RGCs) and amacrine cells in the inner retina are susceptible to ischemia/reperfusion (I/R) [8]. Moreover, vimentin/glial fibrillary acidic protein (GFAP) immunolabelling of Müllers is elevated after ischemia [9]; this is also associated with a reduction in RGC numbers [8]. Overexpression of vascular endothelium growth factor (VEGF), of hypoxia inducible factor (HIF-1α), of pyruvate kinase M2 (PKM2) and of retinoblastoma-binding protein 2 (RBP2) are also known to occur together in the ischemic retina [8, 10–12] and further abnormal NV (late neovessel formation) can lead to visual dysfunction due to edema and hemorrhage. Upregulation of HIF-1α and VEGF has also be observed in the Norrin depleted retina [5]. In addition to VEGF [8, 10, 12], placental growth factor (PLGF) has been reported to be increased when there are defined ischemic disorders of the retina/choroid vasculature; thus, downregulation of this factor is able to be utilized as a biomarker for visual functional outcome and treatment [13]. The present study aims to provide further confirmation regarding these ischemic alterations.

As described in "*An Illustrated Chinese Materia Medica*", DNL (a member of the Orchidae family) is a "vision improving" herbal. DNL has also been used as a tonic and found to have antipyretic/anti-inflammatory effects [14] and anti-angiogenic (e.g. anti-VEGF/HIF-1α) properties [15–17]. DNL has several active ingredients with various action mechanisms, including alkaloids (Tissue necrosis factor receptor 1 protein overexpression via inhibiting the p-p38 mitogen activated protein kinase and NF-κB pathway) [18], flavonal glycosides (α-glucosidase inhibitors) [19], SG-168 and polysaccharides (antioxidative effects) [20, 21]. Furthermore, an anti-angiogenic or anti-oxidative compound moscatilin is one of the active bibenzyl compounds present in DNL and this chemical seems to have a range of effects. These include an anti-VEGF/HIF-1α effect, where it acts as. OH radical scavenger, an anti-inflammation effect and an anti-apoptosis effect [15–17, 22, 23]; there are also other unknown mechanisms of action that are different to those mentioned above. In other words, DNL could possess a number of distinct therapeutic effects that may be shared with its component moscatilin.

The aim of the present study is to examine whether DNL is able to attenuate retinal ischemic injury (see also *Ischemia induction* in the Methods) in the rat. Additionally, the effects of DNL and its mechanisms of action were assessed by electrophysiology, by examining the thickness of various retinal layers, by assessing RGC number, and by examining choline acetyl transferase (ChAT) immuolabeling in amacrine cells and by observing vimentin/GFAP immunoreactivity in Müller cells. Moreover, protein expression levels of HIF-1α, VEGF, PKM2 and RBP2 were analyzed. Furthermore, we for the first time investigated under hypoxia/ischemia the effect of DNL and, of novelty and significance, of its bibenzyl component moscatilin (0.1 μM; non-toxic at the concentration≤1 μM) [23] on vasculogenesis/angiogenesis in relation to the expression levels of NDP (norrin)/PLGF. As part of the NDP study, a RGC-5 cell system (retinal neuronal progenitors; see also in vitro studies in the Methods) model, namely OGD, was used to investigate the mechanisms involved in hypoxic/ischemic-like injury; this part of the study involved the assessment of 3-(4,5-dimethylthiazol-2-yl)-2,5-diphenyl-2H-tetrazolium bromide (MTT) cell viability and the measurement of the expression levels of NDP by the Western blotting assay.

Methods

Chemicals

DNL was purchased from the Ko Da Company (Taipei, Taiwan) and dissolved in ddH_2O. Moscatilin was purchased from EMMX Biotechnology (EN10271, CA, USA) and dissolved in dimethyl sulfoxide (DMSO; vehicle). Various inhibitors/antibodies were purchased from various companies, namely JIB-04 (Sigma-Aldrich), Shikonin (S7576; Sigma-Aldrich), Avastin (Hoffmann-La Roche), or Eylea (Regeneron Pharmaceuticals Inc.).

In vitro studies

Oxygen glucose deprivation and cell treatment

The RGC-5 cells are not transformed rat RGCs but, rather, mouse retinal neuronal precursors [24]. OGD [25] was defined as cells that were maintained in glucose-free Dulbecco's modified Eagle medium (DMEM; Thermo Fisher Scientific Inc.) at 37 °C under the hypoxic (ischemic-like) conditions, namely 1% O_2 (monitored by an analyzer; a Penguin Incubator: control range 1~ 89%; Astec Company, Kukuoka, Japan), 94% N_2 and 5% CO_2. There were different groups (Table 1), consisting of cells that received (i) DMSO in DMEM (control cells; DMSO +DMEM), (ii) DMSO followed by OGD (DMSO+OGD), (iii) OGD and administration of moscatilin (0.1 μM in DMEM) at 1 h pre-OGD (Pre-OGD Mos 0.1 μM), (iv) during OGD (During OGD Mos 0.1 μM), or (v) at 1 h post-OGD (Post-OGD Mos 0.1 μM). At the end of the 1 day OGD period, the cell cultures were returned to fresh DMEM for another 24 h. The MTT (viability) and the Western blotting assays (NDP) were then performed.

MTT cell viability assay

Mitochondria nicotinamide adenine dinucleotide phosphate (NADPH) dependent oxidoreductases are capable of reducing MTT to form formazan [26]. Therefore, an increase in the amount of dark purple formazan corresponds to greater cell viability. MTT (0.5 mg/mL; Sigma-Aldrich) was added for 3 h at 37 °C to the 96-well plates containing the original 100 μL of cells. The reduced MTT was then solubilized by adding 100 μL DMSO. After agitation of the plates, the optical density (OD) of the solubilized formazan was measured using an ELISA reader (Synergy H1 Multi-Mode Reader BioTek Instruments) at 562 nm. Cell viability is expressed as OD values relative to the control (100%).

In vivo studies

Animals

The animal use protocol has been reviewed and approved by the Institutional Animal Care and Use Committee at Cheng Hsin General Hospital (CHGH; Taipei, Taiwan; Approval No: CHIACUC 104–14). A large plastic cage (Shineteh Instruments Co., Ltd., Taipei) was used to keep at most six six-week-old Wistar rats (250–300 g; BioLasco, Taipei) at a humidity of 40 to 60% and a temperature of 19 to 23 °C. For the electroretinogram (ERG) and histopathology [cresyl violet, choline acetyl transferase (ChAT) and vimentin/GFAP] studies, the animals were randomly distributed into various groups (Table 2), i.e. Sham (n = 12), Vehicle+I/R (n = 12), DNL0.5 + I/R (n = 12), DNL1.0 + I/R (n = 12), I/R + Vehicle (n = 10), and I/R + DNL1.0 (n = 10). In addition, for the Western blotting/ ELISA assays, the rats were randomly distributed into following groups (Table 3), namely Sham (n = 10), Vehicle +I/R (n = 10), DNL1.0 + I/R (n = 10), and I/R plus pre-ischemia i.v.i. substances [JIB-04 (n = 4); Shikonin (n = 7); Avastin (n = 4); Eylea (n = 4)]. The number of animals utilized for various defined procedures was 120 (=68 + 49 + 3 = 117 + 3) and this included animals (n = 3) that died during the retinal ischemia. Additionally (n = 16), during the fluorogold retrograde labeling for RGCs, a comparison was made between various groups (Table 4), namely Sham (n = 4), Vehicle+I/R (n = 4), DNL1.0 + I/R

Table 1 Group names and definition of the conditions used to treat the various experimental groups of cells or animals. In vitro MTT/ Western blotting experiments[a]

Group names	Definition of conditions of cells that received
DMSO+DMEM (control)	DMSO in DMEM
DMSO+OGD	OGD and treatment with DMSO at 1 h pre-OGD
Pre-OGD Mos 0.1 μM	OGD and treatment with moscatilin at 1 h pre-OGD
During OGD Mos 0.1 μM	OGD and treatment with moscatilin during OGD
Post-OGD Mos 0.1 μM	OGD and treatment with moscatilin at 1 h post-OGD

[a]The number of experiments in MTT assay for cell viability (n = 6) and Western blot assay for NDP (n = 3). The test compounds were persistently included in the culture medium during the OGD period as defined. Moscatilin (0.1 μM) was kept in DMEM from the administration. *Abbreviations*: *NDP* Norrie disease protein, *DMSO* dimethyl sulfoxide, *OGD* oxygen glucose deprivation

Table 2 Group names and definition of the conditions used to treat the various experimental groups of cells or animals. In vivo eletrophysiological and histopathological experiments[a]

Group names	Definition of conditions of animals that received
i. Sham (*n* = 12; control)	sham procedure
ii. Vehicle+I/R (*n* = 12)	Pre-ischemic treatment with vehicle followed by I/R
iii. DNL0.5 + I/R (*n* = 12)	Pre-ischemic treatment with DNL0.5 followed by I/R
iv. DNL1.0 + I/R (*n* = 12)	Pre-ischemic treatment with DNL1.0 followed by I/R
v. I/R + Vehicle (*n* = 10)	I/R followed by post-ischemic treatment with vehicle
vi. I/R + DNL1.0 (*n* = 10)	I/R followed by post-ischemic treatment with DNL1.0

[a]These animals were evaluated by ERG and sacrificed for histopathological studies, namely cresyl violet, ChAT and vimentin/GFAP labelings. Subtotally, 68 animals were used. Pre−/post-ischemia oral gavage of 0.5 g/kg/day (DNL0.5 + I/R), 1.0 g/kg/day of DNL (DNL1.0 + I/R; I/R + DNL1.0), or the same volume of vehicle was given (Vehicle+I/R; I/R + Vehicle). *Abbreviations*: *ChAT* choline acetyltransferase, *GFAP* glial fibrillary acidic protein

(n = 4), I/R + DNL1.0 (n = 4). In total, the overall number of the animals used was 136 (=120 + 16; Tables 2, 3 and 4). All animals were kept on a 12-h light/dark cycle with 12–15 air changes/hour. The animals were provided with food and water at liberty.

Drug administration

For the electrophysiological, immuohistochemical and molecular biological studies, drug administration was carried out for seven days and involved a number of different groups (Tables 1, 2, 3 and 4), namely a post-ischemic administration (daily high dose of DNL at 1 g/kg/day, I/R + DNL1.0), or pre-ischemic administration (daily high dose of DNL, DNL1.0 + I/R; low dose of DNL at 0.5 g/kg/day, DNL0.5 + I/R) [21]. The rats in the vehicle group that were subjected to ischemia were either post-administrated (I/R + Vehicle) or pre-administrated with a similar volume of vehicle (Vehicle+I/R) as the DNL group. One/seven days after retinal ischemia and pre-ischemic/post-ischemic administration of defined compounds, the rats were sacrificed; this was also done either one or seven days after sham procedure. To reduce the number of the animals used, in these cases only a high dose of DNL (I/R + DNL1.0) were administered after ischemia.

As compared with the Sham, Vehicle+I/R or DNL1.0 + I/R group, the ischemic eyes of other groups (Tables 1, 2, 3 and 4) received intravitreal injections using a 30-gauge needle connected to a 25 μl syringe after the pupil was dilated with 1% tropicamide and 2.5% phenylephrine. Specifically, the ischemic eyes received 1 day pre-ischemia intravitreal administrations of one of the various inhibitors/antibodies, namely 10 μM/5 μl JIB-04, 4 μM/5 μl Shikonin, 125 μg/5 μl Avastin, or 200 μg/5 μl Eylea. One day after retinal I/R and administration of relevant compounds or after a sham procedure, the animals were sacrificed to minimize degradation of the proteins of interest, for example, the occurrence of degradation 7 days after retinal ischemia. Retinal samples were used to measure the protein levels of HIF-1α, RBP2, PKM2, VEGF-A and PLGF by the Western blot analysis or ELISA. Rats were also sacrificed in order to allow analysis of the retina by various methods such as ERG and cresyl violet, flurogold, ChAT, vimentin or GFAP staining histopathology. This was carried out one day after retinal ischemia and pre-ischemic administration of various compounds. On the other hand, the post-ischemia treatment groups were followed up for 7 days in order to observe any long-term (chronic) post-ischemic alterations.

Table 3 Group names and definition of the conditions used to treat the various experimental groups of cells or animals. In vivo Western blotting/ELISA experiment[a]

Group names	Definition of conditions of animals that received
i. Sham (*n* = 10; control)	sham procedure
ii. Vehicle+I/R (*n* = 10)	Pre-ischemic oral vehicle followed by I/R
iii. DNL1.0 + I/R (*n* = 10)	Pre-ischemic oral DNL1.0 followed by I/R
iv. JIB-04 + I/R (*n* = 4)	Pre-ischemic intravitreous JIB-04 followed by I/R
v. Shikonin+I/R (*n* = 7)	Pre-ischemic intravitreous shikonin followed by I/R
vi. Avastin+I/R (*n* = 4)	Pre-ischemic intravitreous avastin followed by I/R
vii. Eylea+I/R (*n* = 4)	Pre-ischemic intravitreous eylea followed by I/R

[a]These animals were evaluated by Western blotting/ELISA assays and sacrificed for the measurement of various proteins, namely HIF-1α, VEGF, PKM2, RBP2 and PLGF. Subtotally, 49 animals were used. The number of animals utilized for various defined procedures was 120 (=68 + 49 + 3) and this included animals (*n* = 3) that died during the retinal ischemia. Pre-ischemia intravitreous injection of 1.0 g/kg/day of DNL (DNL1.0 + I/R), or inhibitors/antibodies of PKM2 (shikonin), RBP2 (JIB-04), VEGF-A (avastin), PLGF (Eylea), or the same volume of vehicle was administered. *Abbreviations*: *HIF-1α* hypoxia inducible factor, *VEGF* vascular endothelium growth factor, *PKM2* pyruvate kinase M2, *RBP2* retinoblastoma-binding protein 2, *PLGF* placental growth factor

Table 4 Group names and definition of the conditions used to treat the various experimental groups of cells or animals. In vivo fluorogold RGC experiment[a]

Group names	Definition of conditions of animals that received
i. Sham ($n = 4$; control)	sham procedure
ii. Vehicle+I/R ($n = 4$)	Pre-ischemic treatment with vehicle followed by I/R
iii. DNL1.0 + I/R ($n = 4$)	Pre-ischemic treatment with DNL1.0 followed by I/R
iv. I/R + DNL1.0 ($n = 4$)	I/R followed by post-ischemic treatment with DNL1.0

[a]These animals were evaluated by the fluorogold retrograde labeling for RGC. Subtotally, 16 animals were used. In total, the overall number of the animals used was 136 (=120 + 16). Pre–/post-ischemia oral gavage of 1.0 g/kg/day of DNL (DNL1.0 + I/R; I/R + DNL1.0), or the same volume of vehicle was applied

In previous reports, higher concentrations of moscatilin (1.25~ 20 μM) have been shown to be able to dose-dependently and time-dependently reduce cell viability with IC_{50} at 7.0 and 6.7 μM for 24 h in two cell lines, respectively [17]; thus, 0.1 μM, which is a non-toxic concentration [23], was presently used to evaluate the compound's protective effect against OGD. Moscatilin (0.1 μM) was administered at 1 h pre-OGD, during OGD, or alternatively at 1 h post-OGD (Tables 1, 2, 3 and 4). The therapeutic effects of the drug were evaluated by MTT and Western blotting analysis.

Establishing retinal ischemia

Anesthesia and euthanasia

An intraperitoneal injection (i.p.) of 100 mg/kg ketamine (Pfizer) and 5 mg/kg xylazine (Sigma-Aldrich) was used to anesthetize the animals. Furthermore, at least 140 mg/kg sodium pentobarbital (SCI Pharmtech) was intraperitoneally given to humanely kill the animals (Scientific Procedures Acts 1986).

Ischemia induction

Each rat was anesthetized with the above anesthetics and placed in a stereotaxic frame. The anterior chamber of one eye was cannulated using a 30-gauge needle linked to an elevated 0.9% saline reservoir; this was used to bring about an increase in intraocular pressure (IOP) to 120 mmHg for 1 h [8]. A whitening of the retina indicated a build-up of ischemic injury. A sham version of the above-mentioned ischemia induction procedure, but without the elevation of the saline bottle connected to the rat's eye, was carried out as a control. Animals were placed on a heating pad at 37°C and kept normothermic during ischemia & the following 3-h reperfusion.

Flash ERG measurements

Flash ERG were recorded from all the animals before the sham procedure or I/R (day 0), and one day after the sham procedure or I/R with pre-administration of the various drugs. In the post-administration group, ERG data were recorded for all the animals pre-ischemia (day 0), and post-ischemia (day 1, 3, 5 or 7 after ischemia and administration of appropriate compounds). Dark adaption was allowed for 8 h and then anesthesia was carried out to allow recording of the ERG after dilation of pupils. A stimulus of 0.5 Hz was provided using a strobe 2 cm before the animal's eye. Fifteen continuous recordings were collected at two-second interval and at 10 kHz; their amplitudes were maximized and calculated to obtain an average; this involved the use of an amplifier (P511), a regulated power supply (RPS 107) and a stimulator (PS22), all obtained from Grass-Telefactor. To allow comparisons between the various groups, the ratio of the b-wave amplitude of one eye (sham or ischemia) to that of the untreated fellow normal eye was measured [8].

Cresyl violet staining

Across all groups, after the rats were sacrificed, they received an intracardial perfusion of physiologic saline. The eyeballs were marked at the 12 o'clock on the cornea using a silk suture and then enucleation was carried out. This was followed by fixation in 4% paraformaldehyde at 4 °C for 24 h, dehydration in a graded ethanol series and embedding in paraffin (Tissue-Tek TEC 5; Sakura). Sectioned samples (5 μm) were obtained along the vertical meridian. These were subjected to cresyl violet labeling and were then observed under a light microscope (Leica). Each retinal section was photographed at the same magnifying power and the retinal thickness of the various different layers was measured from photographs (Ilford Pan-F plus film, 50 ASA). To quantify the degree of retinal ischemic injury, firstly, the whole retinal thicknesses was measured from the internal limiting membrane (ILM) to retinal pigment epithelium (RPE) layer. Secondly, the inner retinal thickness from the ILM to inner nuclear layer (INL) were measured by an expert who was masked to the conditions under which the sectioned samples had been obtained. The various experimental groups were compared to the control group (sham).

RGC retrograde staining

Under anesthesia, a 2-cm incision was created in the animal's scalp and two small holes were drilled into the skull as illustrated [8]. Next, injections of 10-μl of 5% fluorogold (Sigma-Aldrich) were carried out using a micropipette at 3.8, 4.0, and 4.2 mm below the surface.

The fluorogold was injected 3 days before the animals were sacrificed. Retrieval, fixation, dissection and processing of retinal samples were performed as described previously [8]. The RGC density was calculated as the ratio of the total number of RGCs divided by the total area of the retinal sample [8].

Immunofluorescence analysis

After sacrifice of the animals and intracardial perfusion, the eyeballs of the rats were enucleated, fixed for 45 min, dehydrated and finally embedded in paraffin as above-mentioned. Sampling was carried out 1 day after the sham procedure or induction of retinal ischemia with pre-ischemia/post-ischemia administration of DNL or vehicle. Each 5 μm retinal section was incubated overnight with primary antibodies, namely either goat anti-ChAT polyclonal antibody (1:100; AB144p; Chemicon), mouse anti-vimentin monoclonal antibody (1:100; V6630; Sigma-Aldrich), or rabbit anti-GFAP polyclonal antibody (Millipore). Next, retinal sections were incubated with an appropriate secondary antibody, either rhodamine-conjugated rabbit anti-goat antibody (1:500; AP106R; Chemicon), or fluorescein isothiocyanate (FITC)-conjugated goat anti-mouse IgG (1:500; AP124F; Millipore)/anti-rabbit IgG (AP132F; 1:500; Millipore). In parallel, cellular nuclei were labeled using 4′,6-diamidino-2-phenylindole (DAPI; Molecular Probes). Finally, retinal sections were examined using a fluorescence microscope (Olympus BX61) by an expert who was masked to the conditions under which the sectioned samples had been obtained in order to grade the immunolabeling level of various different groups against the control group (sham).

Western blotting assays

Retinal samples or samples of cells were sonicated in lysis buffer, namely mammalian protein extraction reagent (MPER; HyCell). Identical quantities of denatured proteins (40 μg/30 μl/well) then underwent sodium dodecyl sulfate polyacrylamide gel electrophoresis (SDS-PAGE; Bio-Rad) as described previously [10]. After separation, the protein bands were transferred to a polyvinylidene difluoride membrane, which was treated for 12 h at 4 °C with the following primary antibodies, mouse monoclonal anti-β-actin antibody (AC-15; 1:2000; ab6276)/anti-HIF-1α antibody (1:200; H1alpha67-ChIP Grade; Abcam Inc.), rabbit polyclonal anti-VEGF antibody (A-20; 1:200; sc-152)/anti-PKM2 antibody (1:500; ab38237), or rabbit monoclonal anti-RBP2 antibody (ab177486; 1:1000; Abcam Inc.). The blots were next treated with relevant secondary antibody, HRP-conjugated goat anti-rabbit IgG (1:5000; Santa Cruz Biotechnology Inc.) or goat anti-mouse IgG (1:5000; sc-2005) at 37 °C for 1 h. Dilution of primary/secondary antibodies was carried out in 5% fat-free skimmed milk. Finally, the membranes were processed using an enhanced chemiluminescent analysis system (HyCell) and exposed to an X-ray film (Fujifilm). The amount of each protein was then evaluated by scanning densitometry.

Enzyme-linked immunosorbent assay

The level of PLGF was determined using ELISA [27]. One day after ischemia, the retina was separated from the enucleated eye cup, dissociated and then lysed by incubation in MPER (Hycell) for 30 min; the lysate was then centrifuged at 13,000 rpm for another 30 min. The total protein in each sample was determined using a bicinchoninic acid protein kit (Thermo Fisher Scientific) [28]. The PLGF levels in the supernatant were measured using a PLGF ELISA kit (CSB-E07400r; Cusabio Life Scince) accordingly. Anti-PLGF antibody had been previously coated onto the microwell. After twice washing each well with 200 μL wash buffer over 15 min, the PLGF in the samples or various concentrations of PLGF standard protein (100 μL) was allowed to bind to the antibodies coating the microwells at room temperature for 2 h on a shaker (75 rpm). After washing each well twice with 200 μL wash buffer [Phosphate buffered saline with Tween-20 (PBST)], 100 μL of biotin-conjugated anti-PLGF antibody (diluted in assay buffer: PBST and 0.5% BSA) was added to each well for 1 h on a shaker (75 rpm), which allowed the binding to the PLGF captured by the coated antibody. After twice washing to remove unbound biotin-conjugated anti-PLGF, 100 μL avidin- horseradish peroxidase (HRP; diluted in assay buffer) was added; this bound to the biotin conjugated anti-VEGF-A antibody (75 rpm). Following 1-h incubation on a shaker, the unbound avidin-HRP was removed by washing twice. Finally, 90 μL of 3,3′,5,5′-trimethylbenzene (TMB; 100 μM) solution, which is oxidized by HRP, was added to each well for 20 min. The color was then changed to yellow and the reaction was stopped by the addition of 50 μL stop solution (sulfuric acid solution, 100 μM). The maximum absorbance (OD) at 450 nm was detected immediately using a microplate reader (Synergy H1 Hybrid Multi-Mode Reader, Biotek ELx800). The PLGF concentration of each sample was determined by constructing a standard curve using various amounts of PLGF (0, 3.125, 6.25, 12.5, 25, 50, 100 and 200 pg/mL). The instrument was adjusted to zero using a 100 μL sample diluent, which served as the blank. The results are expressed as ODs relative to that of the control group (100%).

Statistical analysis

Comparisons between two groups were made using the unpaired Student's *t*-tests. One-way analysis of variance (ANOVA) was performed to compare three or more independent groups. Following the one-way ANOVA, the Dunnet's test was used to compare the control (e.g. Vehicle+I/

R) with all other groups (e.g. DNL1.0 + I/R). All results were shown as means±SE. A value of $P < 0.05$ was considered significant.

Results

MTT cell viability assay

Firstly, changes in the cell morphology and the number of RGC-5 cells were examined by light microscopy. The cells cultured in the DMEM with pre-administration of DMSO (DMSO+DMEM; Fig. 1a) had a pyramidal shape and exhibited a characteristic neuronal morphology. By way of contrast to the DMSO+DMEM group, the cells subjected to OGD and pre-administrated with DMSO (DMSO+OGD) were deformed (as indicated by white arrows; Fig. 1b); moreover, there was also a considerable reduction in their cell number. Next, the effects of administering moscatilin (0.1 μM to 100 μM) to cells subjected to OGD were observed. Specifically, the protective effect of pre-OGD administration of moscatilin on the OGD was demonstrated by increased cell viabilities at 0.1 (62.65 ± 4.35%; $n = 6$) or 1 μM (66.36±9.35%; $n = 4$); however, a cytotoxic effect, namely a decrease in the cell viability, was shown at 10 (30.60 ± 9.05%; $n = 4$) and 100 μM (12.75 ± 3.34%; n = 4). The latter two concentrations would seem to be beyond the pharmacological protective levels. This is not inconsistent with previous research, which has indicated that moscatilin acts in a time-dependent (1~ 3 days) and dose-dependent manner (1.25~ 20 μM) [17]. The compound seems to have a cytotoxic effect that is probably related to its ability to induce a G2 phase arrest in the mitosis at the concentration of 20 or 50 μM as early as 15 h posttreatment [29]. However, the concentrations of moscatilin equal to or less than 1 μM have been proved to be non-toxic and are able to act as a potent. OH radical scavenger [23]. An investigation into how a low concentration of moscatilin (0.1 μM) is able to increase the cell viability was then carried out. As compared with the DMSO+OGD group (Fig. 1b), administration of 0.1 μM at 1 h pre-OGD (Fig. 1c), during OGD (Fig. 1d), or at 1 h post-OGD (Fig. 1e) was evaluated in order to demonstrate the extent of cytoprotection provided by moscatilin against the OGD. The effect of 0.1 μM moscatilin was found to be greatest when administered at 1 h pre-OGD (Fig. 1c), followed by during OGD

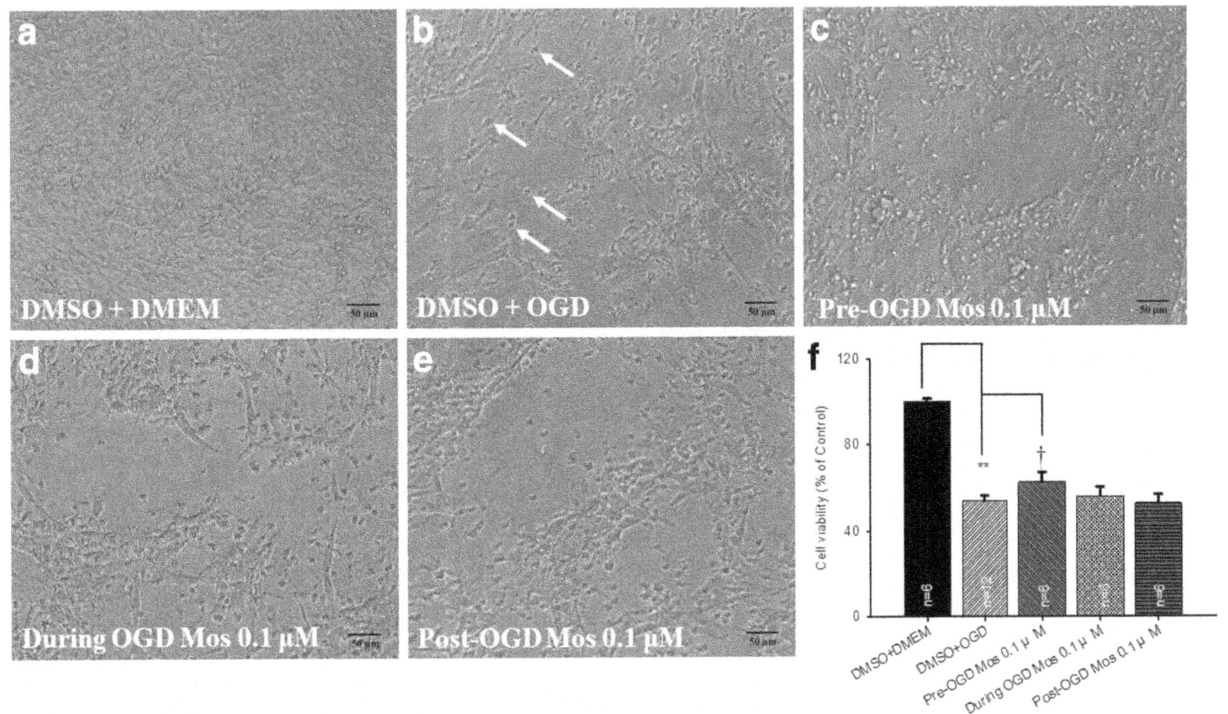

Fig. 1 a~e The cell viability study of the effects of moscatilin on RGC-5 cells subjected to OGD using light microscopy. After pre-administration of DMSO (vehicle) followed by OGD (DMSO+OGD), the cells were found to be less numerous and some were deformed (as indicated by arrows) as compared to the normal control group (cells cultured in DMEM and pre-administration of DMSO; DMSO+DMEM). These OGD-induced alterations were mitigated by pre-administration of moscatilin (Mos) at 1 h pre-OGD (Pre-OGD 0.1 μM Mos). **f** The effects of moscatilin on cells subjected to OGD analyzed quantitatively by MTT assay. ** indicates a significant difference ($P < 0.01$) between the control (DMSO+DMEM) and the "DMSO +OGD" group. † indicates a significant difference ($P = 0.04$) between the "DMSO+OGD" group and the "Pre-OGD 0.1 μM Mos" group. Please refer to Table 1 for definitions of the other two groups, namely "During OGD 0.1 μM Mos" and "Post-OGD 0.1 μM Mos". Results are presented as means±S.E.M. ($n = 6$). DMSO, dimethyl sulfoxide; DMEM, Dulbecco's modified Eagle's medium; OGD, oxygen glucose deprivation; RGC, retinal ganglion cell; MTT, 3-(4,5-dimethylthiazol-2-yl)-2,5-diphenyltetrazolium bromide. Scale = 50 μm

(Fig. 1d). There was no protective effect at 1 h post-OGD (Fig. 1e).

Cell viability was compared against the DMSO+DMEM group (normal control: 100%; $n = 6$) after OGD and pre-administration of DMSO. Cell viability was significantly ($P < 0.001$) reduced (53.66 ± 2.67%) in the group DMSO+OGD (Fig. 1f). Furthermore, as compared with the DMSO+OGD group, administration of 0.1 μM moscatilin 1 h pre-OGD (Fig. 1f; 62.65 ± 4.35%; $P = 0.04$) resulted in a significant protective effect against the OGD. However, administration of 0.1 μM moscatilin during OGD (Fig. 1f; 56.03 ± 4.08%; $P = 0.31$), or at 1 h post-OGD (Fig. 1f; 52.61 ± 4.16%; $P = 0.41$) did not significantly protect cells against the OGD.

As compared to the DMEM alone (10^5 cells/ml = 100%), DMSO (50 μl) did not significantly affect cell numbers (DMSO+DMEM, 97.66±1.66%; n = 6). Similarly, moscatilin (0.1 μM) also did not influence cell numbers (moscatilin+DMEM, 99.25 ± 6.05%; $n = 4$). Likewise, compared to DMEM+OGD (53.85±7.03%; n = 4), DMSO (50 μl) did not induce a significant change in cell numbers (DMSO +OGD, 53.66±2.67%; n = 6) as mentioned above.

The effect of moscatilin on the expression of NDP relative to β-actin in vitro

In order to examine alterations in vasculogenesis related NDP, representative immunoblotting images and an analytical bar chart are presented in Fig. 2. When compared to the DMSO+DMEM group (normal control: 100%; $n = 3$), pre-OGD administration of vehicle followed by OGD (DMSO+OGD; $P < 0.001$) significantly reduced the amount of NDP to 44.54 ± 3.15%. When the DMSO +OGD group was compared to the pre-OGD moscatilin +OGD group, there was a significant ($P = 0.048$) increase in the amount of NDP (108.38 ± 29.33%). This elevation in protein expression was greatest when the moscatilin was administered 1 h before the OGD, followed by 1 h post-OGD (54.36 ± 3.88%), with the least effect occurring during OGD (48.99 ± 9.89%).

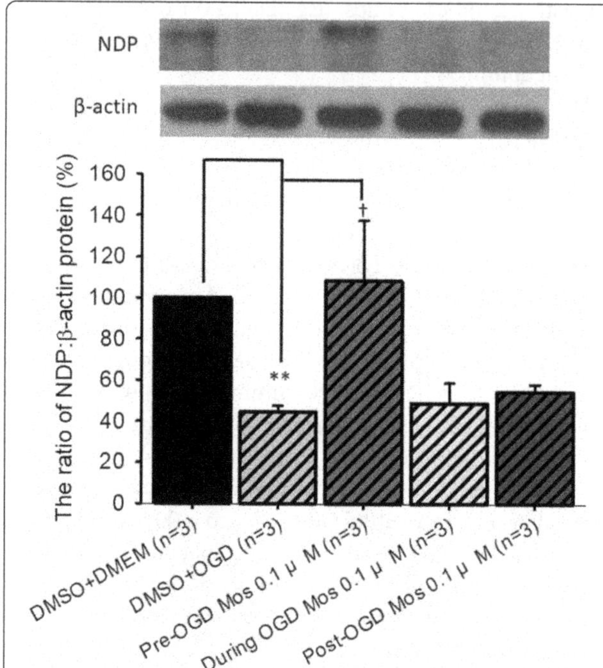

Fig. 2 The effect of moscatilin on the protein expression levels of NDP relative to β-actin. Top: a series representative immunoblotting images. Bottom: bar chart. The protein expression level of NDP vs. β-actin in the normal control (DMSO+DMEM: RGC-5 cells cultured in DMEM and pre-administration of DMSO) was adjusted to 100%. ** indicates a significant difference ($P < 0.01$) between the "DMSO+DMEM" group and the "DMSO+OGD" group. † indicates a significant difference ($P = 0.048$) between the "DMSO+OGD" and "Pre-OGD 0.1 μM Mos" groups (0.1 μM moscatilin given 1 h pre-OGD). The results are presented as means±S.E.M. ($n = 3$). Please refer to definitions of various groups in Table 1. Abbreviations: NDP, Norrie disease protein; DMSO, dimethyl sulfoxide; DMEM, Dulbecco's modified Eagle's medium; OGD, oxygen glucose deprivation; RGC, retinal ganglion cell

The effect of DNL on ERG b-wave

We next examined the retinal electrophysiological functioning. After the sham procedure (Sham, Fig. 3), the ERG b-wave amplitude was measured and found to be 0.41 mV. Following retinal ischemia, there was a drastic reduction in b-wave amplitude and this was not affected by either pre-ischemia or post-ischemia treatment with vehicle (Vehicle+I/R: 0.03 mV, Fig. 3a; I/R + Vehicle: 0.07 mV, Fig. 3b). However, pre-ischemia (DNL0.5 + I/R; DNL1.0 + I/R; Fig. 3a) or post-ischemia treatment with DNL (I/R + DNL1.0 D7; Fig. 3b) was able to alleviate the ischemia-induced b-wave decrease, raising the amplitudes for the three groups to 0.18, 0.22 and 0.15 mV, respectively. Furthermore, pre-ischemia treatment with DNL was also found to dose-dependently attenuate the amplitude decrease.

As shown in Fig. 3c ($n = 12$), compared to the Sham group (1.00 ± 0.08), the b-wave ratio in the Vehicle+I/R group (0.10 ± 0.03) was decreased significantly ($P = 0.002$). Importantly, pre-ischemia treatment with DNL dose-responsively and significantly [DNL1.0 + I/R: 0.57 ± 0.06; DNL0.5 + I/R: 0.45 ± 0.03 ($P < 0.001$)] mitigated the ischemia-induced b-wave ratio decrease following I/R.

In Fig. 3d ($n = 10$), compared to the Sham group, the b-wave ratio was significantly ($P < 0.001$) decreased in the I/R + Vehicle group (day 1: 0.13 ± 0.04; day 3: 0.10 ± 0.02; day 5: 0.09 ± 0.03; day 7: 0.06 ± 0.03). Importantly, post-ischemia administration of DNL (I/R + DNL1.0) significantly [D1: 0.14 ± 0.04; D3: 0.26 ± 0.05 ($P = 0.02$); D5: 0.34 ± 0.05 ($P = 0.003$); D7: 0.40 ± 0.04 ($P < 0.001$)] reduced the ischemia-induced b-wave ratio decrease. The pre-ischemia (day 0) b-wave ratios were 1.00 ± 0.09 (I/R + Vehicle) and 1.00 ± 0.08 (I/R + DNL1.0), respectively. When a comparison between the

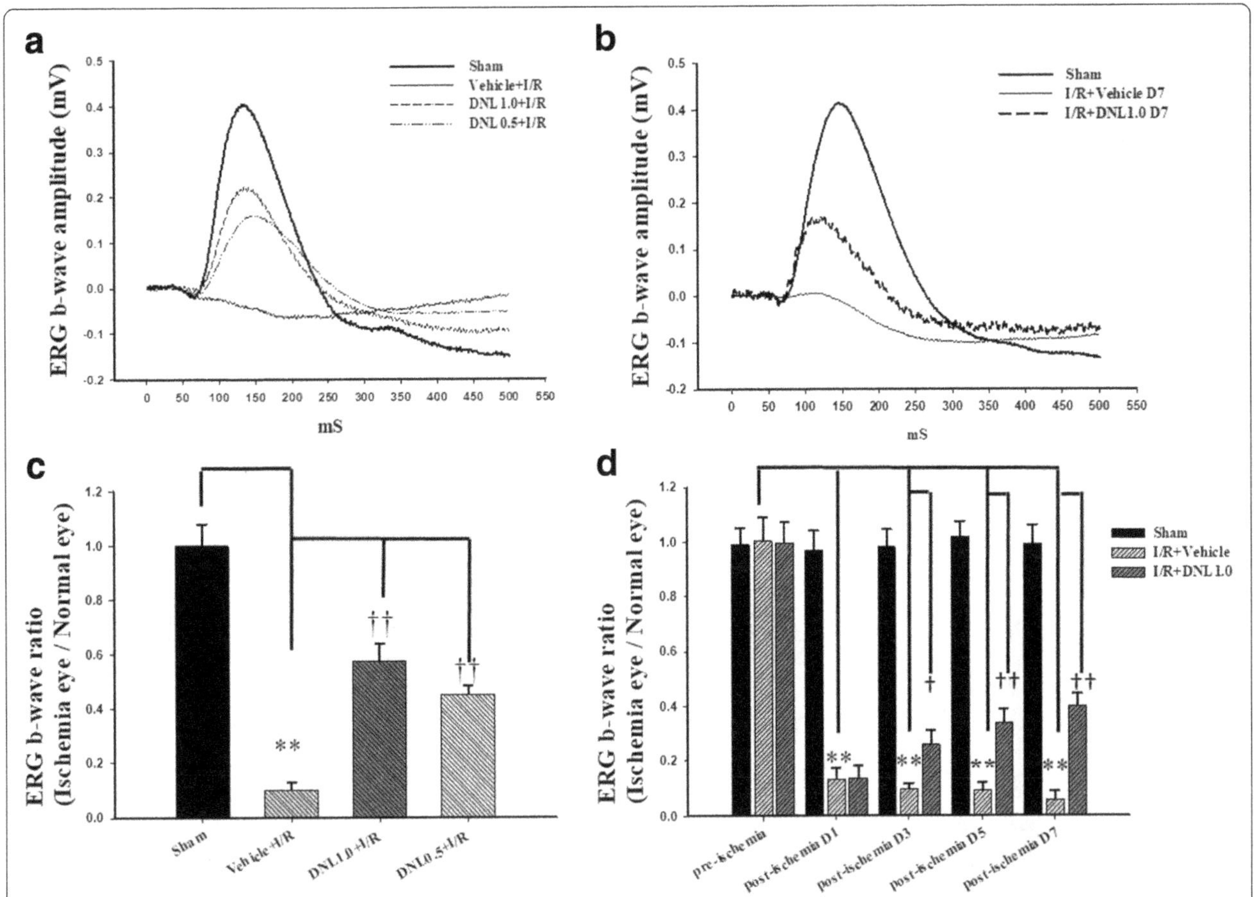

Fig. 3 Electroretinogram (ERG) analysis. **a** and **b** Compared to the control retina (Sham), there was a drastic decrease in the ERG b-wave amplitudes after HIOP-induced retinal I/R and pre-administration (**a**) or post-administration (**b**) of vehicle. This decrease was dose-dependently counteracted by pre-ischemia administration of DNL (DNL1.0 + I/R; DNL0.5 + I/R; **a**) or post-ischemia administration of DNL (I/R + DNL1.0; **b**). **c** Compared to the normal control (Sham), a significant (**; $P < 0.01$) decrease in the ERG b-wave ratio occurred in the "Vehicle+I/R" group after retinal I/R. A significant (††; $P < 0.01$) counteraction of this ischemia-induced reduction was dose-responsive and obtained when there was pre-administration of a high dose (DNL1.0 + I/R) and low dose (DNL0.5 + I/R) of DNL. **d** ERG b-wave amplitude was found to be significantly (**; $P < 0.01$) reduced on day 1, 3, 5 or 7 after retinal I/R and post-ischemia administration of vehicle. A significant (†/††; $P < 0.05/0.01$) alleviation of this reduction in ERG b-wave amplitude was achieved by post-administration of DNL (I/R + DNL1.0). Please refer to definitions of various groups in Table 2. Abbreviations: HIOP, high intraocular pressure; I/R, ischemia plus reperfusion. DNL, Dendrobium nobile Lindley. The results are present as means±S.E.M. (n = 10~ 12)

ERG b-wave ratios of the Sham group on days 0, 1, 3, 5 and 7 (0.99 ± 0.06, 0.97 ± 0.07, 0.98 ± 0.06, 1.02 ± 0.01 and 0.99 ± 0.07) was made and they were not significantly different.

The effect of DNL on the thickness of the retinal layers labeled with cresyl violet

Retinal thickness was assessed by sectioning retinal samples at the same distance (1.5 mm) from disc across various groups (n = 10~ 12; Fig. 4). Compared to retinas that had received the sham procedure (Sham, Figs. 4a and g: 225.50 ± 3.26 μm for the whole retina, 112.08 ± 2.58 μm for the inner retina), the retinal thicknesses of the animal pre-administrated with vehicle and subjected to I/R (Vehicle+I/R, Fig. 4b and g: 110.83 ± 1.85 μm for the whole retina, 62.50 ± 3.06 μm for the inner retina) were significantly ($P < 0.001$) decreased. Moreover, this decrease was dose-dependently and significantly ($P < 0.001$) counteracted when the animal received I/R and pre-administration of DNL (DNL1.0 + I/R, Fig. 4c and g: 190.08 ± 4.48 μm for the whole retina, 94.92 ± 2.27 μm for the inner retina; DNL0.5 + I/R, Fig. 4d and g: 148.58 ± 2.80 μm for the whole retina, 78.25 ± 1.53 μm for the inner retina).

In contrast to retinas subjected to the sham procedure (Sham, Fig. 4a), the retinal thicknesses of the rats that were given I/R and post-administration of vehicle (I/R + Vehicle, Fig. 4e and h: 115.00 ± 2.04 μm for the whole retina, 63.92 ± 3.30 μm for the inner retina) were significantly ($P < 0.001$) reduced. Moreover, post-administration of DNL blunted this ischemia-induced reduction significantly [I/R + DNL1.0; Fig. 4f and h: 125.25 ± 2.66 μm for the whole retina (P = 0.006); 71.50 ± 1.51 μm for the inner retina (P = 0.048)].

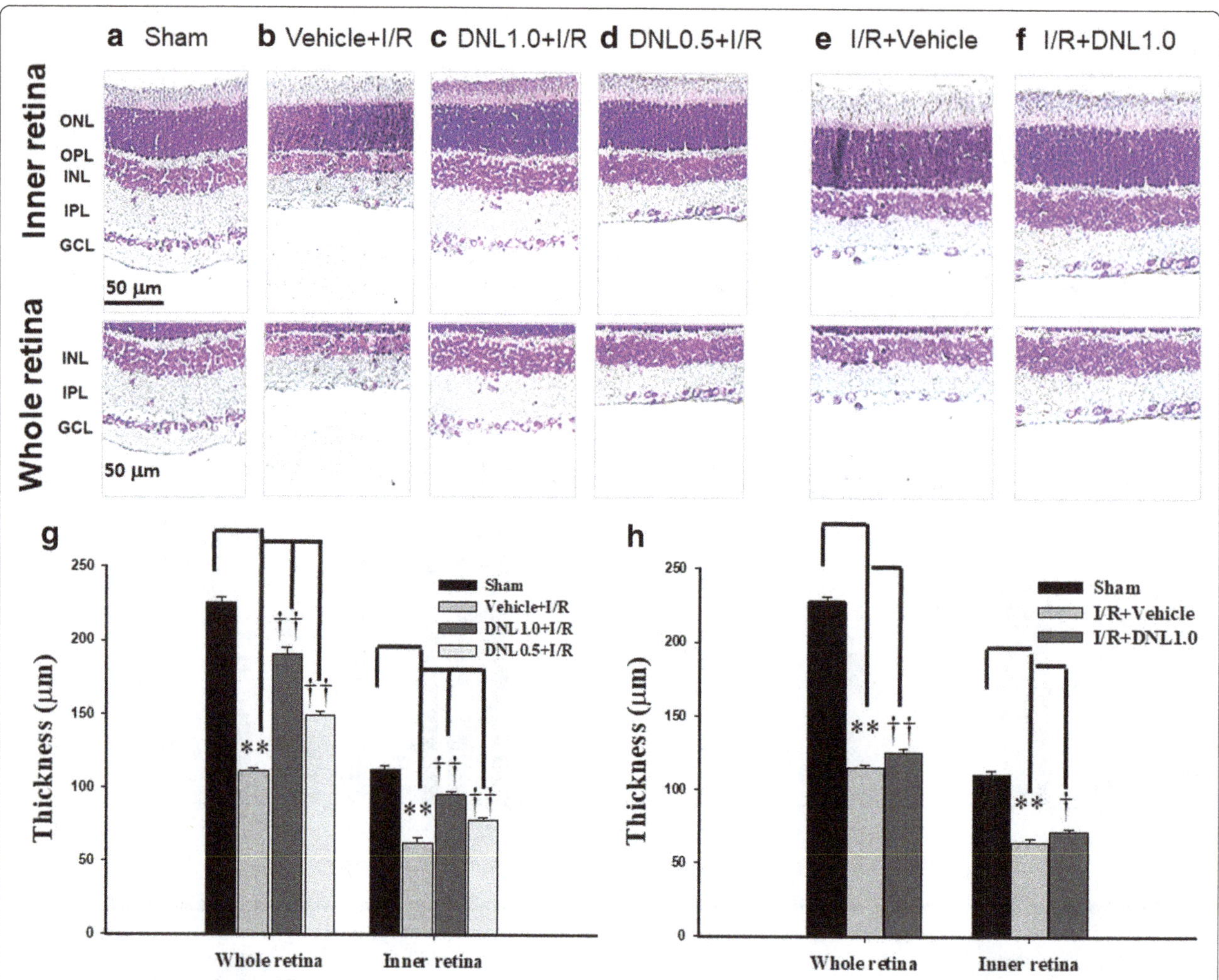

Fig. 4 Analysis of the thickness of the whole or inner retina labeled with cresyl violet. **a**, **b**, **e** Shows a retina that received the sham procedure (Sham), or I/R and pre-administration (**b**)/post-administration of vehicle (**e**). **c**, **d**, **f** Are retinas that have undergone I/R and pre-administration of 0.5 g/kg/day (**c**, DNL0.5 + I/R), or 1.0 g/kg/day (**d**, DNL1.0 + I/R), or post-administration of 1.0 g/kg/day (**f**, I/R + DNL1.0) of DNL. The thickness of the whole or inner retina obtained from sections of equal eccentricity that were morphometrically analyzed (**g**, **h**). The results are presented as means±S.E.M. (n = 10~ 12). ** represents a significant difference ($P < 0.01$) from the Sham retina. † or †† represents a significant difference ($P < 0.05$ or $P < 0.01$) from the Vehicle +I/R or I/R + Vehicle. Abbreviations: I/R, ischemia plus reperfusion; DNL, Dendrobium nobile Lindley; ONL, outer nuclear layer; OPL, outer plexiform layer; INL, inner nuclear layer; IPL, inner plexiform layer; GCL, ganglion cell layer. Scale bar = 50 μm

The effect of DNL on the density of retrograde fluorogold immunolabeled RGCs

When RGC density was assessed (Fig. 5; $n = 4$), the density of the sham group (Sham, Figs. 5a and e) was 363.23 ± 2.84 cells/field. Compared to the Sham group, there was a significant ($P < 0.001$) reduction in RGC density (192.06 ± 23.53 cells/field) in animals that underwent retinal ischemia and pre-administration of vehicle (Vehicle+I/R, Figs. 5b and e). Furthermore, this decrease was significantly ($P = 0.006$ or 0.045) mitigated when the animals received either retinal ischemia and pre-administration of DNL (DNL1.0 + I/R; Figs. 5c and e: 295.15 ± 7.14 cells/field), or post-ischemia administration of DNL (I/R + DNL1.0; Figs. 5d and e: 256.26 ± 9.46 cells/field).

The effect of DNL efficacy on ChAT immunoreactivity

ChAT immunoreactivity in the retina after the sham procedure (Sham; Fig. 6a) is able to pinpoint ChAT (red) immunolabeling of the amacrine cell bodies (short arrows) present in the INL and ganglion cell layer (GCL). This procedure also demonstrates the presence of two distinct strata (long arrow) within the inner plexiform layer (IPL). In retinas that had undergone ischemia and pre–/post-administration of vehicle (Vehicle+I/R; Fig. 6b; I/R + Vehicle, Fig. 6e), the numbers of CHAT-immunolabeled amacrine cell bodies were drastically decreased; furthermore, their IPL immunolabeling was considerably reduced. It is clinically important to note that these changes were nullified in a dose-dependent manner when the ischemic retinas had received pre-administration of DNL (DNL0.5 + I/R, Fig. 6c;

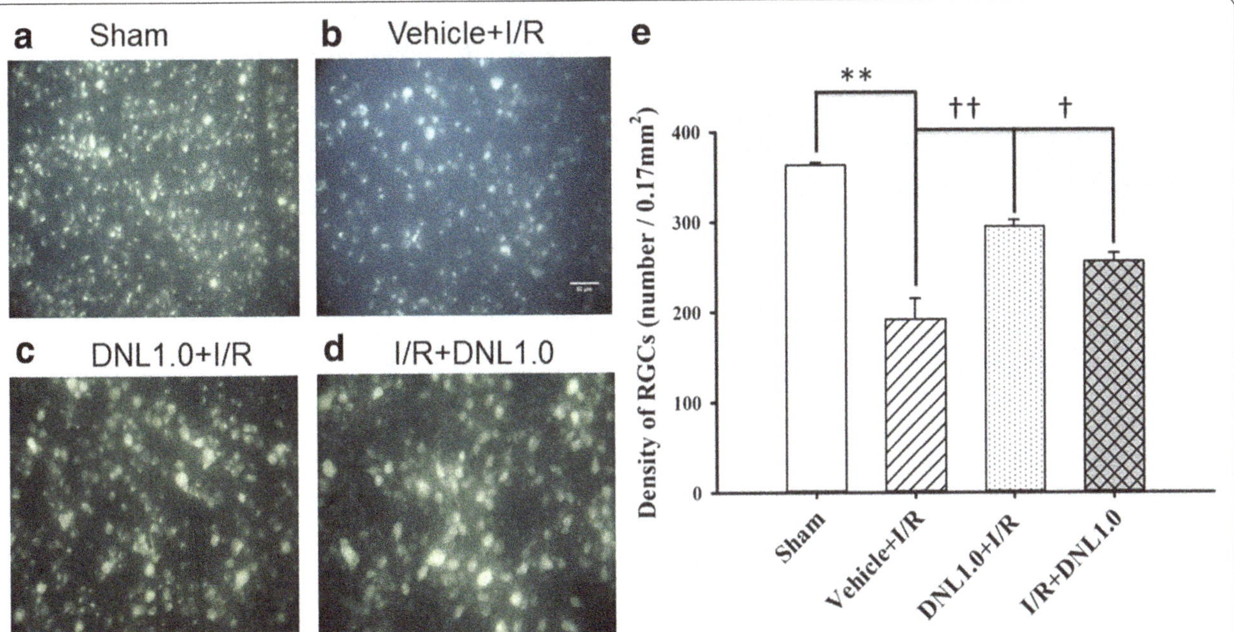

Fig. 5 Fluorogold labeling. The micrographs shows the retinal ganglion cell (RGC) density after the sham procedure (**a**, Sham), or after ischemia followed by reperfusion (I/R) plus pre-ischemia administration of vehicle (**b**, Vehicle+I/R) or pre–/post-ischemia administration of DNL at 1.0 g/kg/day (**c**, DNL1.0 + I/R; **d**, I/R + DNL1.0). The RGC density was quantitatively analyzed (**e**). As indicated by each bar, the results were means±S.EM. ($n = 4$). ** indicates a significant difference from the sham retina ($P < 0.01$; Sham vs. Vehicle+I/R); †† or † indicates a significant difference from the Vehicle+I/R ($P < 0.01$ or $P < 0.05$; Vehicle+I/R vs. DNL1.0 + I/R or I/R + DNL1.0). DNL, Dendrobium nobile Lindley. Scale bars = 50 μm

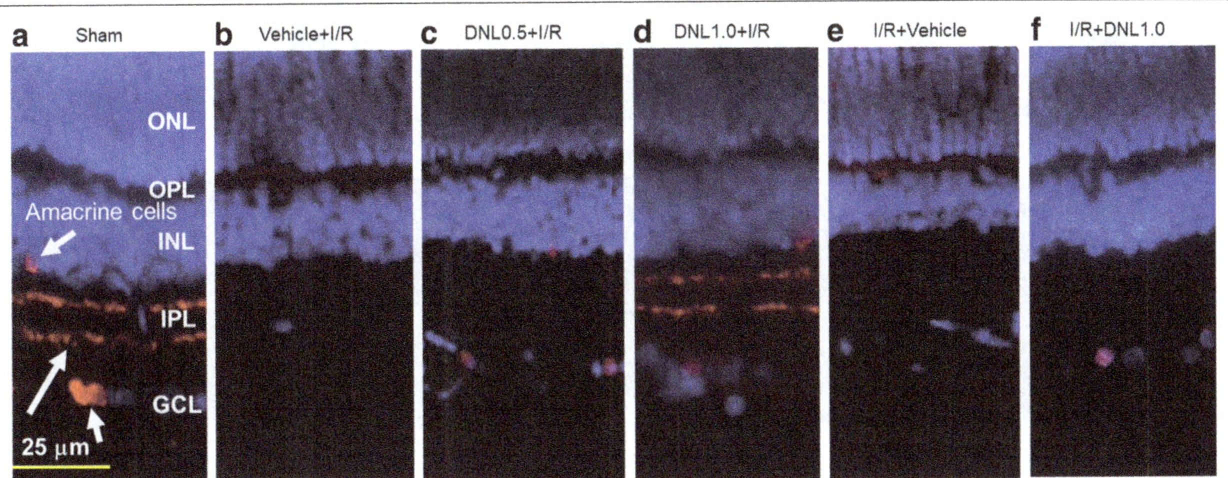

Fig. 6 Choline acetyltransferase (ChAT, red) immunohistochemical studies. **a** Shows a retina that have undergone the sham procedure (Sham); cell nuclei are counterstained with 4,6-diamidine-2-phenylindole dihydrochloride (DAPI, blue). Amacrine cell bodies (Sham; short arrows) can be seen in the INL and GCL and their neuronal processes (long arrow) display a two-band pattern in the IPL. **b**, **e** Show retinas that have undergone I/R together with pre–/post-administration of vehicle (Vehicle+I/R or I/R + Vehicle). A considerable reduction in the IPL immunoreactivity can be seen together with a great reduction in the number of amacrine cell bodies. **c**, **d**, **f** show sectioned retinas that have received I/R and pre-administration of 0.5 g/kg/day (c, DNL0.5 + I/R), or 1.0 g/kg/day of DNL (d, DNL1.0 + I/R), or that have received I/R and post-administration of 1.0 g/kg/day of DNL (f, I/R + DNL1.0). In these groups, the ischemia-induced changes can be seen to be obviously and dose-dependently mitigated when the ischemic retinas have received pre-administration of 0.5 and 1.0 g/Kg/day of DNL. Post-administration of 1.0 g/Kg/day of DNL can also be seen to obviously mitigate these ischemia-induced changes. Abbreviations: ONL, outer nuclear layer, OPL, outer plexiform layer, INL, inner nuclear layer, IPL, inner plexiform layer, GCL, ganglion cell layer. DNL, Dendrobium nobile Lindley. Scale bar = 25 μm

DNL1.0 + I/R, Fig. 6d). Additionally, post-administration of DNL (I/R + DNL1.0, Fig. 6f) also obviously mitigated these ischemia-induced changes. Merge images of ChAT immunolabeling and DAPI staining of cellular nuclei are used for all presented pictures.

The effect of DNL on vimentin and GFAP immunoreactivity

Immunohistochemical investigations were carried out with the aim of investigating the vimentin immunoreactivity and GFAP immunoreactivity.

Vimentin immunohistochemistry

In the control retina (Sham, Fig. 7b), the Müller cell processes showed vimentin immunolabeling at the end feet (arrow heads; see also Figs. 7c and f) in the GCL as well as at the processes that extended into the IPL (arrows; see also Figs. 7c and f), INL and ONL. Compared to the control retina (Sham, Fig. 7b), an increase in the anti-vimentin immunoreactivity was found after retinal I/R and pre–/post-administration of vehicle (Vehicle+I/R, Fig. 7c; I/R + Vehicle, Fig. 7f). This increase was considerably and dose-dependently blunted by pre-administration of DNL (DNL0.5 + I/R, Fig. 7d; DNL1.0 + I/R, Fig. 7e). Furthermore, post-administration of DNL (I/R + DNL1.0, Fig. 7g) also drastically nullified this ischemia-induced change.

GFAP immunohistochemistry

Compared to the control retina (Sham, Fig. 7i), an increase of the anti-GFAP immunolabeling was observed in the ischemic retina pre/post-administrated with vehicle (Vehicle+I/R, Fig. 7j; I/R + Vehicle, Fig. 7m). Moreover, this change was obviously and dose-responsively reduced when the ischemic retinas were preadministered with DNL (DNL0.5 + I/R, Fig. 7k; DNL1.0 + I/R, Fig. 7l). Post-administration of DNL (I/R + DNL1.0, Fig. 7n) also obviously reduced this ischemia-induced change. DAPI (blue; Figs. 7a and h) was used to stain cellular nuclei of the Sham retina.

The effects of DNL on the levels of various proteins in the rat retina

The levels of various proteins in the control retinas (Sham; Table 3; $n = 4\sim 10$) were measured and the results are shown in Fig. 8a1 and a2 (HIF-1α = 51.17

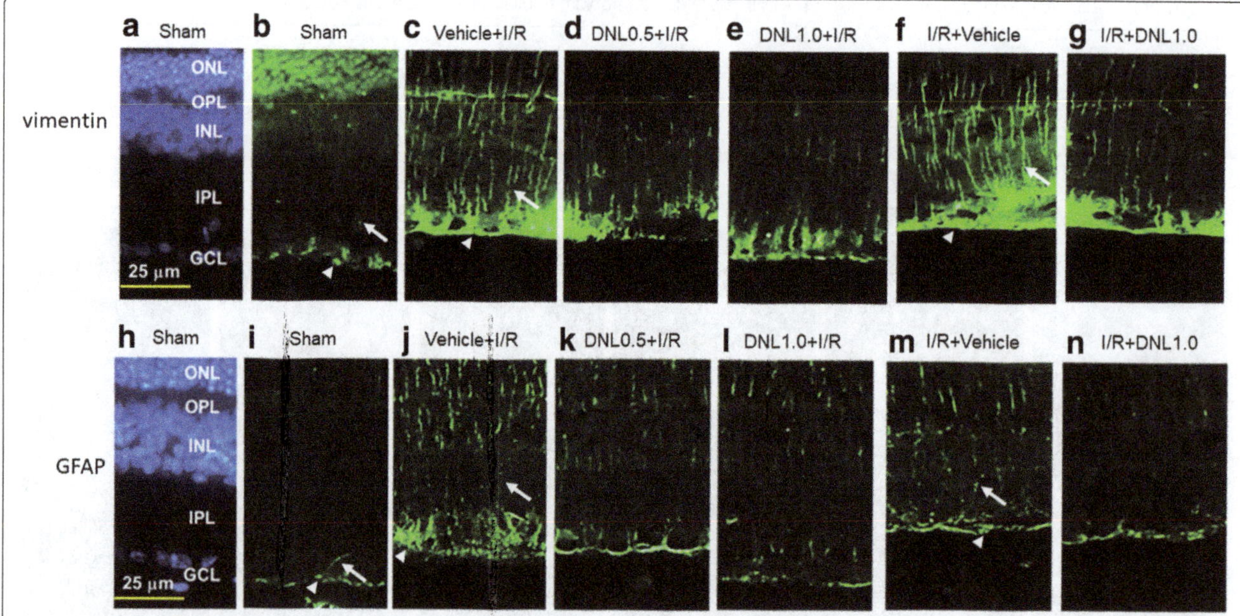

Fig. 7 Vimentin immunohistochemistry. **b** After the sham procedure (Sham), anti-vimentin (green) immunoreactivity can be seen in the end feet of Müller cells (arrow heads; see also **c** and **f**) within the ganglion cell layer (GCL) as well as their processes are also immunolabeled in the IPL (arrows; see also c and f), INL and ONL. **c**, **f** Compared to the sham retina, there was a considerable enhancement of the anti-vimentin immunolabeling after ischemia and pre-administration or post-administration of vehicle (Vehicle+I/R or I/R + Vehicle). **d**, **e**, **g** This enhancement was obviously counteracted by pre-administration of 0.5 g/kg/day (DNL0.5 + I/R), or 1 g/kg/day of DNL (DNL1.0 + I/R), or post-administration of 1 g/kg/day of DNL (I/R + DNL1.0). GFAP immunohistochemical study. After the sham procedure (Sham; **i**), the Müller cells displayed GFAP immunoreactivity at their end feet within the GCL (arrow heads; see also **j** and **m**), and at their processes in the IPL (arrows; see also **j** and **m**), INL and ONL. Compared to the Sham retina, anti-GFAP immunolabeling was enhanced after ischemia and pre-administration/post-administration of vehicle (Vehicle+I/R, **j**; I/R + Vehicle, **m**). This enhancement was mitigated by pre-administration of 0.5 g/kg/day (DNL0.5 + I/R; **k**) or 1 g/kg/day of DNL (DNL1.0 + I/R; **l**), or post-administration of 1 g/kg/day of DNL (I/R + DNL1.0; **n**). **a**, **h** DAPI (blue) was used to counterstain cell nuclei in the sham retina. DNL, Dendrobium nobile Lindley. GFAP, glial fibrillary acidic protein; IPL, inner plexiform layer; INL, inner nuclear layer; ONL, outer nuclear layer; DAPI, 4,6-diamidine-2-phenylindole dihydrochloride. Scale bar = 25 μm

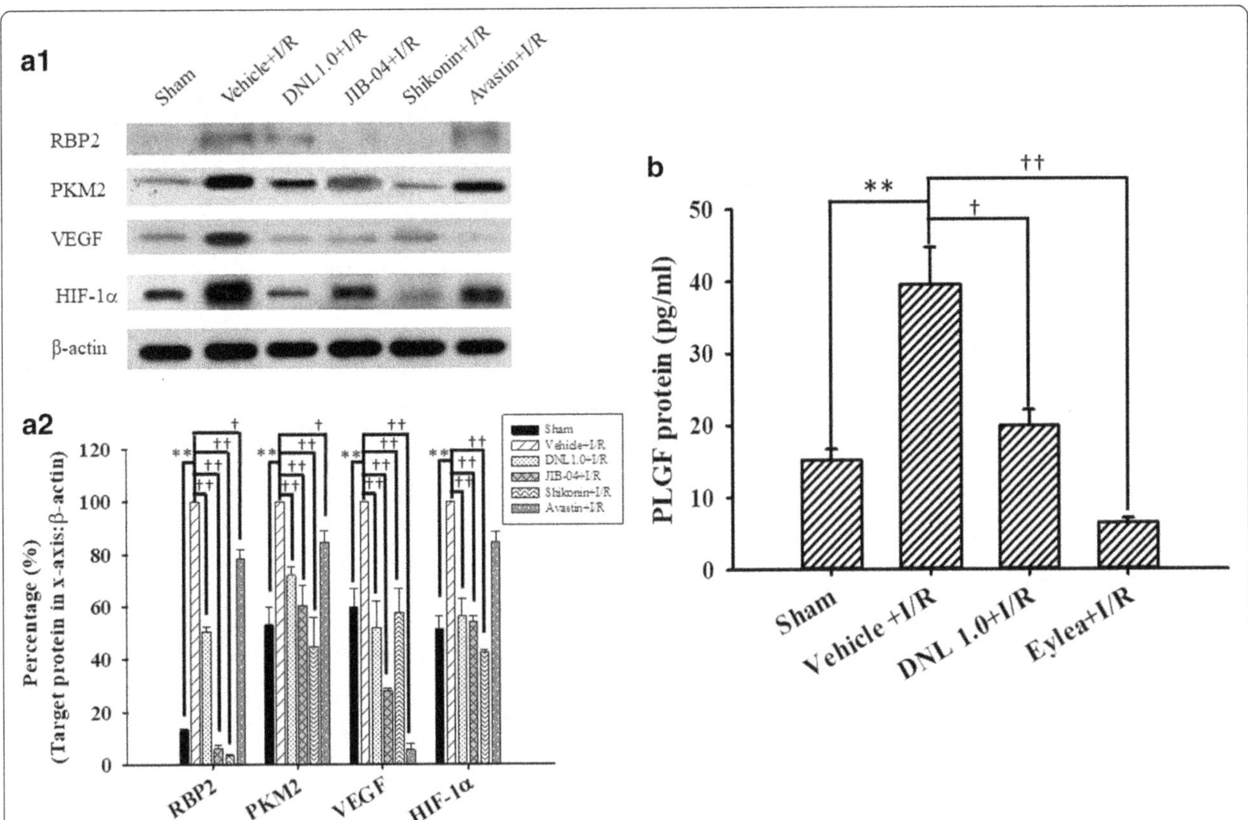

Fig. 8 Western blot analysis showing the expression levels of β-actin, HIF-1α, VEGF, PKM2 and RBP2. Lane 1 or 2 of picture **a1** shows a sham retina subjected to the sham procedure (Sham), or a ischemic retina pre-administered with vehicle (Vehicle+I/R), respectively. Lane 3 shows a retina that received ischemia together with pre-ischemia administration of 1 g/kg/day DNL (DNL1.0 + I/R). Lanes 4~ 6 show retinas that underwent ischemia together with pre-ischemia administration of 10 μM/5 μl JIB-04 (RBP2 inhibitor), 4 μM/5 μl shikonin (PKM2 inhibitor), or 125 μg/5 μl avastin (anti-VEGF), respectively. Each bar in picture **a2** represented the ratio of RBP2, PKM2, VEGF and HIF-1α to β-actin. ** indicates a significant ($P < 0.01$) difference between the Sham retina and the ischemic retina pre-administered with vehicle (Vehicle+I/R). † or †† indicated a significant ($P < 0.05$ or $P < 0.01$) difference between the "Vehicle+I/R" group and the ischemic retina pre-administered with DNL1.0, JIB-04, shikonin or avastin. The results are presented as means±S.E.M. ($n = 4$~ 10). The results of the ELISA assay are presented in picture **b**. The concentration of PLGF was measured in the retinas obtained from various groups, namely Sham, Vehicle+I/R, DNL1.0 + I/R or Eylea+I/R. Rats that received I/R plus pre-ischemia administration of 200 μg/5 μl Eylea was defined as the "Eylea+I/R" group. ** indicates a significant difference ($P < 0.01$) between the Sham retina and Vehicle+I/R. † or †† indicated a significant ($P < 0.05$ or $P < 0.01$) difference between Vehicle+I/R and DNL1.0 + I/R or between Vehicle+I/R and Eylea+I/R. Results are presented as means±S.E.M. (n = 4). Abbreviations: DNL, Dendrobium nobile Lindley. HIF-1α, hypoxia inducible factor-1α; VEGF, vascular endothelium factor; PKM2: pyruvate kinase M2, RBP2: retinoblastoma-binding protein 2; PLGF, placental growth factor

± 5.14%; VEGF = 59.72 ± 6.94%; PKM2 = 52.93 ± 7.01%; RBP2 = 12.81 ± 0.55%). After I/R and preadministration of vehicle, significant (all $P \leq 0.001$) elevations were observed in the levels of HIF-1α, VEGF, PKM2 and RBP2 (normalized to 100%). Furthermore, these elevations were significantly (all $P < 0.001$; HIF-1α = 56.08 ± 6.76; VEGF = 51.87 ± 9.89; PKM2 = 71.99 ± 3.05; RBP2 = 50.64 ± 1.48) inhibited when the ischemic retinas were preadministered with 1.0 g/Kg/day of DNL. Additionally, there was a significant ($P \leq 0.002$ except those for avastin) attenuation of the ischemia-induced increase in the levels of HIF-1α [JIB-04 = 53.98 ± 2.29; shikonin = 42.65 ± 0.76; avastin = 84.61 ± 3.96 ($P = 0.07$)], VEGF (JIB-04 = 27.82 ± 1.21; shikonin = 57.55 ± 9.40; avastin = 5.38 ± 2.51), PKM2 [JIB-04 = 60.36 ± 7.59; shikonin = 44.94 ± 10.91; avastin = 84.44 ± 4.53 ($P = 0.01$)], and RBP2 (JIB-04 = 5.83 ± 1.43; shikonin = 3.40 ± 0.23; avastin = 78.35 ± 3.29 ($P = 0.02$)] after pre-administration of each inhibitor/antibody JIB-04 (RBP2 inhibitor), shikonin (PKM2 inhibitor) and avastin (VEGF antibody).

As shown in Fig. 8b (n = 4), in contrast to the control retinas (Sham = 15.11 ± 1.58 pg/ml), after I/R and preadministration of vehicle, there was a significant ($P = 0.004$) elevation in the level of PLGF (Vehicle+I/R = 39.53 ± 5.25). Moreover, this elevation was significantly ($P = 0.01$ or $P < 0.001$) blunted when the ischemic retinas were pre-administrated with DNL (DNL1.0 + I/R = 19.93 ± 2.24), or anti-PLGF antibody Eylea (Eylea +I/R = 6.44 ± 0.60).

Discussion

As mentioned in the Introduction, many of DNL's various active components, including alkaloids, flavonal glycosides, SG-168 and polysaccharides, have known action mechanisms [18–21]; on the other hand, moscatilin is also an active ingredient (bibenzyl) of DNL seems to have a novel mode of action. In the present study, we found that the protein levels of HIF-1α, VEGF, PKM2 and RBP2 were significantly upregulated in the ischemic retinas, which agrees with previous studies [8, 10–12], but importantly the significant upregulation events affecting these proteins were significantly mitigated by administration of DNL; furthermore, this did not happen with vehicle alone (Fig. 8a). As shown in Fig. 8b, the ischemia-induced elevation of PLGF [13] was also significantly blunted when ischemic retinas were pre-administrated with the VEGF trap/anti-PLGF Eylea. This is similar to the effect of 1.0 g/Kg/day of DNL. This finding suggests that DNL might have a novel and clinical significant anti-angiogenesis/VEGF (PLGF) trapping effect. This is not inconsistent with previous reports where a bibenzyl component of DNL, moscatilin, has been shown to act as an anti-angiogenesis agent and inhibit HIF-1α and VEGF [15, 16, 22].

Up to the present, it has been believed that ischemia is likely to be very similar in mode of action to various diseases such as CRVO/BRVO/CRAO/BRAO, nvAMD and DR, as well as various developmental retinal vasculopathies such as familial exudative vitreoretinopathy and Norrie disease. Over the past twenty years, anti-VEGF antibodies have been used to clear ocular hemorrhage and macular edema effectively in many cases; however, disappointingly, poor visual results do occur in some patients. An increasing body of evidence supports a role of the norrin-dependent Wnt-signaling pathway in both the early normal development of retinal vessels and in the late progression of defined developmental retinal vascular diseases [1–5, 7]. The latter condition may possibly further aggravate ischemia/hypoxia and form NV. Consistently, NDP (norrin) seems to protect the eye from abnormal angiogenesis and retinopathy and it does this by modulating the norrin-dependent Wnt signaling pathway [30]. Moreover, overexpression of NDP has been shown to protect photoreceptors and RGCs from cell death via activation of the norrin-dependent Wnt signaling pathway [31, 32]. Presently, hypoxia (OGD) is known to lead to a significant decrease in the level of NDP (Fig. 2) as well as to cause a significant decrease in the cell viability (Fig. 1). Furthermore, a significant nullification in the OGD induced reduction in the NDP level (Fig. 2) and cultured cell number (Fig. 1) in the presence of moscatilin (0.1 μM), implies that this bibenzyl ingredient of DNL is to be able to significantly alleviate hypoxic/ischemic-like (OGD) injury. As supported by the present results and by various previous reports [5, 7, 15, 16, 22, 30–32], DNL and/or moscatillin would seem to be able to activate the NDP (norrin)-dependent Wnt signaling pathway (Graphical Abstract for DNL & moscatilin as anti-PLGF & NDP stimulator; Additional file 1) and thus provide neuroprotection against retina ischemia (Figs. 1, 3, 4, 5, 6 and 7). This presumably occurs via an inhibition of VEGF-A/PLGF (Fig. 8) and an upregulation of NDP (Fig. 2). This approach seems to be a novel promising way of protecting against retinal ischemia that should further terminate abnormal vasculogenesis, ischemia associated neovascularization (angiogenesis), and the progression of various developmental vascular disorders that are associated with persistent ischemia/hypoxia [5, 7].

After ischemic insult and the administration of vehicle, the inner retinal thickness (Fig. 4), the number of RGCs (Fig. 5) and the ChAT immunoreactivity of amacrine cells (Fig. 6) were significantly/obviously decreased, which is not inconsistent with a previous report [8]. Importantly, our findings in the present study also confirm that these ischemia induced changes were significantly or obviously blunted by pre- administration or post-administration of a high dose of DNL (at 1 g/kg/day). Moreover, in the ischemic retinas with pre–/post-administration of vehicle, vimentin/GFAP immunolabeling overexpression (Fig. 7) was found to parallel the decrease in b-wave (Fig. 3). This is of clinical importance because the present results also show that these ischemic alterations are significantly or obviously counteracted by pre-administration or post-administration of DNL at 1 g/kg/day.

The present results demonstrate that ischemia/hypoxia (ischemia-mimetic OGD), significantly or obviously affects the retina electrophysiologically (Fig. 3), morphometrically (Fig. 4), and immunohistochemically (Figs. 5, 6 and 7) as well as affect at the level of molecular biology and cellular viability (Figs. 1, 2 and 8). In terms of clinical situation, all of these changes following ischemia/OGD are effectively attenuated by pre-treatment or post-treatment with DNL or its bibenzyl component moscatilin (Figs. 1, 2, 3, 4, 5, 6, 7 and 8). This is the first study to show that the Chinese herb DNL (and its bibenzyl ingredient moscatilin) [22, 33] might be able to electrophysiologically, morphometrically, immunohistochemically and molecular biologically protect against the retinal ischemic/ischemic-like injury. These protective mechanisms are presumed to act by suppressing the upregulation of HIF-1α, VEGF-A, PKM2, RBP2, and, above all, PLGF, as well as, possibly, by upregulating the level of NDP (Figs. 2 and 8).

Taking the above findings as a whole, DNL and/or moscatilin seems to be able to protect against or even prevent defined retinal ischemic/ischemic-like alterations and this is likely to occur via the inhibition of the PLGF and also probably via the upregulation of NDP. DNL treatment (and/or moscatilin) might be an useful way of providing a complementary approach that helps to prevent and/or manage the developmental vascular disorders such as Norrie disease in patients where the diseases might progress due to the presence of persistent ischemia/hypoxia [5, 7].

Conclusions

The present study has that demonstrated various ischemic/hypoxic (OGD) alterations that occur in the retina or in retinal cells and these can be monitored by electroretinography, immunohistochemistry (RGCs, amacrine cells, Müller cells), histopathology (retinal thickness), cell viability and measurement of expression levels of various proteins (PLGF, HIF-1α, VEGF-A, PKM2, RBP2 and NDP). Of clinical significance and novel to this study, the protein concentration of PLGF (Fig. 8) was found to be upregulated in such circumstances and that of NDP (Fig. 2) was downregulated. Moreover, and importantly, treatment with DNL/moscatillin (DNL's bibenzyl ingredient) significantly counteracted these alterations. Furthermore, neither moscatilin nor DMSO has an effect on cell numbers in the control groups [moscatilin (0.1 μM) + DMEM or DMSO (50 μl) + DMEM]. DNL/moscatillin might safely provide an alternative way to prevent and/or manage patients with the persistent hypoxia/ischemia associated progression that occurs in various developmental vascular disorders such as Norrie disease; this might occur via a downregulation of the level of PLGF and an upregulation of the concentration of NDP.

Abbreviations

AMD: Age-related macular degeneration; ANOVA: Analysis of variance; ARVO: Association for research in vision and ophthalmology; BCA: Bicinchoninic acid; BRAO: Branch retinal artery occlusion; BRVO: Branch retinal vein occlusion; BSA: Bovine serum albumin; ChAT: Choline acetyltransferase; CHGH: Cheng Hsin General Hospital; CHIACUC: Institutional Animal Care and Use Committee at CHGH; CRAO: Central retinal artery occlusion; CRVO: Central retinal vein occlusion; DAPI: 4,6-diamidine-2-phenylindole dihydrochloride; DMEM: Dulbecco's modified eagle's medium; DMSO: Dimethyl sulfoxide; DNL: Dendrobium nobile Lindley; ECL: Enhanced chemiluminescent; ERG: Electroretinogram; FEVR: Familial exudative vitreoretinopathy; FITC: Fluorescein isothiocyanate; FITC: Fluorescein isothiocyanate; Fzd-4: Frizzled-4; GCL: Ganglion cell layer; GFAP: Glial fibrillary acidic protein; HIF-1α: Hypoxia-inducible factor-1α; HIOP: High intraocular pressure; HRP: Horseradish peroxidase; I/R: Ischemia/reperfusion; ILM: Internal limiting membrane; INL: Inner nuclear layer; IPL: Inner plexiform layer; MPER: Mammalian protein extraction reagent; MTT: 3-(4,5-dimethylthiazol-2-yl)-2,5-diphenyltetrazolium bromide; NADPH: Nicotinamide adenine dinucleotide phosphate hydrogen; NDP: Norrie disease protein; NV: Neovascularization; OD: Optical density; OGD: Oxygen glucose deprivation; PBS: Phosphate-buffered saline; PBST: Phosphate buffered saline containing 0.05% Tween 20; PDR: Proliferative diabetic retinopathy; PHPV: Persistent hyperplastic primary vitreous disease; PKM2: Pyruvate kinase M2; PLGF: Placental growth factor; PVDF: Polyvinylidene difluoride; RBP2: Retinoblastoma-binding protein 2; RGCs: Retinal ganglion cells; RPE: Retinal pigment epithelium; SDS-PAGE: Sodium dodecyl sulfate polyacrylamide gel electrophoresis; SE: Standard error; TMB: Tetramethylbenzidine; VEGF: Vascular endothelium growth factor

Acknowledgements

Sincere grateful thanks are conveyed for the financial support provided by the Ministry of Science and Technology, Taiwan [104-2320-B-350-001-]. We also thank Ms. Yu-Chun Wang for her skillful technical help with the animal experiments and molecular biological assays as well as Professor Ralph Kirby for his expertise in correcting the manuscript.

Authors' contributions

HMC was the main designer of this research. WHC and MIL were involved in performing the experiments and writing the manuscript. HTP, HWS, MMC and HMC carried out the analysis of the data and the revision of the manuscript. All authors have read and approved the final draft of the manuscript. All authors unanimously endorse the final manuscript.

Ethics approval

Methods

In vivo studies

Animals (1st sentence)

The animal use protocol has been reviewed and approved by the Institutional Animal Care and Use Committee at Cheng Hsin General Hospital (CHGH; Taipei, Taiwan; Approval No: CHIACUC 104–14).

Competing interests

The authors declare that they have no competing interests.

Author details

[1]Institute of Pharmacology, School of Medicine, National Yang-Ming University, Taipei, Taiwan. [2]Department of Ophthalmology, Cheng Hsin General Hospital, Taipei, Taiwan. [3]Department of Ophthalmology, Taipei Medical University-Shuang Ho Hospital, New Taipei City, Taiwan. [4]Department of Chinese Medicine, School of Chinese Medicine, China Medical University, Taichung, Taiwan.

References

1. Xu Q, Wang Y, Dabdoub A, Smallwood PM, Williams J, Woods C, et al. Vascular development in the retina and inner ear: control by Norrin and Frizzled-4, a high-affinity ligand-receptor pair. Cell. 2004;116(6):883–95. 15035989
2. Nikopoulos K, Venselaar H, Collin RW, Riveiro-Alvarez R, Boonstra FN, Hooymans JM, et al. Overview of the mutation spectrum in familial exudative vitreoretinopathy and Norrie disease with identification of 21 novel variants in FZD4, LRP5, and NDP. Hum Mutat. 2010;31(6):656–66. https://doi.org/10.1002/humu.21250.
3. Wu JH, Liu JH, Ko YC, Wang CT, Chung YC, Chu KC, et al. Haploinsufficiency of RCBTB1 is associated with coats disease and familial exudative vitreoretinopathy. Hum Mol Genet. 2016;25(8):1637–47. https://doi.org/10.1093/hmg/ddw041.
4. Wang Y, Rattner A, Zhou Y, Williams J, Smallwood PM, Nathans J. Norrin/Frizzled4 signaling in retinal vascular development and blood brain barrier plasticity. Cell. 2012;151:1332–44. https://doi.org/10.1016/j.cell.2012.10.042.
5. Luhmann UFO, Lin J, Acar N, Lammel S, Feil S, Grimm C, et al. Role of the Norrie disease pseudoglioma gene in sprouting angiogenesis during development of the retinal vasculature. Invest Ophthalmol Vis Sci. 2005;46:3372–82. https://doi.org/10.1167/iovs.05-0174.

6. Chao HM, Chuang MJ, Liu JH, Liu XQ, Ho LK, Pan WH, et al. Baicalein protects against retinal ischemia by antioxidation, antiapoptosis, downregulation of HIF-1α, VEGF, and MMP-9 and upregulation of HO-1. J Ocul Pharmacol Ther. 2013; 29(6):539–49. https://doi.org/10.1089/jop.2010.0063.
7. Beck SC, Feng Y, Sothilingam V, Garrido MG, Tanimoto N, Acar N, et al. Long-term consequences of developmental vascular defects on retinal vessel homeostasis and function in a mouse model of Norrie disease. PLoS One. 2017;12(6):e0178753. https://doi.org/10.1371/journal.pone.0178753.
8. Tan S, Geng S, Liu JH, Pan WH, Wang LX, Liu HK, et al. Xue-Fu-Zhu-Yu decoction protects rats against retinal ischemia by downregulation of HIF-1α and VEGF via inhibition of RBP2 and PKM2. BMC Complement Altern Med. 2017;17(1):365. https://doi.org/10.1186/s12906-017-1857-2.
9. Wurm A, Iandiev I, Uhlmann S, Wiedemann P, Reichenbach A, Bringmann A, et al. Effects of ischemia-reperfusion on physiological properties of Müller glial cells in the porcine retina. Invest Ophthalmol Vis Sci. 2011;52(6):3360–7. https://doi.org/10.1167/iovs.10-6901.
10. Liu JH, Wann H, Chen MM, Pan WH, Chen YC, Liu CM, et al. Baicalein significantly protects human retinal pigment epithelium cells against H_2O_2-induced oxidative stress by scavenging reactive oxygen species and downregulating the expression of matrix metalloproteinase-9 and vascular endothelial growth factor. J Ocul Pharmacol Ther. 2010;26(5):421–9. https://doi.org/10.1089/jop.2010.0063.
11. Luo W, Hu H, Chang R, Zhong J, Knabel M, O'Meally R, et al. Pyruvate kinase M2 is a PHD3-stimulated coactivator for hypoxia-inducible factor 1. Cell. 2011;145(5):732–44. https://doi.org/10.1016/j.cell.2011.03.054.
12. Qi L, Zhu F, Li SH, Si LB, Hu LK, Tian H. Retinoblastoma binding protein 2 (RBP2) promotes HIF-1α-VEGF-induced angiogenesis of non-small cell lung cancer via the Akt pathway. PLoS One. 2014;9(8):e106032. https://doi.org/10.1371/ journal.pone.0106032.
13. Mesquita J, Castro-de-Sousa JP, Vaz-Pereira S, Neves A, Passarinha LA, Tomaz CT. Vascular endothelial growth factors and placental growth factor in retinal vasculopathies: current research and future perspectives. Cytokine Growth Factor Rev. 2018;39:102–15. https://doi.org/10.1016/j.cytogfr.2017.11.005.
14. Lam Y, Ng TB, Yao RM, Shi J, Xu K, Sze SC, et al. Evaluation of chemical constituents and important mechanism of pharmacological biology in dendrobium plants. Evid Based Complement Alternat Med. 2015;2015: 841752. https://doi.org/10.1155/2015/841752.
15. Liu YN, Pan SL, Peng CY, Huang DY, Guh JH, Chen CC, et al. Moscatilin repressed lipopolysaccharide-induced HIF-1alpha accumulation and NF-kappaB activation in murine RAW264.7 cells. Shock. 2010;33(1):70–5. https://doi.org/10.1097/shk.0b013e3181a7ff4a.
16. Tsai AC, Pan SL, Liao CH, Guh JH, Wang SW, Sun HL, et al. Moscatilin, a bibenzyl derivative from the India orchid Dendrobrium loddigesii, suppresses tumor angiogenesis and growth in vitro and in vivo. Cancer Lett. 2010;292(2):163–70. https://doi.org/10.1016/j.canlet.2009.11.020.
17. Chen CA, Chen CC, Shen CC, Chang HH, Chen YJ. Moscatilin induces apoptosis and mitotic catastrophe in human esophageal cancer cells. J Med Food. 2013;16(10):869–77. https://doi.org/10.1089/jmf.2012.2617.
18. Li Y, Li F, Gong Q, Wu Q, Shi J. Inhibitory effects of dendrobium alkaloids on memory impairment induced lipopolysaccharide in rats. Planta Med. 2011; 77(2):117–21. https://doi.org/10.1055/s-0030-1250235.
19. Sun J, Zhang F, Yang M, Zhang J, Chen L, Zhan R, et al. Isolation of α-glucosidase inhibitors including a new flavonol glycoside from Dendrobium devonianum. Nat Prod Res. 2014;28(21):1900–5. https://doi.org/10.1080/14786419.2014.955495.
20. Yoon MY, Hwang JH, Park JH, Lee MR, Kim HJ, Park E, et al. Neuroprotective effects of SG-168 against oxidative stress-induced apoptosis in PC12 cells. J Med Food. 2011;14(1–2):120–7. https://doi.org/10.1089/jmf.2010.1027.
21. Pan LH, Li XF, Wang MN, Zha XQ, Yang XF, Liu ZJ, et al. Comparison of hypoglycemic and antioxidative effects of polysaccharides from four different Dendrobium species. Int J Biol Macromol. 2014;64:420–7. https://doi.org/10.1016/j.ijbiomac.2013.12.024.
22. Gong CY, Lu B, Yang L, Wang L, Ji LL. Bibenzyl from Dendrobium inhibits angiogenesis and its underlying mechanism. Yao Xue Xue Bao. 2013;48(3): 337–42. PMID: 23724644
23. Kowitdamrong A, Chanvorachote P, Sritularak B, Pongrakhananon V. Moscatilin inhibits lung cancer cell motility and invasion via suppression of endogenous reactive oxygen species. Biomed Res Int. 2013;2013:765894. https://doi.org/10.1155/2013/765894.
24. Van Bergen NJ, Wood JP, Chidlow G, Trounce IA, Casson RJ, Ju WK, Weinreb RN, Crowston JG. Recharacterization of the RGC-5 retinal ganglion cell line. Invest Ophthalmol Vis Sci. 2009;50(9):4267–72. https://doi.org/10.1167/iovs.09-3484.
25. Tasca CI, Dal-Cim T, Cimarosti H. In vitro oxygen-glucose deprivation to study ischemic cell death. Methods Mol Biol. 2015;1254:197–210. https://doi.org/10.1007/978-1-4939-2152-2_15.
26. Mosmann T. Rapid colorimetric assay for cellular growth and survival: application to proliferation and cytotoxicity assays. J Immunol Methods. 1983;65(1–2):55–63. https://doi.org/10.1016/0022-1759(83)90303-4.
27. Engvall E, Perlmann P. Enzyme-linked immunosorbent (ELISA). Quantitative assay of immunoglobulin G. Immunochemistry. 1971;8:871–4. PMID: 5135623
28. Smith PK, Krohn RI, Hermanson GT, Mallia AK, Gartner FH, Provenzano MD, et al. Measurement of protein using bicinchoninic acid. Anal Biochem. 1985; 150:76–85. PMID: 3843705
29. Ho C, Chen C. Moscatilin from the orchid Dendrobrium loddigesii is a potential anticancer agent. Cancer Investig. 2003;21(5):729–36. https://doi.org/10.1081/CNV-120023771.
30. Drenser KA. Wnt signaling pathway in retinal vascularization. Eye Brain. 2016;8:141–6. https://doi.org/10.2147/EB.S94452.
31. Braunger BM, Ohlmann A, Koch M, Tanimoto N, Volz C, Yang Y, et al. Constitutive overexpression of Norrin activates Wnt/β-catenin and endothelin-2 signaling to protect photoreceptors from light damage. Neurobiol Dis. 2013;50:1–12. https://doi.org/10.1016/j.nbd.2012.09.008.
32. Dailey WA, Drenser KA, Wong SC, Cheng M, Vercellone J, Roumayah KK, et al. Norrin treatment improves ganglion cell survival in an oxygen-induced retinopathy model of retinal ischemia. Exp Eye Res. 2017;164:129–38. https://doi.org/10.1016/j.exer.2017.08.012.
33. Miyazawa M, Shimamura H, Nakamura S, Sugiura W, Kosaka H, Kameoka H. Moscatilin from Dendrobium nobile, a naturally occurring bibenzyl compound with potential antimutagenic activity. J Agric Food Chem. 1999; 47(5):2163–7. PMID: 10552513

12

Determination of the volatile and polyphenol constituents and the antimicrobial, antioxidant, and tyrosinase inhibitory activities of the bioactive compounds from the by-product of *Rosa rugosa Thunb. var. plena Regal* tea

Guixing Ren[1,4*†], Peng Xue[2,4†], Xiaoyan Sun[4] and Gang Zhao[3*]

Abstract

Background: The phytochemical constituents and biological activities of *Rosa rugosa Thunb. var. plena Regal* flower cell sap (RFCS) were investigated.

Methods: Volatile constituent, such as linalool, phenylethyl alcohol, citronellol, α-bisabolol, were identified by GC-MS. The contents of hyperoside, kaempferol-3-O-rutinosid, rutin, and luteolin as well as the total flavonoid content in RFCS were determined by HPLC and HPLC-MS. The total polyphenol content was evaluated by the Folin-Ciocalteu colorimetric method. The antioxidant activities of RFCS and the standards were evaluated by DPPH and ABTS radical scavenging assays. The tyrosinase inhibitory activities of the rose samples and standard substance were determined by a spectrophotometric method. The antimicrobial effects of RFCS were evaluated in terms of minimum inhibitory concentrations (MICs) and minimum bactericidal concentrations (MBCs) or minimum Fungicidal concentrations (MFCs).

Results: The rose fraction exhibited a high content of biologically active ingredients. The total content of volatile compounds in RFCS was approximately 48.21 ± 2.76 ng/mL. The total phenolic acid content and total flavonoid content were 0.31 ± 0.01 mg/mL and 0.43 ± 0.01 mg/mL, respectively. Its IC_{50} value in the DPPH assay was 1120 ± 42 μg/mL, and its IC_{50} value for ABTS radical scavenging activity was 1430 ± 42 μg/mL.RFCS strongly inhibited L-tyrosine oxidation with an IC_{50} value of 570 ± 21 μg/mL. Every compound identified in RFCS exhibited broad-spectrum antimicrobial activity. *F. nucleatum* was most susceptible to RFCS with an MIC of 64 μg/mL and MBC of 250 μg/mL.

Conclusions: Due to its rose-like aroma, phenylethyl alcohol may be combined with linalool for use as a natural skin-whitening agent and skin care additive in the and pharmaceutical industries.

Keywords: RFCS, Phytochemical constituents, Antioxidant, Antimicrobial, Tyrosinase inhibitory activities

* Correspondence: renguixing@cdu.edu.cn; zhaogang@cdu.edu.cn
[†]Guixing Ren and Peng Xue contributed equally to this work.
[1]College of Pharmacy and Biological Engineering, Chengdu University, Chengdu 610000, People's Republic of China
[3]Key Laboratory of Coarse Cereal Processing, Ministry of Agriculture, No.2025 Chengluo Road, Longquanyi District, Chengdu 610106, People's Republic of China
Full list of author information is available at the end of the article

Background

The flower of *Rosa rugosa Thunb. var. plena Regal* is not only used in perfume production but has also been used as a health food and medicine in Asian countries for thousands of years. Additionally, roses contain active materials, such as essential oils, polyphenols, flavonoids and anthocyanin, which are known for their antimicrobial, anti-inflammatory, hypoglycemic, and antioxidant activities [1–4]. Roses can be consumed in many forms, such as rose teas, rose cookies, and rose oils. The production of rose tea or dried flower petals via low-temperature drying of rose flowers (*Rosa rugosa cv. Plena*) yields a condensate called "rose flower cell sap" (RFCS). The disposal of RFCS represents a great waste of resources due to its high content of polyphenols and rose essential oil, which has very high biological activity. In addition, environmental pollution may be caused by the improper disposal of RFCS because it is difficult to decompose. In addition, essential oils and polyphenols are active ingredients in the pharmaceutical, cosmetic, and food industries. The drying of 1 kg of raw rose petals or flower bud material can produce approximately 0.2 L of condensate. Approximately 40,000 kg of rose flower buds and 20,000 kg of petals are used per cycle of industrial microwave-drying in Pingyin alone. To date, no studies have reported a suitable method for the disposal of RFCS and the bioactive compounds contained therein.

Rose oil distillation wastewater (RODW) is another by-product of the steam distillation of dried rose flowers to product rose oil. In previous studies, RODW has been concentrated to generate a polyphenol-enriched residue containing non-volatile phenolic compounds [5]. Moreover, the polyphenol fraction of RODW can strongly inhibit mushroom tyrosinase (IC_{50} value of 0.41 μg/mL) [6]. Thus, the polyphenols in RODW may be used as a bioactive substance to relieve hyperpigmentation.

Food-related pathogenic bacteria cause foodborne illnesses in millions of people and even hundreds of deaths every year in the USA alone, and the associated cost total approximately $ 2.4 billion [7]. Thus, the increasing demand for healthy, non-toxic, and effective antimicrobial agents has inspired research on multifunctional, naturally produced food additives. Although rose oil primarily contains essential oils known for their antimicrobial activities [8], the antimicrobial effects of RFCS have not been investigated.

The phenolic compounds and volatile substances in flowers have strong biological activities such as antioxidant and tyrosinase inhibitory effects [9]. The development of additional methods for inhibiting tyrosinase activity is an active area of research in the functional cosmetics and food industries due to tyrosinase's whitening effect and ability to control browning [10, 11]. Antioxidants may lower the risks of health concerns such as cancer, aging, and atherosclerosis by reducing the level of reactive oxygen species (ROS) [12]. Some antioxidants, such as ascorbic acid, also have been reported to have whitening effects [11].

In our preliminary test, antimicrobial, antioxidant, and tyrosinase inhibitory activities of RODW from *Rosa rugosa Thunb. var. plena Regal* were evaluated [13]. However, there are no reports in the literature investigating the phytochemical composition and biological activities of RFCS from *Rosa rugosa cv. Plena*. In this study, (1) contents of the total phenolics, flavonoids, total solid and volatile contents were investigated; (2) the antibacterial (six strains) and anti fungal (one strain) activity, antioxidant, and tyrosinase inhibitory activities of each active compound and RFCS were examined. Our results will help to improve the value of roses in the fields of medicinal and cosmetic products [13–16].

Methods

Chemicals

Phenylethyl alcohol, α-bisabolol, α-terpineol, citronellol, miconazole nitrate, hydrochloride tetracycline, menthol and camphor were purchased from J&K Scientific Ltd. (Beijing). Kojic acid, hyperoside, quercetin, gallic acid, kaempferol-3-O-acetylglucosylrhamnoside and kaempferol-3-O-glucoside were purchased from Sigma (Shanghai, China). Anaerobic blood agar base medium (CDC), actinomycete broth medium (GAM broth), brain heart infusion (BHI) broth, and nutrient agar were obtained from Suolaibao Biotech Co., Ltd. (Beijing, China). The remaining chemicals were analytical or chromatographic grade.

Sample preparation

RFCS of *Rosa rugosa Thunb. var. plena Regal* was obtained from Fragrant Rose Biological Technology Co., LTD in Pingyin. The samples were filtered through a 0.42 μm microfiltration membrane prior to analyses. The total solid content of RFCS was evaluated by freeze-drying. The identification of *Rosa rugosa Thunb. var. plena Regal* was identificated by senior agronomist Guo and confirmed in voucher sample (Ser. No. 0712) deposited at Herbarium, Pingyin Institute of Rose Sciences.

HPLC analyses

The concentration of polyphenol constituents in the extract was determined by HPLC and UV analyses. The HPLC apparatus was an LC-20A HPLC system (Shimadzu Corporation, Kyoto, Japan), and it was equipped with an Ultrasphere 5 C_{18} column (4.6 mm × 250 mm, Ultrasphere Co., Ltd., Berkshire, UK). The mobile phase was a gradient elution of water (A) and acetonitrile (B) and was programmed as follows: starting with 10% B for 10 min, 10–25% B between 15 and 20 min, 25–30% B between

20 and 25 min, 30–60% B between 25 and 50 min, 60–10% B between 50 and 51 min, and 10% B between 51 and 55 min. The flow rate of the mobile phase was maintained at 1 mL/min, the detector wavelength was set at 350 nm, the column oven was set at 25 °C, and the sample injection volume was 10 μL.

HPLC-ESI-MS conditions

The electrospray ionization (ESI) mass spectrometry (MS) data were recorded on an Agilent-LC-1100 instrument (Agilent, USA). The HPLC conditions for the HPLC-ESI-MS analysis were as described above. The ESI parameters were as follows: the collision gas (N_2) flow rate was maintained at 10 mL/min, the column oven was 25 °C, data were acquired in negative ionmode $[M-H]^-$, scans were conducted over m/z 50–2000, the spray voltage was 4.5 kV, the capillary voltage was 10 V, and the capillary temperature was 250 °C. The components in the sample were identified based on their mass spectral data and retention time.

GC/MS analysis

The volatile constituents in RFCS were determined by a Shimadzu GC/MS model QP2010 Ultra system equipped with an Rtx-5MS (30 m × 0.25 mm, film thickness 0.25 μm) capillary column. The oven program was as follows: starting at 60 °C, heating to 120 °C at a rate of 1.7 °C/min, heating to 200 °C at 2.5 °C/min, heating to 260 °C at a rate of 8 °C/min, and finally holding at 260 °C for 2 min. Helium was used as the carrier gas, and the flow rate was 1.0 mL/min. The injector and detector temperatures were held at 250 °C and 280 °C, respectively. A split injection was conducted in splitless mode. The ion source temperature was 250 °C and its ionization energy was 70 eV. The mass range was 35–500 Da. The components in the sample were identified based on their mass spectral data and retention time.

Preparation of standard curves

Solutions of phenylethyl alcohol (2.23 mg), α-bisabolol (2.1 mg), α-terpineol (5.23 mg), citronellol (1.52 mg), menthol (1.32 mg), and camphor were separately prepared in 1 mL of acetonitrile. Next, the stock solutions were diluted by factors of ten thousand to one billion with ethyl acetate, and 1 μL of each sample was analyzed by GS/MS. Solutions of kojic acid (1.12 mg), hyperoside (1.07 mg), quercetin (1.07 mg), gallic acid (1.29 mg), and kaempferol-3-O-acetylglucosylrhamnoside (1.15 mg) were separately prepared in 1 mL of methyl alcohol. The stock solutions were diluted by factors of 2 with methyl alcohol, and 10 μL of each solution was analyzed by HPLC. Each concentration of working solution was analyzed in three times. The calibration curves were plotted as the peak areas against the concentration of each standard. The content of the reference substance in each sample was calculated using the calibration curves.

Determination of total phenolics, flavonoids and total solid content

The total phenolic contents of the RFCS were evaluated by the Folin-Ciocalteu colorimetric method [17]. The total content of phenolic substance was determined by comparison to a standard curve of gallic acid. The total flavonoid contents of the RFCS samples were evaluated by HPLC, which provided the total amount of all tested flavonoid compounds. A 10-mL sample of RFCS was freeze-dried to determine the total solid content. Every determination was carried out in triplicate.

Antioxidant properties

DPPH radical scavenging activity

The antioxidant activity of RFCS and the standards were evaluated by DPPH radical scavenging activity using a slightly modified version of a previously reported method [18]. Briefly, 10 μL aliquots of the rose samples (1000 μg/mL to 62.5 μg/mL) were mixed with 190 μL of 50% ethanol containing 0.4 mM DPPH and incubated in the dark for 30 min. Aliquots (100 μL) of the supernatants were transferred into a 96-well microplate, and the absorbance of each was recorded at 517 nm using a Spectramax Plus384 UV-Vis spectrophotometer (Molecular Devices, Sunnyvale, California, USA). Ascorbic acid (1000 μg/mL to 0.05 μg/mL) was used as a positive control, and DPPH solution without sample was used as the negative control. The IC_{50} values, which represent the concentrations of rose samples and standard substance at which 50% of the DPPH radical was inhibited, were determined. The tests were performed in triplicate, and the percentage of DPPH scavenging was calculated using the following equation.

$$\text{Inhibition } (\%) = \{(H_0 - H)/H_0\} \times 100$$

H : Absorbance of RFCS and the standards;
H_0 : Absorbance of the blank

Determination of ABTS radical scavenging

The ABTS assay of RFCS was performed according to a modified version of a previously reported method [19]. Briefly, the stock solutions were generated by mixing equal quantities of 7.4 mM $ABTS^{\bullet+}$ solution and 2.6 mM potassium persulfate solution, and the mixture was incubated at room temperature for 12 h in the dark. Then, the solution was equilibrated with 1 mL of $ABTS^{\bullet+}$ solution with 50% ethanol serving as a positive control. The absorbance of the solution at 734 nm was 1.17 ± 0.02 units. Aliquots (10 μL) of the rose samples

(1000 μg/mL to 62.5 μg/mL) were mixed with 1.0 mL of the diluted $ABTS^{•+}$ solution. The mixture was mixed vigorously and incubated at 30 °C for 30 min. The absorbance was then measured at 520 nm with an excitation wavelength of 734 nm using the spectrophotometer. The positive standard was Trolox (2000 μg/mL to 0.05 μg/mL).

$$\text{Inhibition } (\%) = \{(\text{Absorbance of blank} - \text{Absorbance of sample}) / \text{Absorbance of blank}\} \times 100$$

Determination of the Tyrosinase inhibitory activity

The tyrosinase inhibitory activities of the rose samples and standard substance were determined by a spectrophotometric method [17]. First, 300 μL aliquots of different concentrations (1000 μg/mL to 62.5 μg/mL) of each sample were diluted with 700 μL of 0.175 M sodium phosphate buffer (pH 6.8), then 1.0 mL of 10 mM DOPA solution and 1.0 mL of mushroom tyrosinase (220 units/mL) were added. Ethanol (300 μL, 50%) and kojic acid (2000 μg/mL to 0.1 μg/mL) were used as the blank reference and positive standard, respectively. The reaction mixture was vortexed and maintained at 37 °C for 15 min, and then the absorption maximum of dopachrome (set at 479 nm) was measured using a microplate reader (Molecular Devices, Sunnyvale, California, USA). The tests were performed in triplicate, and the value of tyrosinase inhibition activity was calculated as described above.

Antimicrobial properties

Antibacterial and antifungal assays

The antimicrobial activity was measured by the method described by Xue [20]. All standard strains were obtained from the Guangdong Microbiology Culture Center (Guangzhou, China). *Listeria ivanovii* (ATCC 19119) was cultured in BHI, *Salmonella enteritidis enteritidis* (ATCC 14028) *Staphylococcus aureus* (ATCC 25923) and *Escherichia coli* (ATCC 25922) were cultured in nutrient agar (NA) for 24 h and at 37 °C. *candida albicans* (ATCC 10231) was cultured in PHB at 37 °C for 24 h. *Propionibacterium acnes* (ATCC 6919) and *Fusobacterium nucleatum* (ATCC 10953) were cultured in CDC agar at 37 °C for 48 h in a YQX-II anaerobic incubator (Shanghai, China). The final cell counts in 1 mL of broth were approximately 10^6 colony-forming units (CFU/mL). A 10 mg/mL solution of miconazole nitrate and hydrochloride tetracycline in water was used as a positive control against fungi and bacteria, respectly.

Determination of minimum inhibitory concentration (MIC) and minimum bactericidal concentration (MBC) or minimum fungicidal concentration (MFC)

The MIC and MBC or MFC values were determined as described previously by Xue. Briefly, 100 μL dilutions (approximately 100,000 CFU/mL) of *Staphylococcus aureus, Escherichia coli, Salmonella enteritidis enteritidis, Fusobacterium nucleatum*, and *Candida albicans* in nutrient broth and *Listeria ivanovii* and *Propionibacterium acnes* in GMA broth were inoculated into microtiter plates. Then, 100 μL aliquots of the solutions of the test compound were added after a two-fold serial dilution with nutrient broth (from 2 mg/mL to 3 μg/mL). Broths with 5% (*v*/v) DMSO were used as controls. The petri dishes were incubated at 37 °C for 24 h with the exception of *Propionibacterium acnes* and *Fusobacterium nucleatum*, which were incubated at 37 °C for 48 h. The MIC was recorded as the lowest concentration of sample showing no detectable growth. To determine the MBC or MFC values for no bacterial or fungus growth, 10 μL of sub-inhibitory concentrations of the test compounds were incubated on CDC or GMA agar plates for 24 or 48 h. Every determination was carried out in triplicate.

Date analysis

Data are presented as the mean of three replicates ± standard deviation. One-way ANOVA with Duncan's multiple range test was used to analyze the results with SPSS 13.0 and Sigma Plot 10.0, respectively, using a computer (Lenovo, Yangtian B 41) equipped with the Win 7 operating system. A p value of < 0.05 was determined to be statistically significant.

Results and discussion

The contents of volatile substance

Since the RFCS samples had a specific rose fragrance, we analyzed and compared the volatile components of its ethyl acetate extract. The contents of the volatile components of the ethyl acetate extract of RFCS were determined by GC/MS and analyzed by comparison to four standard curves, and the results are expressed as ng/mL.

Six principal components were simultaneously identified according to their standard retention times and MS ion fragments. The GC chromatograms of the reference substance in RFCS are shown in Fig. 1. The content of each element in every sample is presented in Table 1. As shown in Fig. 1, six compounds were successfully separated under the gradient temperature program. The total content of volatile compounds in RFCS was approximately 48.21 ± 2.76 ng/mL, and six major kinds of volatile compounds, including phenylethyl alcohol (40.48 ± 2.24 ng/mL), citronellol (7.83 ± 0.77 ng/mL), α-bisabolol (0.08 ± 0.01 ng/mL) and phenylethyl acetate (11.20 ± 0.89 ng/mL) were identified (two peaks have not been identified and the content of linalool is rare). In previous studies on the volatile compounds in RODW, GC-MS, more specifically HS-SPME/GC/MS, techniques have been widely utilized [13, 21–24]. In

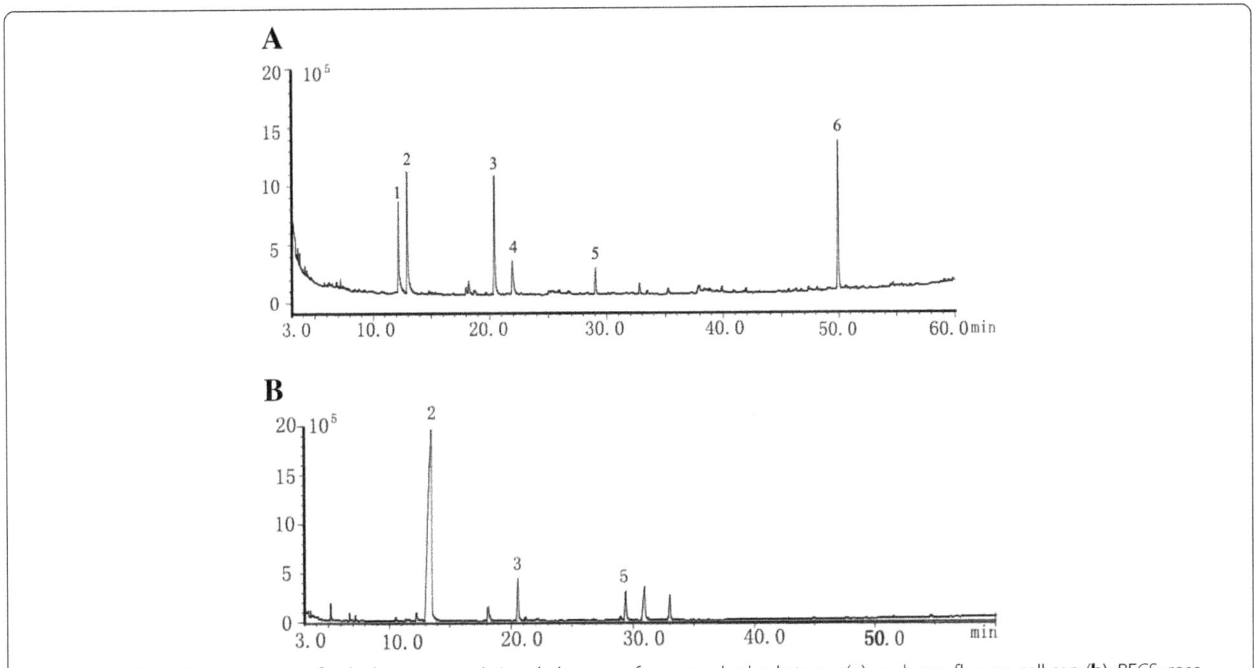

Fig. 1 a Total ion chromatogram of volatile compounds in ethyl acetate from standard substance (**a**), and rose flowers cell sap (**b**). RFCS: rose flower cell sap. Identification of peaks. 1, linalool; 2, phenylethyl alcohol; 3, citronellol; 4, ester phenylethyl acetate; 5, citronellol acetate; 6, α-bisabolol

contrast to these previous studies, our study reports the absolute contents of the components. Although there was a broad range of volatile compounds, there were no differences in the dominant components. The major volatile compounds in RFCS were monoterpene alcohols (citronellol, linalool, and phenylethyl alcohol, which is specific to small roses). The types of dominant components in RFCS are similar to those of RODW, but there is a significant difference in the contents of the components [13]. One possible reason for these differences is that most of the volatile components were lost in the rose tea drying process.

Total phenolic, flavonoid and soild contents

The flavonoids, their retention times, and the calibration curves of standard compounds in RFCS, as determined

Table 1 Analytical characteristics of volatile substances in rose waste. (ng/mL)

Compound	RT	Formula structure	Weight	RFCS
Linalool	12.163	$C_{10}H_{18}O$	154.25	n.d
Phenylethyl alcohol	12.921	$C_8H_{10}O$	122.16	40.48 ± 2.24
Citronellol	20.393	$C_{10}H_{20}O$	156.27	7.83 ± 0.77
Phenylethyl acetate	21.923	$C_{10}H_{12}O_2$	164.2	11.20 ± 0.89
Citronellol acetate	29.029	$C_{12}H_{22}O_2$	198.3	n.d
α-bisabolol	49.909	$C_{15}H_{26}O$	222.36	0.08 ± 0.01
Total content				48.21 ± 2.76

nd not detected; Data are expressed as mean ± standard deviation of triplicate samples; *RFCS* rose flower cell sap

using HPLC, are showen in Fig. 2. Four compounds were successfully separated under the gradient temperature program, as showen in Fig. 2. The linearity of calibration curves and regression coefficients of flavonoids were demonstrated in Table 2. It was found that the reference compounds showed good linearity ($R^2 \geq 0.997$). RFCS was found to contain three main components, namely, hyperoside (0.18 ± 0.01 mg/mL), kaempferol-3-O-rutinosid (0.12 ± 0.01 mg/mL), and rutin (0.23 ± 0.01 mg/mL). The total phenolic content and total flavonoid content were 0.31 ± 0.01 mg/mL and 0.43 ± 0.01 mg/mL, respectively. The total solid content in RFCS was 1.45 ± 0.04 mg/mL.

Previous studies have reported that the dominant phenolic and flavonoid compounds in rose rugosa tea were gallic acid, catechin, epicatechin, and quercetin and the total polyphenol content and flavonoid content in the *Rosa rugosa* tea polyphenol extract were 875.2 mg/g and 610.3 mg/g, respectively [1]. In addition, rutin, multiflorin B, hyperoside, kaepferol, and ellagic acid were also found in the resin fractions of RODW [6]. Furthermore, unlike previous studies, although our study used HPLC-MS to determine the phenol and flavonoid compounds in RODW, only one of the dominant compounds, kaempferol-3-O-rutinosid, was found in this study and in previous studies [6, 13]. Neither of the phenol compounds was detected in RFCS by HPLC primarily because the concentrations of phenols and flavonoids in RFCS are very low, and thus they are undetectable by HPLC. Those solids in RFCS were mixture of small molecules.

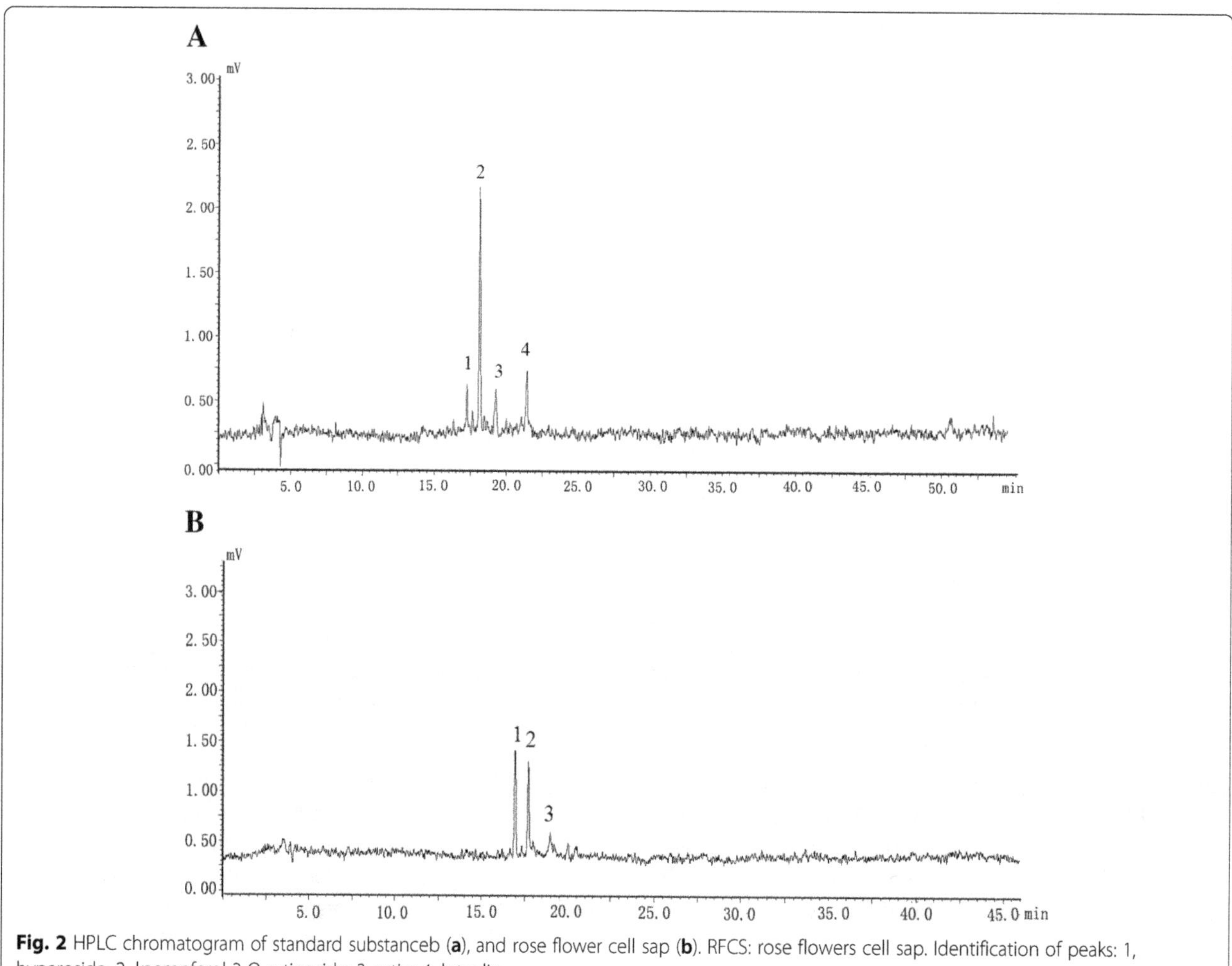

Fig. 2 HPLC chromatogram of standard substanceb (**a**), and rose flower cell sap (**b**). RFCS: rose flowers cell sap. Identification of peaks: 1, hyperoside; 2, kaempferol-3-O-rutinoside; 3, rutin; 4, luteolin

Antioxidant capacity

Table 3 presents the DPPH IC_{50} values of RFCS and the standard compounds. The flavonoids with IC_{50} values < 1 μg/mL, including hyperoside (IC_{50} value of 0.695 ± 0.021 μg/mL), kaempferol-3-O-rutinoside (IC_{50} value of 0.808 ± 0.024 μg/mL), rutin (IC_{50} value of 0.715 ± 0.017 μg/mL), and luteolin (IC_{50} value of 0.507 ± 0.015 μg/mL), showed stronger DPPH radical scavenging activities than RFCS (IC_{50} value of 1120 ± 42 μg/mL). Single volatile compounds, such as linalool, phenylethyl alcohol, citronellol, and α-bisabolol, showed weak radical scavenging activity with IC_{50}values of > 10,000 μg/mL. In previous reports, the antioxidant activities of various natural products, including those from rose, have been attributed to the contents of phenolic compounds [25, 26]. The ABTS radical assay is also used to evaluate the radical scavenging activity of hydrogen-donating and chain-breaking antioxidants in

Table 2 Analytical characteristics of compounds in rose waste. (mg/mL)

Peak	Ginsenoside	Retention time	Calibration curve	R^2	RFCS
1	hyperoside	16.981	y = 14,955x-5214	0.9989	0.18 ± 0.01
2	kaempferol-3-O-rutinoside	17.737	y = 7102x + 3256	0.9984	0.12 ± 0.01
3	rutin	19.01	y = 41,285x-43,792	0.9979	0.23 ± 0.01
4	luteolin	22.01	y = 31,527x-5241	0.9991	n.d
	total phenolic content				0.31 ± 0.01
	total flavonoid content				0.43 ± 0.01
	total solid content				1.45 ± 0.04

nd not detected; Data are expressed as mean ± standard deviation of triplicate samples; *RFCS* rose flower cell sap

Table 3 Total solid content and IC_{50} values of single compounds in rose products. (μg/mL)

	DPPH radicalscavenging activity	Tyrosinase inhibition	ABTS radicalscavenging activity
RFCS	1120 ± 42 b	570 ± 21 ab	1430 ± 49 b
Linalool	> 10,000 a	730 ± 44 a	> 10,000 a
Phenylethyl alcohol	> 10,000 a	315 ± 13 b	> 10,000 a
Citronellol	> 10000a	825 ± 31 a	> 10,000 a
α-bisabolol	> 10,000 a	635 ± 22 a	> 10,000 a
Hyperoside	0.695 ± 0.021 c	0.762 ± 0.018 d	0.526 ± 0.014 c
Kaempferol-3-O-Rutinoside	0.808 ± 0.024 c	0.908 ± 0.021 d	0.719 ± 0.016 c
Rutin	0.715 ± 0.017 c	0.856 ± 0.014 d	0.621 ± 0.024 c
Luteolin	0.507 ± 0.015 c	0.613 ± 0.016 d	0.436 ± 0.026 c
Positive control	0.449 ± 0.013 c	80 ± 17 c	0.324 ± 0.019 c

Data are expressed as mean ± standard deviation of triplicate samples; *RFCS* rose flower cell sap
Values in each column followed by different letters are significantly different ($P < 0.01$)

many natural products [27, 28]. As shown in Table. 3, the ABTS radical scavenging activities of single compounds and RFCS are expressed as μg/mL. Consistent with previous works, flavonoids exhibited significantly higher antiradical activities and antioxidant capacities than volatile compounds [8, 13]. In the present study, the results of ABTS scavenging were similar to those of DPPH; flavonoid compounds with IC_{50} values < 1 μg/mL, including hyperoside (IC_{50} value of 0.526 ± 0.014 μg/mL), kaempferol-3-O-rutinoside (IC_{50} value of 0.719 ± 0.016 μg/mL), rutin (IC_{50} value of 0.621 ± 0.024 μg/mL), and luteolin (IC_{50} value of 0.436 ± 0.026 μg/mL), showed stronger ABTS radical scavenging activities than RFCS (IC_{50} value of 1430 ± 49 μg/mL). Single volatile compounds, such as linalool, phenylethyl alcohol, citronellol, and α-bisabolol, exhibited weak antiradical activities (IC_{50} values of > 10,000 μg/mL).

Tyrosinase inhibitory activities

Tyrosinase is a multifunctional copper-containing enzyme found in fungi, mammals, and plants [29]. Tyrosinase has two distinct enzyme activities, namely, monophenolase activity and diphenolase activity [30]. We conducted an initial study of the tyrosinase inhibitory activities of mushroom tyrosinase. As per this assay, RFCS showed strongly tyrosinase inhibitory activities with an IC_{50} value of 570 ± 21 μg/mL (Table 3). The volatile compounds, including linalool, phenylethyl alcohol, citronellol, and α-bisabolol, also showed dose-dependent tyrosinase inhibitory effects with IC_{50} values of 730 ± 44 μg/mL, 315 ± 13 μg/mL, 825 ± 31 μg/mL, and 635 ± 22 μg/mL, respectively. All the flavonoid compounds, namely, hyperoside, kaempferol-3-O-rutinosid, and even rutin were more potent than kojic acid (80 ± 17 μg/mL), and they all had IC_{50} values bellow 1 μg/mL.

Similar to the report by Solimine, the polyphenol-enriched fraction of RODW, which contains flavonoid compounds, exhibits obvious tyrosinase inhibitory activity with an IC_{50} value of 0.41 ± 0.01 μg/mL [6]. Meanwhile, the tyrosinase inhibitory effects of RFCS is stonger than RODW from Pingyin [13]. The flavonoid content contributes to the overall tyrosinase inhibitory effect of RODW.

Antimicrobial activities

The results of the antimicrobial activity studies of the different rose fractions, RFCS, and the standard antibiotics (tetracycline and hydrochloride) are presented in Table 4. *F. nucleatum* was most susceptible to RFCS and showed an MIC of 64 μg/mL and MBC of 250 μg/mL. The MIC values for RFCS against both *P. acnes* and *S. aureus* were 125 μg/mL. The MIC values against other bacteria were 250 μg/mL. The MIC and MBC or MFC values of the nine components of RFCS were determined to identify the constituents responsible for the antimicrobial effects of RFCS. *L. ivanovii* and *F. nucleatum* were found to be the most susceptible to α-bisabolol, and it showed MIC values of 8 μg/mL and MBC values of 32 μg/mL against these species (Table 4). After α-bisabolol, phenylethyl alcohol showed the lowest MIC and MBC or MFC values among all the constituents of RFCS. Overall, the volatile constituents played a more important role than the flavonoid compounds in the antimicrobial activity of RFCS.

Previous investigations of the antimicrobial effects of the various fractions of rose have reported similar results [8, 28, 31]. The essential oil and various extracts of rose, including the aqueous extract, ethanol extract, chloroform extract, ethyl acetate fraction, and butanol fraction, exhibit broad-spectrum antimicrobial activities. With the exception of the ethyl acetate fraction, rose essential oil is comparatively more active against the tested bacteria [28]. The absolute and essential oils of rose contain high levels of polyphenols and phenylethyl alcohol, which result in outstanding antimicrobial properties [8]. Because

Table 4 MIC and MBC or MFC of RFCS and different monomers against pathogenic bacteria (μg/mL)

Compound	*L. ivanovii*		*S. enteritidis enteritidis*		*S. aureus*		*E. coli*		*C. albicans*		*P. acnes*		*F. nucleatum*	
	MIC	MBC	MIC	MBC	MIC	MBC	MIC	MBC	MIC	MFC	MIC	MBC	MIC	MBC
RFCS	500	> 1000	500	> 1000	125	1000	500	1000	1000	> 1000	125	500	64	250
Linalool	500	> 1000	500	> 1000	250	1000	250	1000	250	1000	250	1000	250	1000
Phenylethyl alcohol	250	500	125	500	125	250	250	1000	250	500	125	500	8	32
Citronellol	250	500	250	1000	125	500	250	500	250	500	125	500	250	1000
α-bisabolol	8	32	500	> 1000	250	1000	500	1000	1000	> 1000	125	500	8	32
Hyperoside	250	500	250	500	250	1000	250	1000	250	1000	250	1000	250	500
Kaempferol-3-O-rutinosid	500	1000	500	> 1000	250	1000	500	> 1000	250	1000	500	1000	500	> 1000
Rutin	500	1000	125	500	250	500	250	1000	500	1000	125	250	62	500
Luteolin	500	1000	250	1000	500	> 1000	250	1000	250	500	250	500	125	500
Miconazole Nitrate	–	–	–	–	–	–	–	16	8	–	–	–	–	–
Hydrochloride tetracycline	< 0.1	< 0.1	8	16	16	16	16	–	–	16	8	16	2	2

Data are expressed as mean ± standard deviation of triplicate samples
MIC minimum inhibitory concentration, *MBC* minimum bactericidal concentration, *MFC* minimum Fungicidal concentration, *RFCS* rose flower cell sap, *L. ivanovii Listeria ivanovii, S. enteritidis subspecies enteritidis: Salmonella enteritidis enteritidis, S. aureus Staphylococcus aureus, E. coli Escherichia coli, C. albicans Candida albicans, P. acnes Propionibacterium acnes, F. nucleatum Fusobacterium nucleatum*

the content of volatile oil in RODW is higher than RFCS, the antimicrobial effect of RODW better than RFCS [13]. The polyphenolic-enriched fraction from rugosa tea could inhibit *Escherichia coli* and *Pseudomonas aeruginosa* quorum sensing and biofilm formatiosignificancen [1]. The antimicrobial effects of some of the active ingredients of rose oil such as linalool, citronellol, and geraniol have been confirmed [32, 33]. To date, the antimicrobial activity of RFCS of *R. fenghua* has not been evaluated. This result explicitly supports the fact that high contents of phenylethyl alcohol and other volatile components contribute to the antimicrobial activities of RFCS [34].

Conclusions

Our study demonstrated the strong antioxidant, antimicrobial, and tyrosinase inhibitory activities of RFCS. Due to the rose-like aroma of phenylethyl alcohol in combination with the tyrosinase inhibitory activities and antimicrobial effect against *S. enteritidis subspecies enteritidis*, *C. albicans*, and *P. acnes*, RFCS may be used as a natural skin-whitening and skin care additive in the cosmetics industry. Additionally, due to its antioxidant activities and antimicrobial effects against *L. ivanovii, S. subspecies, E. coli,* and *S. aureus*, RFCS can be used as a natural preservative and antimicrobial agent in the food and pharmaceutical industries.

Abbreviations

BHI: Brain heart infusion; CDC: Anaerobic blood agar base medium; ESI: Electrospray ionization; GAM broth: Actinomycete broth medium; MBC: Minimum bactericidal concentration; MFC: Minimum fungicidal concentration; MIC: Minimum inhibitory concentration; MS: Mass spectrometer; RFCS: *Rosa rugosa Thunb. var. plena Regal* flower cell sap; RODW: Rose oil distillation wastewater; ROS: Reactive oxygen species

Acknowledgments

Thank you to the Fragrant Rose Biological Technology Co., LTD in Pingyin for providing the RFCS.

Funding

This work was supported by the Ginseng Planting Resource Collection and Innovation (No. 20151FDA31290).

Authors' contributions

GR, GZ and PX conceived the study. GR and GZ were responsible for data collection and data entry. PX and XS analyzed data and wrote the manuscript. All authors read and approved the final manuscript.

Competing interests

The authors declare that they have no competing interests.

Author details

[1]College of Pharmacy and Biological Engineering, Chengdu University, Chengdu 610000, People's Republic of China. [2]Social Risk Prediction and Management, School of Public Health and Management, Weifang Medical University, No.7166 Baotong West Street Weicheng District, Weifang 261053, People's Republic of China. [3]Key Laboratory of Coarse Cereal Processing, Ministry of Agriculture, No.2025 Chengluo Road, Longquanyi District, Chengdu 610106, People's Republic of China. [4]Institute of Crop Sciences, Chinese Academy of Agricultural Sciences, No.80 XUEYUAN South Road, Handian District, Beijing 100081, People's Republic of China.

References

1. Zhang JM, Rui X, Wang L, Guan Y, Sun XM, Dong MS. Polyphenolic extract from *Rosa rugosa* tea inhibits bacterial quorum sensing and biofilm formation. Food Control. 2014;42:125–31.
2. Tursun X, Zhao YX, Talat Z, Xin XL, Tursun A, Abdulla R, Akber AH. Anti-inflammatory effect of *Rosa rugosa* flower extract in lipopolysaccharide -stimulated RAW264.7 macrophages. Biomol Ther. 2016;24:184–90.
3. Thao NP, Luyen BTT, Tai BH, Yang SY, Jo SH, Cuong NX, Nam NH, Kwon YI, Minh CV, Kim YH. Rat intestinal sucrase inhibition of constituents from the roots of *Rosa rugosa* Thunb. Bioorg Med Chem Lett. 2014;24:1192–6.
4. Lee HJ, Ahn JW, Lee BJ, Moon SG, Seo Y. Antioxidant activity of *Rosa rugosa*. Ksbb J. 2004;19:67–71.
5. Kovacheva N, Rusanov K, Atanassov I. Industrial cultivation of oil bearing rose and rose oil production in Bulgaria during 21st century, directions and challenges. Biotechnol Biotec Eq. 2010;24:1793–8.

6. Solimine J, Garo E, Wedler J, Rusanov K, Fertig O, Hamburger M, Atanassov I, Butterweck V. Tyrosinase-inhibitory constituents from a polyphenol enriched fraction of rose oil distillation wastewater. Fitoterapia. 2016;108:13–9.
7. Callaway TR, Edrington TS, Anderson RC, Byrd JA, Nisbet DJ. Gastrointestinal microbial ecology and the safety of our food supply as related to salmonella. J Anim Sci. 2008;86:163–72.
8. Shohayeb M, Abdel-Hameed ESS, Bazaid SA, Maghrabi I. Antibacterial and antifungal activity of *Rosa damascena* MILL.Essential oil, different extracts of rose petals. Global J Pharmac. 2014;8:01–7.
9. Kim S, Lee S, Gwak K, Lee J, Choi I. Whitening effect and antioxidant activity of essential oils from *Cryptomeria japonica*. Planta Med. 2011;77:1301.
10. Baek SH, Nam IJ, Kwak HS, Kim KC, Lee SH. Cellular anti-melanogenic effects of a *euryale ferox* seed extract ethyl acetate fraction via the lysosomal degradation machinery. Int J Mol Sci. 2015;16:9217–35.
11. Roh JS, Han JY, Kim JH, Hwang JK. Inhibitory effects of active compounds isolated from safflower (*Carthamus tinctorius* L.) seeds for melanogenesis. Biol Pharm Bull. 2004;27:1976–8.
12. Takaki A, Yamamoto K. Control of oxidative stress in hepatocellular carcinoma: helpful or harmful? World J Hepatol. 2015;7:968–79.
13. Xue P, Sun XY, Zhang WY, Wang QC, Ren GX. Phytochemical constituents, antioxidant, antimicrobial, Tyrosinase inhibitory activities of RODW. Modern Food Sci Tech. 2017;33:105–10.
14. Briehl MM. Oxygen in human health from life to death - an approach to teaching redox biology and signaling to graduate and medical students. Redox Bio. 2015;5:124–39.
15. Ellinsworth DC. Arsenic, reactive oxygen, and endothelial dysfunction. J Pharmacol Exp Ther. 2015;353:458–64.
16. Balaguer A, Chisvert A, Salvador A. Environmentally friendly LC for the simultaneous determination of ascorbic acid and its derivatives in skin-whitening cosmetics. J Sep Sci. 2008;31:229–36.
17. Fawole OA, Makunga NP, Opara UL. Antibacterial, antioxidant and tyrosinase-inhibition activities of pomegranate fruit peel methanolic extract. BMC Complem Altern Med. 2012;12:1–11.
18. Park KM, Kwon KM, Lee SH. Evaluation of the antioxidant activities and tyrosinase inhibitory property from *Mycelium Culture* extracts. Evid-Based Compl Alt Med. 2015;2015:616298–304.
19. Thaipong K, Boonprakob U, Crosby K. Comparison of ABTS, DPPH, FRAP, and ORAC assays for estimating antioxidant activity from guava fruit extracts. J Food Compos Anal. 2006;19:669–75.
20. Xue P, Yao Y, Yang XS, Feng J, Ren GX. Improved antimicrobial effect of ginseng extract by heat transformation. J Gins Res. 2016;41:180–7.
21. Rusanov KE, Kovacheva NM, Atanassov II. Comparative gc/ms analysis of rose flower and distilled oil volatiles of the oil bearing rose. Biotechnol Biotec Eq. 2014;25:2210–6.
22. Koksal N, Saribas R, Kafkas E, Aslancan H, Sadighazadi S. Determination of volatile compounds of the first rose oil and the first rose water by hs-spme/gc/ms techniques. Afr J Tradit Complem Alt Med. 2015;1212:145–50.
23. Mahboubifar M, Shahabipour S, Javidnia K. Evaluation of the valuable oxygenated components in iranian rose water. Intern Int J Chemtech Res. 2014;6:4782–8.
24. Lei G, Wang L, Liu X, Zhang A. Fast quantification of phenylethyl alcohol in rose water and chemical profiles of rose water and oil of and from Southeast China. J Liq Chromatogr Rela Tech. 2015;38:823–32.
25. Wong PY, Kitts DD. Studies on the dual antioxidant and antibacterial properties of parsley (*petroselinum crispum*) and cilantro (*coriandrum sativum*) extracts. Food Chem. 2006;97:505–15.
26. Li L, Ham H, Sung J, Kim Y, Lee H. Antioxidant activities of methanolic extracts from four different rose cultivars. J Food Nutr Res. 2014;2:69–73.
27. Netzel M, Strass G, Bitsch I, Konitz R, Christmann M, Bitsch R. Effect of grape processing on selected antioxidant phenolics in red wine. J Food Eng. 2003; 56:223–8.
28. Joo SS, Kim YB, Lee DI. Antimicrobial and antioxidant properties of secondary metabolites from white rose flower. Plant Pathol J. 2010;26:57–62.
29. Saanchez-Ferrer A, Rodríguez-López JN, García-Cánova F, García-Carmona F. Tyrosinase: a comprehensive review of its mechanism. Bioch Et Biophy Acta. 1995;1247:1–11.
30. Kim YJ, Uyama H. Tyrosinase inhibitors from natural and synthetic sources: structure, inhibition mechanism and perspective for the future. Cell Mol Life Sci. 2005;62:1707–23.
31. Said BOS, Haddadi-Guemghar H, Boulekbache-Makhlouf L, Rigou P, Remini H, Adjaoud A. Essential oils composition, antibacterial and antioxidant activities of hydrodistillated extract of *eucalyptus globulus* fruits. Ind Crop Prod. 2016;89:167–75.
32. Aridogan BC, Baydar H, Kaya S, Demirci M, Mumcum E. Antimicrobial activity and chemical composition of some essential oils. Arch Pharml Res. 2002;25:860–4.
33. Gochev V, Wlcek K, Buchbauer G, Stoyanova A, Dobreva A, Schmidt E, Jirovetz L. Comparative evaluation of antimicrobial activity and composition of rose oils from *various geographic* origins, in particular Bulgarian rose oil. Nat Prod Commun. 2008;3:1063–8.
34. Etschmann MMW, Bluemke W, Sell D, Schrader J. Biotechnological production of 2-phenylethanol. Appl Microbiol Biot. 2002;59:1–8.

13

An assessment of the use of complementary and alternative medicine by Korean people using an adapted version of the standardized international questionnaire (I-CAM-QK)

Ju Ah Lee[1†], Yui Sasaki[2†], Ichiro Arai[3], Ho-Yeon Go[4], Sunju Park[5], Keiko Yukawa[6], Yun Kung Nam[3], Seong-Gyu Ko[2], Yoshiharu Motoo[7], Kiichiro Tsutani[8] and Myeong Soo Lee[9*]

Abstract

Background: In Korea, there are two types of medical doctors: one practises conventional medicine (hereafter called a physician), and the other practises traditional medicine (hereafter called a Korean medical doctor). This study aimed to compare the provision of complementary and alternative medicine (CAM) by these providers to CAM use per self-judgement in Korea.

Methods: We analysed 1668 Korean people via an internet survey with the Korean adopted version of the I-CAM-Q, namely, the International Questionnaire to measure use of CAM, to understand whether respondents used CAM based either on a prescription or advice from a physician or a Korean medical doctor or on self-judgement.

Results: In the previous 12 months, the proportions of respondents who were treated by a physician, who were treated by a Korean medical doctor and who were not treated by anyone were 67.9, 20.7 and 14.2%, respectively. Among the respondents who received CAM based on a prescription or advice from a physician, traditional Korean medicine practices and dietary supplements were commonly used; only a small percentage used other CAM therapies. Respondents who received CAM based on a prescription or advice from a Korean medical doctor showed similar results. Acupuncture and moxibustion, traditional Korean medicines (decoction), or cupping were more commonly used. Korean traditional medicines as over-the-counter (OTC) drugs were more commonly used by respondents who received CAM therapy based on a prescription or advice from a physician than by those who received CAM therapy based on a prescription or advice from a Korean medical doctor. A total of 74% of the responders used any CAM by self-judgement in the previous 12 months.

Conclusions: For the use of CAM in Korea, in addition to the Korean traditional medical care provided by Korean medical doctors, general physicians advised people regarding Korean traditional medical care and dietary supplements.

Keywords: Complementary and alternative medicine, Korea, I-CAM-Q

* Correspondence: drmslee@gmail.com; mslee@kiom.re.kr
[†]Ju Ah Lee and Yui Sasaki contributed equally to this work.
[9]Clinical Medicine Division, Korea Institute of Oriental Medicine, 1672 Yuseong-daero, Yuseong-gu, Daejeon 34054, Republic of Korea
Full list of author information is available at the end of the article

Background

Traditional medicine is classified as complementary and alternative medicine (CAM) in many countries. However, in East Asian countries, such as Korea, Japan, and China, traditional medicine is now used not as CAM but as official medicine; nevertheless, in previous surveys of CAM use in these countries, almost all studies classified traditional medicine as CAM [1–17].

The reports on the utilization of CAM in South Korea (hereafter Korea) through 2011 have been reviewed by Kim SG et al. [1]. There have also been several other reports since 2011 [2–11]. However, most studies either report on the utilization of CAM in patients with specific diseases (e.g., cancer) or provide an indirect report. According to a direct survey on the utilization of CAM throughout Korea (performed by Ock SM et al. [12]) in 2006, 74.8% of Koreans had used some type of CAM therapy in the past 12 months.

The results of the survey on the utilization of CAM may be significantly influenced by the manner of questioning; moreover, the results of the surveys may vary greatly depending on the contents of the questionnaires, even if the surveys are conducted in the same country [18]. Therefore, in an international group of CAM researchers, a standardized questionnaire, the International Questionnaire to measure use of Complementary and Alternative Medicine (I-CAM-Q), was developed to reduce questionnaire-related bias and to conduct an international comparison of the utilization of CAM [19]. The use of the I-CAM-Q was originally limited; then, several surveys on the utilization of CAM were conducted using this questionnaire in several countries [20–30]. As the type and circumstances of CAM may vary greatly according to differences in the cultural backgrounds of each country, an adapted version of the I-CAM-Q may be developed before implementation in a survey [23, 27].

This paper describes the results of a survey in Korea on the use of CAM that includes Korean traditional medicine. This survey was carried out using the I-CAM-Q for the first time and included CAM providers' viewpoints.

Methods

Development of draft questionnaire

Using the original I-CAM-Q for a survey of CAM without adapting it to the environment of Korea makes the I-CAM-Q not suitable. Therefore, we first developed the adapted version of the I-CAM-Q for Korea by referring to the I-CAM-QJ, the adapted version of the I-CAM-Q for Japan [31]. We referred to the I-CAM-QJ because Japan uses traditional medicine derived from ancient China as the official medicine, and the cultural background for CAM is similar to that of Korea. To develop the I-CAM-QK (Korean version of I-CAM-Q; Additional file 1), the most important revision from the original I-CAM-Q was the addition of "Korean medical doctor" as a healthcare provider. In Korea, there are two types of medical doctors' licences: one is for conventional medicine, and the other is for traditional medicine. Korean medical doctors can prescribe traditional Korean medicines and practice acupuncture and moxibustion and provide other traditional remedies. In addition, in the option list, CAM treatments that are used frequently, such as "Cupping", in Korea were added. The herbal medicines listed in the options were changed to the most commonly used ones in Korea by referring to the documents of the National Health Insurance Service of Korea [32]. Additionally, we changed the options in dietary supplements by referring to the documents of the Ministry of Food and Drug Safety of Korea [33].

Validation and revision of questionnaire by a pilot interview survey

Using the draft questionnaire according to the above-mentioned policies, an interview survey was conducted involving 30 Korean people at Daejeon University and Semyung University (Semyung University, IRB No. 1608–07) in Korea between September 2016 and December 2016. Based on the results of this survey, we slightly revised some terms of the questionnaires to prevent misunderstanding by the respondents.

Internet survey

Between February 24 and March 3, 2017, a survey company in Japan (ANTERIO Inc.) conducted an internet survey using the I-CAM-QK.

The survey method was as follows. A tie-ups company of Anterio has over 500,000 panels (willing partners for internet interviews) in Korea. For each generation, namely, people in their twenties, thirties, forties, and fifties/sixties, approximately 200 samples of both males and females were needed ($200 \times 2 \times 4 = 1600$). We excluded people who were over 69 years old because most of them in Korea might not use the internet and were not registered in the panel. We also excluded people who were under 20 years old because they might answer the questions incorrectly and were not registered in our panel. We collected the same number of answers from each generation/sex for comparisons to surveys in other countries that we plan to perform.

The survey implementation date was February 24, 2017. The database of internet addresses included those of the general population. No specific group of people was over-represented. There was no stratification such as according to the region of the country. The internet survey began by requesting 200 samples as the target number for each sex and generation group via e-mail. The questionnaire was e-mailed again to groups that had not been reached. People working in any of the following areas were excluded from the survey: medicine, media, advertising and market research. We excluded these people because they may have presumed the purpose of the survey and not answered honestly. The average time to answer was 28 min (median 7 min).

This internet survey was performed after obtaining the approval of the ethics committee of Nihon Pharmaceutical University (approved number: 28–05) and of the institutional review board (IRB) of the Second Affiliated Korean Medical Hospital in Chungju, Semyung University (Semyung University IRB No. 1702–01). Before initiation, this survey was registered in the University Hospital Medical Information Network in Japan (UMIN000026399).

Results

Demographics

Table 1 shows the attributes of the respondents. A total of 1668 people were enrolled as respondents, who were equally distributed in each age group and sex group. For their current health condition, approximately 15% of respondents indicated that they were in 'bad' and 'very bad' health, while the rest indicated that they were at least in 'acceptable' health. Regarding educational background, the percentage of respondents who graduated from a university was approximately 60%. In terms of long-term disease/disorders, 32.3% of the respondents indicated that they had at least one; hypertension, gastrointestinal disease, dental disease and skin disease were commonly found in high proportions (> 20% for each).

Healthcare providers

As shown in Table 2, 67.9% of respondents indicated that they received medical care/health services from physicians in the last 12 months. On average, participants visited 2.2 different health providers in the last 12 months. In contrast, 20.7% of respondents indicated that they received medical care/health services from Korean medical doctors in the last 12 months, which was equivalent to one-third of the respondents who received the services from physicians. Regarding services from providers other than physicians, the respondents received services from dentists, pharmacists and nurses (35.9, 43.5, and 43.5%, respectively). In terms of the services from CAM providers other than Korean medical doctors, the percentage of respondents who received services from massage practitioners or acupressure therapists was relatively high, at 9.7%. However, the percentage of respondents who received CAM therapies from other providers was low, at < 4%.

For the reasons provided by respondents for seeing a Korean medical doctor, the percentage of those who reported improved well-being was high, while the percentage of those who reported acute illness was low. The percentages of respondents who were satisfied with the services provided by physicians and Korean medical doctors were 94.8 and 89.5%, respectively.

CAM treatments received from physicians

The respondents who received medical services from physicians (1132 respondents) were asked to answer a question regarding 'medical/healthcare services that were used based on the advice of physicians in the last 12 months' (Table 3). The most common CAM used by these respondents was over-the-counter (OTC) traditional Korean medicine, which was used by 26.7% of the 1132 respondents, equivalent to 18.1% of all 1668 respondents. This was followed by dietary supplementation (18.5% of 1132 respondents; 12.6% of all respondents), acupuncture and moxibustion (15.9%; 10.8%), manufactured traditional Korean medicine for prescription (11.4%; 7.7%) and traditional Korean medicines (decoction) (9.0%; 6.1%). Of the respondents who received traditional Korean medicines, the number of respondents who used OTC traditional Korean medicine was highest, whereas the number of respondents who used decoctions was lowest.

CAM treatments received from Korean medical doctors

The respondents who received services from Korean medical doctors (345 respondents) were asked to answer a question regarding 'medical/healthcare services that were used based on the advice of Korean medical doctors in the last 12 months' (Table 4). The CAM used most commonly, by 69.0% of the 345 respondents, which was equivalent to 14.3% of all 1668 respondents, was acupuncture and moxibustion. This was followed by traditional Korean medicine (decoction) (36.2% of 345 respondents; 7.5% of all respondents) and cupping (32.5%; 6.7%). Of the respondents who received traditional Korean medicine, the number of respondents who used decoction was highest, while the number of those who used OTC traditional Korean medicine was lowest. The helpfulness of these CAM treatments was largely reported as similar to the results regarding the CAM therapies that the respondents used based on a prescription or advice from a physician. For medical care/health services

Table 1 Demographics

	Number	%
Total Number (Male/Female)	1668	
Male / Female	831 / 837	49.8 / 50.2
Age (Male/Female)		
20's Male / 20's Female	205 / 210	12.3 / 12.6
30's Male / 30's Female	210 / 217	12.6 / 13.0
40's Male / 40's Female	209 / 210	12.6 / 12.6
50~ 60's Male / 50~ 60's Female	207 / 200	12.4 / 12.0
Profession		
Agriculture, fisheries, forestry, mining	16	1.0
Productions	242	14.6
Retails	86	5.2
Civil engineering and construction, Real Estate, Building Services, Transportation, Warehouse Logistics related	181	10.9
Communication industry, Software, Information processing, Other information service	105	6.3
Electricity, Gas, Heat supply Water supply	26	1.6
Finance, Insurance	39	2.3
Food, Accommodation, Travel services	26	1.6
Education, Learning support	155	9.3
Welfare	32	1.9
Housewife	281	16.8
Student	158	9.5
Unemployed	123	7.4
Others	198	11.8
Final Education		
Middle school	15	0.9
High school	321	19.2
Special college	226	13.5
University	965	57.9
Graduate school	134	8.0
Others	7	0.4
Health condition		
Very good	141	8.5
Good	562	33.7
Acceptable	708	42.4
Bad	241	14.4
Long-term diseases and disorders		
Yes	539	32.3
Hypertension	140	26.0
Stroke (cerebral hemorrhage, cerebral infarction, etc.)	12	2.2
Heart disease	15	2.8
Diabetes	54	10.0
Dyslipidemia (hyperlipidemia)	54	10.0
Respiratory illness	65	12.1
Diseases of the gastrointestinal tract (gastrointestinal, liver, gall bladder, pancreas, etc.)	139	25.8
Kidney and urological diseases	43	8.0
Musculoskeletal diseases (osteoporosis, arthropathy, back pain, etc.)	103	19.1
Trauma (falls, fractures, etc.)	13	2.4
Cancer (including blood cancer and sarcoma)	12	2.2
Blood disease (other than tumor)	14	2.6
Immune disease (such as collagen disease)	18	3.3
Mental disorders such as depression / dementia	54	10.0
Nose disease	94	17.4
Eye disease	80	14.8
Ear disease	39	7.2
Skin disease	114	21.2
Tooth disease	123	22.8
Others	51	9.5
No	1129	67.7
Subscribing to private medical insurance		
Subscribe	1109	66.5
Not subscribe	559	33.5

that the respondents used based on a prescription or advice from a Korean medical doctor, the availability of CAM other than traditional Korean medicine was low.

Self-help practices

All 1668 respondents were asked to answer a question regarding whether they engaged in 'self-help practices in the last 12 months' (Table 5). The respondents who did not engage in such practices in the last 12 months made up 26.3% of the respondents; the rest engaged in some type of self-help practice. The most common self-help practice that the respondents reported was walking (54.9%). The least common self-help practices that at least 10% of the respondents reported were yoga, use of an electric massage machine and spa therapy (13.2, 10.1 and 10.0%, respectively). The proportion of respondents who engaged in self-help practices to improve their well-being was higher than that of the respondents who used CAM per a prescription or advice from physicians/Korean medical doctors.

Table 2 Visiting health care providers

Health care providers	Visited[a] (%)	Motivation[a] (%)				Helpfulness[a] (%) (Very and somewhat)	Number of visit[b]
		Acute illness[c]	Long-term illness[d]	Improvement of well-being	Others		
Physicians	67.9	35.1	30.0	27.7	7.2	94.8	2.6
Korean medical doctor	20.7	26.7	29.6	38.3	5.5	89.6	3.0
Dentist	35.9	23.1	22.2	46.5	8.2	97.0	1.7
Pharmacist	43.5	42.0	20.7	33.1	4.3	93.2	3.0
Nurse	22.4	41.4	19.8	31.8	7.0	93.6	2.9
Maternity nurse	0.1	0.0	0.0	0.0	100.0	100.0	1.0
Massage practitioner / Acupressure therapist	9.7	6.8	14.8	75.3	3.1	89.5	2.8
Acupuncturist / Moxibustionist	2.0	21.2	42.4	36.4	0.0	90.9	2.9
Judo therapist (Bonesetter)	0.3	40.0	40.0	20.0	0.0	100.0	2.2
Nutritionist	1.6	3.7	0.0	92.6	3.7	77.8	4.9
Yoga instructor	3.6	0.0	6.7	90.0	3.3	88.4	11.5
Chiropractor	1.4	20.8	37.5	41.7	0.0	83.4	2.2
Manual therapist	3.7	24.6	34.4	39.3	1.6	88.6	2.8
Aromatherapist / Herb therapist	3.2	11.3	7.5	75.5	5.7	84.9	2.3
Spiritual therapist	0.8	0.0	61.5	38.5	0.0	92.3	1.6
Homeopathy therapist	0.6	30.0	40.0	30.0	0.0	90.0	3.0
Others	0.8	0.1	0.2	0.3	0.1	80.0	2.4
Not received medical / health services	14.2	NA	NA	NA	NA	NA	1.0

Number of respondents: 1668
NA Not Applicable
[a] in the last 12 months, [b] in the last 3 months, [c] lasted less than 1 month, [d] lasted more than 1 month

Use of dietary supplements

All 1668 respondents were asked to answer a question regarding which dietary supplements they used (Table 6). The most common dietary supplement that the respondents used was vitamin C (35.1%), followed by red ginseng (30.8%), omega-3 fatty acids (29.3%) and multivitamins (22.0%). These were all used to improve well-being. However, the percentage of respondents who indicated that it was helpful was < 80% (except in cases of dietary supplements, which few respondents used).

The respondents (1326) who indicated that they used dietary supplements were asked about their purchasing methods; pharmacy was most common (47.5%), followed by internet shopping (45.9%), drugstore (12.8%), supermarket (8.2%) and mail order (4.8%), which suggested that half or more of the respondents bought their dietary supplements at actual stores (table not shown).

Use of traditional Korean medicine

All 1668 respondents were asked to answer a question regarding the type of traditional Korean medicine that they used in the last 12 months. The most common type was OTC manufactured Korean medicinal products (32.1%), followed by prescribed manufactured Korean medicinal products (18.5%) and decoctions dispensed by a Korean medical doctor (18.2%) (data not shown).

The 831 respondents who indicated that they had used traditional Korean medicine in the last 12 months were asked to recall the names of the specific medications (Table 7). The most common type that they used was galguentang (kakkonto in Japanese, ge-gen-tang in Chinese; 30.0%); the percentage of each other prescription that was used was < 6%.

Discussion

The I-CAM-Q used for our survey was not a questionnaire to gain factual information on various kinds of CAM but a questionnaire regarding utilization, motivation and helpfulness by distinguishing 'CAM provided by whom'.

In Korea, unlike Western countries and Japan, a licence to practise traditional medicine, as well as a general physician's licence, is authorised; thus, observing how both types of licensed physician are involved in the use of CAM is interesting. Generally, the term 'integrative medicine' is used to combine medical care with CAM. However, in Korea, there may be multiple integrations, including an integration of 'CAM,

Table 3 CAM treatments received by practice or advices of physicians

CAM treatments	Received[b] (%)		Motivation[b] (%)				Helpfulness[b] (%) (Very and somewhat)	Number of visit[c]
	among the visitors to physicians (1132)	among total respondents[a] (1668)	Acute illness[d]	Long-term illness[e]	Improvement of well-being	Others		
Acupuncture and moxibustion	15.9	10.8	28.9	33.3	35.6	2.2	88.9	4.6
Massage	8.1	5.5	13.0	22.8	60.9	3.3	85.9	3.7
Bone-setting	1.0	0.7	45.5	36.4	9.1	9.1	81.9	2.9
Bodywork	6.2	4.2	25.7	34.3	37.1	2.9	81.5	3.2
Chiropractic	2.4	1.6	29.6	33.3	37.0	0.0	92.6	2.1
Cupping	6.1	4.1	33.3	21.7	39.1	5.8	85.5	3.0
Diet therapy	8.0	5.4	9.9	33.0	57.1	0.0	83.5	4.1
Starvation diet	1.3	0.9	26.7	20.0	46.7	6.7	73.4	2.3
Dietary supplement	18.5	12.6	3.8	21.5	73.7	1.0	80.4	12.4
Herb therapy	1.2	0.8	7.1	28.6	64.3	0.0	71.4	2.0
Aromatherapy	2.4	1.6	11.1	18.5	63.0	7.4	96.3	4.1
Hyperthermia	7.6	5.2	29.1	32.6	34.9	3.5	89.5	4.1
Magnet therapy	1.8	1.2	30.0	25.0	45.0	0.0	95.0	3.4
Spa therapy	3.4	2.3	5.1	17.9	76.9	0.0	89.7	3.3
Music therapy	1.2	0.8	14.3	35.7	50.0	0.0	78.6	2.4
Forest therapy	1.0	0.7	0.0	18.2	81.8	0.0	72.8	1.5
Homeopathy	0.7	0.5	50.0	12.5	37.5	0.0	87.5	1.4
Ayurveda	0.3	0.2	33.3	33.3	33.3	0.0	100.0	1.3
Yoga	3.4	2.3	5.3	7.9	81.6	5.3	81.6	10.0
Qigong	1.1	0.7	15.4	38.5	46.2	0.0	92.3	6.2
Traditional Korean medicines (decoction)	9.0	6.1	24.5	31.4	42.2	2.0	90.2	1.8
Manufactured traditional Korean medicines for prescription	11.4	7.7	30.2	26.4	41.1	2.3	88.3	2.1
OTC traditional Korean medicines	26.7	18.1	36.4	24.2	36.4	3.0	84.8	2.5
Spiritual therapy	1.8	1.2	5.0	50.0	45.0	0.0	80.0	2.9
Other	35.6	24.2	16.3	42.9	32.7	8.2	85.8	6.3

CAM Complementary and Alternative Medicine, *NA* Not Applicable
Number of parent population except [(a)] is the visitors to physicians (1132)
[b] in the last 12 months, [c] in the last 3 months, [d] lasted less than 1 month, [e] lasted more than 1 month

Western medicine and traditional medicine', which is provided by physicians, or an integration of 'traditional medicine and other CAMs', which is provided by Korean medical doctors.

When Korean people receive treatment by physicians, they determine whether to consult a physician or a Korean medical doctor according to their disease and symptoms based on their own judgement. In this survey, 67.9% of respondents consulted a physician, and 20.7% consulted a Korean medical doctor in the last 12 months (Table 2). Considering that institutions for Korean medical care made up 21.9% of all medical institutions in Korea in 2015 [34], these results were consistent with the proportion of respondents who consulted Korean medical doctors. The most common reason the respondents consulted a physician was acute illness, while the most common reason they consulted a Korean medical doctor was to improve well-being, which suggested that respondents used both types of specialists properly.

The CAM therapies that respondents used based on a prescription or advice from a physician or Korean medical doctor were traditional Korean medicine and dietary supplements (Tables 3 and 4). Notably, the

Table 4 CAM treatments received by practice or advices of Korean medical doctors

CAM treatments	Received[b] (%)		Motivation[b] (%)				Helpfulness[b] (%) (Very and somewhat)	Number of visit[c]
	among the visitors to Korean medical doctors (345)	among total respondents[a] (1668)	Acute illness[d]	Long-term illness[e]	Improvement of well-being	Others		
Acupuncture and moxibustion	69.0	14.3	33.6	33.6	29.8	2.9	89.1	4.6
Massage	11.6	2.4	20.0	27.5	50.0	2.5	95.0	2.7
Bone-setting	2.0	0.4	42.9	14.3	42.9	0.0	100.0	5.3
Bodywork	6.7	1.4	43.5	34.8	21.7	0.0	95.6	3.3
Chiropractic	7.5	1.6	30.8	50.0	11.5	7.7	88.5	2.3
Cupping	32.5	6.7	29.5	31.3	33.0	6.3	84.9	3.8
Diet therapy	7.0	1.4	8.3	29.2	62.5	0.0	91.6	8.2
Starvation diet	1.7	0.4	33.3	16.7	33.3	16.7	66.6	3.0
Dietary supplement	8.4	1.7	3.4	17.2	79.3	0.0	68.9	12.4
Herb therapy	1.7	0.4	0.0	33.3	66.7	0.0	83.4	2.0
Aromatherapy	2.9	0.6	0.0	20.0	80.0	0.0	80.0	3.0
Hyperthermia	15.4	3.2	24.5	39.6	30.2	5.7	90.6	4.2
Magnet therapy	4.3	0.9	26.7	46.7	26.7	0.0	93.3	5.8
Spa therapy	3.5	0.7	0.0	50.0	50.0	0.0	100.0	2.2
Music therapy	2.0	0.4	0.0	42.9	57.1	0.0	100.0	4.1
Forest therapy	2.0	0.4	28.6	28.6	42.9	0.0	100.0	2.1
Homeopathy	0.3	0.1	0.0	100.0	0.0	0.0	100.0	0.0
Ayurveda	0.9	0.2	0.0	33.3	66.7	0.0	66.6	2.3
Yoga	2.0	0.4	14.3	14.3	71.4	0.0	85.7	3.3
Qigong	2.0	0.4	28.6	57.1	14.3	0.0	71.4	7.1
Traditional Korean medicines (decoction)	36.2	7.5	19.2	30.4	48.8	1.6	87.2	2.8
Manufactured traditional Korean medicines for prescription	19.7	4.1	25.0	33.8	35.3	5.9	85.3	3.1
OTC traditional Korean medicines	10.4	2.2	19.4	36.1	44.4	0.0	91.7	5.4
Spiritual therapy	1.4	0.3	20.0	80.0	0.0	0.0	80.0	3.8
Other	4.7	1.0	50.0	50.0	0.0	0.0	100.0	1.0

CAM Complementary and Alternative Medicine, *NA* Not Applicable
Number of parent population except [(a)] is the visitors to Korean medical doctors (345)
[b] in the last 12 months, [c] in the last 3 months, [d] lasted less than 1 month, [e] lasted more than 1 month

availability of other CAM therapies was lower. One can expect Korean medical doctors to provide prescriptions and advice regarding traditional Korean medicine. However, physicians were shown to also provide prescriptions and advice regarding traditional Korean medicine. In Korea, as physicians cannot prescribe traditional Korean medicine directly, the previous understanding was that physicians would advise people to receive traditional Korean medical care.

By expressing CAM therapy based on a prescription or advice from a physician or Korean medical doctor as the percentage of all 1668 respondents, comparisons could be made regarding whether CAM therapy was used based on a prescription or advice from a physician or a Korean medical doctor (Tables 3 and 4). The respondents who received acupuncture and moxibustion from physicians and/or Korean medical doctors made up 10.8 and 14.3% of all respondents, respectively, which indicated that the number of respondents who received a prescription or advice from a Korean medical doctor was higher. Similarly, 4.1 and 6.7% of all respondents received cupping from a physician or Korean medical doctor, respectively; 6.1 and 7.5% received traditional Korean medicine (decoction) based

Table 5 Self-help practices

CAM treatments	Used[a] (%)	Motivation[a] (%)				Helpfulness[a] (%) (Very and somewhat)	number of times practice[b]
		Acute illness[c]	Long-term illness[d]	Improvement of well-being	Others		
Meditation	9.6	3.1	10.6	85.0	1.3	88.8	12.7
Yoga	13.2	3.6	10.9	82.3	3.2	93.2	15.2
Qigong	1.6	7.4	25.9	63.0	3.7	96.3	14.0
Tai Chi	0.7	25.0	25.0	50.0	0.0	100.0	12.0
Relaxation techniques	2.5	12.2	31.7	56.1	0.0	85.4	4.9
Music therapy	4.2	1.4	18.6	71.4	8.6	94.3	15.5
Picture therapy	1.1	5.6	22.2	50.0	22.2	88.9	4.3
Attend traditional healing ceremony	1.1	5.6	22.2	72.2	0.0	94.5	1.9
Praying for own health	5.9	5.1	10.2	82.7	2.0	85.8	25.7
Electric massage machine	10.1	14.8	16.6	66.9	1.8	82.9	11.0
Other health appliances	7.1	5.0	16.8	78.2	0.0	89.9	22.6
Walking	54.9	1.5	5.9	91.4	1.2	88.3	27.9
Forest therapy	4.6	1.3	13.0	85.7	0.0	85.7	4.2
Aromatherapy	5.5	7.7	12.1	76.9	3.3	81.3	8.0
Hyperthermia	7.1	16.0	26.9	56.3	0.8	89.9	9.4
Magnet therapy	2.7	15.6	35.6	48.9	0.0	86.7	9.6
Spa therapy	10.0	6.0	11.4	81.3	1.2	86.2	5.2
Bath additive	8.3	3.6	8.7	81.9	5.8	73.9	6.2
Others	1.2	0.0	15.0	80.0	5.0	100.0	35.0
Not received	26.3	NA	NA	NA	NA	NA	NA

Number of respondents: 1668
CAM Complementary and Alternative Medicine, *NA* Not Applicable
[a] in the last 12 months, [b] in the last 3 months, [c] lasted less than 1 month, [d] lasted more than 1 month

on a prescription or advice from a physician or Korean medical doctor, respectively, which also indicated that the number of respondents who received a prescription or advice from a Korean medical doctor was higher. Although both manufactured traditional Korean medicines for prescription and OTC Korean medicines are classified as traditional Korean traditional medical care, the percentage of respondents who received them from physicians was higher than that of respondents who received them from Korean medical doctors; 7.7 and 4.1% of all respondents received manufactured traditional Korean medicine for a prescription from a physician and a Korean medical doctor, respectively, and 18.1 and 2.2% of all respondents received OTC Korean medicines from a physician and a Korean medical doctor, respectively.

Notably, OTC Korean medicine was used predominately based on the advice from physicians. Thus, Korean medical doctors originally provided direct prescriptions and procedures for legal traditional Korean medicine, but they did not provide advice for OTC Korean medicine that they did not prescribe themselves, as that role was filled by general physicians. By calculating the proportion of dietary supplement use across all respondents in the same manner, we observed that Korean medical doctors were largely uninvolved in the dietary supplement regimens of the respondents: 12.6 and 1.7% of respondents used supplements based on a prescription or advice from a physician and Korean medical doctor, respectively. The proportion of respondents who used all CAM therapies, other than acupuncture and moxibustion, cupping or traditional Korean medicines (decoction), based on a prescription or advice from a physician was higher than the proportion of respondents who used these CAM therapies based on a prescription or advice from a Korean medical doctor. However, because the absolute availability of CAM therapies other than Korean medicine and dietary supplements was lower, assessing the data precisely was difficult.

This study has several limitations. The study involved an internet survey and excluded people who were over 69 years old because they were not accustomed to internet use. We also excluded people who were under 20 years old because they might answer the questions incorrectly and were not registered in

Table 6 Use of dietary supplements

Dietary supplements	Used[a] (%)	Use now (%)	Motivation[a] (%)				Helpfulness[a] (%) (Very and somewhat)
			Acute Illness[b]	Long-term Illness[c]	Improvement of well-being	Others	
Vitamin A	8.9	5.2	4.7	8.1	86.5	0.7	76.4
Vitamin B_1	5.0	2.8	4.8	14.5	80.7	0.0	78.4
Vitamin B_2	5.1	3.0	7.1	8.2	84.7	0.0	78.8
Vitamin B_6	3.3	1.9	0.0	9.1	90.9	0.0	74.6
Vitamin B_{12}	3.9	1.9	9.2	9.2	81.5	0.0	70.8
Vitamin C	35.1	27.1	1.4	5.0	92.3	1.4	74.0
Vitamin D	15.9	11.3	1.9	12.4	83.8	1.9	72.2
Vitamin E	3.8	2.0	3.1	6.3	90.6	0.0	78.1
Vitamin K	1.9	0.7	6.5	3.2	90.3	0.0	70.9
Multiple vitamin	22.0	18.8	0.5	5.2	92.9	1.4	73.6
Pantothenic acid	0.6	0.4	10.0	0.0	90.0	0.0	90.0
Biotin	1.9	1.1	3.1	18.8	78.1	0.0	59.4
Niacin	0.9	0.5	13.3	13.3	73.3	0.0	60.0
Folic acid	6.7	3.9	2.7	9.9	72.1	15.3	74.8
Iron	5.7	3.5	8.4	16.8	69.5	5.3	78.9
Calcium	11.9	7.6	2.0	11.1	85.4	1.5	68.7
Copper	0.4	0.2	0.0	0.0	100.0	0.0	50.0
Zinc	4.9	2.8	3.7	7.4	88.9	0.0	61.7
Magnesium	9.5	5.6	9.4	5.7	83.6	1.3	63.5
Potassium	4.1	2.0	7.4	11.8	80.9	0.0	70.6
Multi-mineral	6.1	3.7	2.0	6.9	91.1	0.0	67.3
Glucosamine	5.3	3.4	2.2	12.4	84.3	1.1	69.7
Chondroitin	0.2	0.1	0.0	0.0	100.0	0.0	100.0
Saw palmetto	0.2	0.2	0.0	75.0	25.0	0.0	75.0
Green juice	3.3	1.9	7.3	14.5	78.2	0.0	80.0
Collagen	3.5	1.7	6.8	15.3	78.0	0.0	67.8
Placenta	0.4	0.2	16.7	50.0	33.3	0.0	50.0
Blueberry	8.0	4.7	1.5	3.0	92.5	3.0	59.4
Red ginseng	30.8	21.5	1.0	5.1	91.8	2.1	75.7
Ginseng	4.6	2.8	1.3	3.9	94.8	0.0	77.9
Omega-3 fatty acid	29.2	21.0	1.2	9.9	87.7	1.2	67.4
Probiotic	15.8	11.2	3.0	13.3	83.3	0.4	78.1
Others	3.0	2.6	0.0	6.0	90.0	4.0	78.0
Not used	18.3	25.0	NA	NA	NA	NA	NA

Number of respondents: 1668
NA Not Applicable
[a] in the last 12 months, [b] lasted less than 1 month, [c] lasted more than 1 month

our panel. Thus, this internet survey does not completely reflect the demographics of the Korean population. Because we understand the difficulty in reflecting the Korean demographics in this study, we changed the primary aim to a comparison among East Asian countries, and we are now surveying the same generations in these countries. In the future, this study will be useful with this outlook. For the survey to reflect genuine demographics, other methods, such as direct interviews, will be required. However, the direct interview may have many other difficulties, such as variations in the personality of the interviewer. Therefore, an actual conditional survey of CAM should be conducted from many standpoints.

Table 7 Use of Korean medicines

Korean medicines	Used[a] (%)	Use now (%)	Motivation[a] (%)				Helpfulness[a] (%) (Very and somewhat)
			Acute illness[b]	Long-term Illness[c]	Improvement of well-being	Others	
Ojeogsan	5.5	2.0	19.6	23.9	56.5	0.0	78.2
Gunghatang	2.4	1.3	15.0	50.0	35.0	0.0	95.0
Ijintang	3.1	1.9	19.2	34.6	46.2	0.0	76.9
Gumiganghwaltang	3.0	1.9	8.0	32.0	60.0	0.0	88.0
Pyeongwisan	3.5	1.7	24.1	34.5	41.4	0.0	96.5
Hyangsapyeongwisan	3.5	1.9	24.1	34.5	41.4	0.0	89.6
Bojungikgitang	5.7	4.2	8.5	34.0	57.4	0.0	87.2
Socheongryongtang	4.2	2.5	14.3	22.9	60.0	2.9	82.9
Galguentang	30.0	15.5	36.5	14.1	47.8	1.6	82.4
Samsoeum	3.1	1.4	23.1	19.2	57.7	0.0	88.4
Others	7.6	3.2	14.3	11.1	63.5	11.1	80.9
Not know / Not remember	47.4	17.6	NA	NA	NA	NA	NA
Not used	0.0	51.7	NA	NA	NA	NA	NA

Number of respondents: 831
NA Not Applicable
[a] in the last 12 months, [b] lasted less than 1 month, [c] lasted more than 1 month

Conclusions

For the use of CAM in Korea, in addition to the traditional Korean medical care that is provided by Korean medical doctors, general physicians advised people regarding traditional Korean medical care and dietary supplements.

Funding
This research was supported by a Grant from the Japan Agency for Medical Research Development, Japan 2016 (16lk0310024h0001). MSL was supported by the Korea Institute of Oriental Medicine (K18043).

Authors' contributions
IA, KT and MSL conceptualized this study. IA, YS, KY, and YL drafted the I-CAM-QK from the I-CAM-QJ. JL, HG, SP, SG and ML validated the draft version of the I-CAM-QK by interview survey, made the revisions and created the final version. JAL, IA, YS, and ML made the web version and performed the internet survey. JAL, IA, YS, KY, YM, KT and ML wrote the manuscript. All authors critically commented on the manuscript and approved the final version.

Ethics approval and consent to participate
This internet survey was performed after obtaining the approval of the ethics committee of Nihon Pharmaceutical University (approved number: 28-05) and of the institutional review board (IRB) of the Second Affiliated Korean Medical Hospital in Chungju, Semyung University (Semyung University IRB No. 1702-01). Written informed consent was obtained from each study participant prior to participation in the survey. All participants in the survey were asked on the first page of the questionnaire whether they agreed to participate in the study.

Competing interests
The authors declare that they have no competing interests.

Author details
[1]Department of Korean Internal Medicine, College of Korean Medicine, Gachon University, Incheon, Republic of Korea. [2]Institute of Safety and Effectiveness Evaluation for Korean Medicine, Department of Preventive Medicine, College of Korean Medicine, Kyung Hee University, Seoul, Republic of Korea. [3]Department of Pharmaceutical Sciences, Nihon Pharmaceutical University, Saitama, Japan. [4]Department of Internal Medicine, College of Korean Medicine, Semyung University, Jecheon, Republic of Korea. [5]Department of Preventive Medicine, College of Korean Medicine, Daejeon University, Daejeon, Republic of Korea. [6]Department of Health Policy and Technology Assessment, National Institute of Public Health, Saitama, Japan. [7]Department of Medical Oncology, Kanazawa Medical University, Ishikawa, Japan. [8]Faculty of Health Sciences, Tokyo Ariake University of Medical and Health Sciences, Tokyo, Japan. [9]Clinical Medicine Division, Korea Institute of Oriental Medicine, 1672 Yuseong-daero, Yuseong-gu, Daejeon 34054, Republic of Korea.

References
1. Kim SM, Lee SH, Seo HJ, Baek SM, Choi SM. Research trend analysis of the prevalence of complementary and alternative medicine in Korea. J Korean Oriental Med. 2012;33:24–41. Korean
2. Kang E, Yang EJ, Kim SM, Chung IY, Han SA, Ku DH, et al. Complementary and alternative medicine use and assessment of quality of life in Korean breast cancer patients: a descriptive study. Support Care Cancer. 2012;20: 461–73. https://doi.org/10.1007/s00520-011-1094-z.
3. Kim JH, Nam CM, Kim MY, Lee DC. The use of complementary and alternative medicine (CAM) in children: a telephone-based survey in Korea. BMC Complement Altern Med. 2012;12:46. https://doi.org/10.1186/1472-6882-12-46.
4. Choi WS, Song SH, Son H. Epidemiological study of complementary and alternative medicine (CAM) use for the improvement of sexual function in young Korean men: the Korean internet sexuality survey (KISS), part II. J Sex Med. 2012;9:2238–47. https://doi.org/10.1111/j.1743-6109.2012.02790.x.
5. Kim GW, Park JM, Chin HW, Ko HC, Kim MB, Kim JY, et al. Comparative analysis of the use of complementary and alternative medicine by Korean patients with androgenetic alopecia, atopic dermatitis and psoriasis. J Eur Acad Dermatol Venereol. 2013;27:827–35. https://doi.org/10.1111/j.1468-3083.2012.04583.x.
6. Choi JY, Chang YJ, Hong YS, Heo DS, Kim S, Lee JL, et al. Complementary and alternative medicine use among cancer patients at the end of life: Korean national study. Asian Pac J Cancer Prev. 2012;13:1419–24.
7. Baek SM, Choi SM, Seo HJ, Kim SG, Jung JH, Lee M, et al. Use of complementary and alternative medicine by self- or non-institutional therapists in South Korea: a community-based survey. Integr Med Res. 2013; 2:25–31. https://doi.org/10.1016/j.imr.2013.02.001.
8. Kim SY, Kim KS, Park JH, Shin JY, Kim SK, Park JH, et al. Factors associated with discontinuation of complementary and alternative medicine among Korean cancer patients. Asian Pac J Cancer Prev. 2013;14:225–30.

9. Seo HJ, Baek SM, Kim SG, Kim TH, Choi SM. Prevalence of complementary and alternative medicine use in a community-based population in South Korea: a systematic review. Complement Ther Med. 2013;21(3):60–71. https://doi.org/10.1016/j.ctim.2013.03.001.
10. Jeong MJ, Lee HY, Lim JH, Yun YJ. Current utilization and influencing factors of complementary and alternative medicine among children with neuropsychiatric disease: a cross-sectional survey in Korea. BMC Complement Altern Med. 2016;16:91. https://doi.org/10.1186/s12906-016-1066-4.
11. Jang A, Kang DH, Kim DU. Complementary and alternative medicine use and its association with emotional status and quality of life in patients with a solid tumor: a cross-sectional study. J Altern Complement Med. 2017;23: 362–9. https://doi.org/10.1089/acm.2016.0289.
12. Ock SM, Choi JY, Cha YS, Lee J, Chun MS, Huh CH, et al. The use of complementary and alternative medicine in a general population in South Korea: results from a national survey in 2006. J Korean Med Sci. 2009;24:1–6.
13. Yamashita H, Tsukayama H, Sugishita C. Popularity of complementary and alternative medicine in Japan: a telephone survey. Complement Ther Med. 2002;10:84–93.
14. Togo T, Urata S, Sawazaki K, Sakuraba H, Ishida T, Yokoyama K. Demand for CAM practice at hospitals in Japan: a population survey in Mie prefecture. Evid Based Complement Alternat Med. 2011;591868 https://doi.org/10.1093/ecam/neq049
15. Fukui T. The Health and Labour Sciences Research in 2010. Research on the way of information dissemination of integrative medicine. Available at: http://hospital.luke.ac.jp/about/approach/pdf/ra16/research_activities_16_1.pdf. Accessed 3 Aug 2018.
16. Chang MY, Liu CY, Chen HY. Changes in the use of complementary and alternative medicinein Taiwan: a comparison study of 2007 and 2011. Complement Ther Med. 2014;22:489–99. https://doi.org/10.1016/j.ctim.2014.03.001.
17. Yeh ML, Lin KC, Chen HH, Wang YJ, Huang YC. Use of traditional medicine and complementary and alternative medicine in Taiwan: a multilevel analysis. Holist Nurs Pract. 2015;29:87–95. https://doi.org/10.1097/HNP.0000000000000071.
18. Eardley S, Bishop FL, Prescott P, Cardini F, Brinkhaus B, Santos-Rey K, et al. A systematic literature review of complementary and alternative medicine prevalence in EU. Forsch Komplementmed. 2012;19(Suppl 2):18–28. https://doi.org/10.1159/000342708.
19. Quandt SA, Verheor MJ, Arcury TA, Lewith GT, Steinsbekk A, Kristoffersen AE, et al. Development of an international questionnaire to measure use of complementary and alternative medicine (I-CAM-Q). J Altern Complement Med. 2009;15:331–9.
20. Bains SS, Egede LE. Association of health literacy with complementary and alternative medicine use: a cross-sectional study in adult primary care patients. BMC Complement Altern Med. 2011;11:138. https://doi.org/10.1186/1472-6882-11-138.
21. Quandt SA, Ip EH, Saldana S, Arcury TA. Comparing two questionnaires for eliciting CAM use in a multi-ethnic US population of older adults. Eur J Integr Med. 2012;4:e205–11.
22. Opheim R, Bernklev T, Fagermoen MS, Cvancarova M, Moum B. Use of complementary and alternative medicine in patients with inflammatory bowel disease: results of a cross-sectional study in Norway. Scand J Gastroenterol. 2012;47:1436–47. https://doi.org/10.3109/00365521.2012.725092
23. Re ML, Schmidt S, Güthlin C. Translation and adaptation of an international questionnaire to measure usage of complementary and alternative medicine (I-CAM-G). BMC Complement Altern Med. 2012;12:259. https://doi.org/10.1186/1472-6882-12-259.
24. Eardley S, Bishop FL, Cardini F, Santos-Rey K, Jong MC, Ursoniu S, et al. A pilot feasibility study of a questionnaire to determine European Union-wide CAM use. Forsch Komplementmed. 2012;19:302–10. https://doi.org/10.1159/000345839.
25. AlBedah AM, Khalil MK, Elolemy AT, Al Mudaiheem AA, Al Eidi S, Al-Yahia OA, et al. The use of and out-of-pocket spending on complementary and alternative medicine in Qassim province, Saudi Arabia. Ann Saudi Med. 2013;33:282–9. https://doi.org/10.5144/0256-4947.2013.282.
26. Shumer G, Warber S, Motohara S, Yajima A, Plegue M, Bialko M, et al. Complementary and alternative medicine use by visitors to rural Japanese family medicine clinics: results from the international complementary and alternative medicine survey. BMC Complement Altern Med. 2014;14:360. https://doi.org/10.1186/1472-6882-14-360.
27. Esteban S, Vázquez Peña F, Terrasa S. Translation and cross-cultural adaptation of a standardized international questionnaire on use of alternative and complementary medicine (I-CAM-Q) for Argentina. BMC Complement Altern Med. 2016;16:109. https://doi.org/10.1186/s12906-016-1074-4.
28. Bryden GM, Browne M. Development and evaluation of the R-I-CAM-Q as a brief summative measure of CAM utilisation. Complement Ther Med. 2016; 27:82–6. https://doi.org/10.1016/j.ctim.2016.05.007.
29. von Conrady DM, Bonney A. Patterns of complementary and alternative medicine use and health literacy in general practice patients in urban and regional Australia. Aust Fam Physician. 2017;46:316–20.
30. Wemrell M, Merlo J, Mulinari S, Hornborg AC. Two-thirds of survey respondents in southern Sweden used complementary or alternative medicine in 2015. Complement Med Res. 2017;24:302–9. https://doi.org/10.1159/000464442.
31. Arai I. Survey on the actual situation of utilization/provision of integrative medicine and its health damage in Japan and other countries, and analysis from the viewpoint of social determinants of health. Research and Development Result Report of Grant from Japan Agency for Medical Research Development, Japan, 2016 (16lk0310024h0001). https://www.amed.go.jp/content/files/jp/houkoku_h28/0501051/h28_001.pdf. Accessed 3 Aug 2018.
32. Main Statistics of Ethical drug. Health Insurance Review and Assessment Service, News & Information, Statistics data. Korean. 2013. https://www.hira.or.kr/bbsDummy.do?pgmid=HIRAA020045010000&brdScnBltNo=4&brdBltNo=2275. Accessed 3 Aug 2018.
33. Production results of health functional foods was 1.8 Trillion won, 12% increase from the previous year. Ministry of Food and Drug Safety, News & Notice. Korean. 2015. http://www.mfds.go.kr/index.do?mid=675&pageNo=2&seq=32955&cmd=v. Accessed 3 Aug 2018.
34. Year Book of Traditional Korean Medicine. Korea Institute of Oriental Medicine, Korea Oriental Medicine Association, Korean Traditional Medicine Foundation, Graduate School of Oriental Medicine, Pusan National University, 2015. Korean. 2015. https://www.kiom.re.kr/brdartcl/boardarticleView.do?menu_nix=WUNNW2Aq&brd_id=BDIDX_o9YEVvNb40b134N1Rt17aq&cont_idx=9. Accessed 3 Aug 2018.

14

Reducing antibiotic use for uncomplicated urinary tract infection in general practice by treatment with uva-ursi (REGATTA)

Kambiz Afshar[1†], Nina Fleischmann[2†], Guido Schmiemann[3], Jutta Bleidorn[1], Eva Hummers-Pradier[2], Tim Friede[4], Karl Wegscheider[5], Michael Moore[6] and Ildikó Gágyor[7*]

Abstract

Background: Uncomplicated urinary tract infections (UTI) are common in general practice and usually treated with antibiotics. This contributes to increasing resistance rates of uropathogenic bacteria. A previous trial showed a reduction of antibiotic use in women with UTI by initial symptomatic treatment with ibuprofen. However, this treatment strategy is not suitable for all women equally. *Arctostaphylos uva-ursi* (UU, bearberry extract arbutin) is a potential alternative treatment. This study aims at investigating whether an initial treatment with UU in women with UTI can reduce antibiotic use without significantly increasing the symptom burden or rate of complications.

Methods: This is a double-blind, randomized, and controlled comparative effectiveness trial. Women between 18 and 75 years with suspected UTI and at least two of the symptoms dysuria, urgency, frequency or lower abdominal pain will be assessed for eligibility in general practice and enrolled into the trial. Participants will receive either a defined daily dose of 3 × 2 arbutin 105 mg for 5 days (intervention) or fosfomycin 3 g once (control). Antibiotic therapy will be provided in the intervention group only if needed, i.e. for women with worsening or persistent symptoms. Two co-primary outcomes are the number of all antibiotic courses regardless of the medical indication from day 0–28, and the symptom burden, defined as a weighted sum of the daily total symptom scores from day 0–7. The trial result is considered positive if superiority of initial treatment with UU is demonstrated with reference to the co-primary outcome number of antibiotic courses and non-inferiority of initial treatment with UU with reference to the co-primary outcome symptom burden.

Discussion: The trial's aim is to investigate whether initial treatment with UU is a safe and effective alternative treatment strategy in women with UTI. In that case, the results might change the existing treatment strategy in general practice by promoting delayed prescription of antibiotics and a reduction of antibiotic use in primary care.

Trial registration: EudraCT: 2016–000477-21. Clinical trials.gov: NCT03151603 (registered: 10 May 2017).

Keywords: Comparative effectiveness design, *Arctostaphylos uva-ursi*, Antibiotic prescription, General practice, Herbal remedy

* Correspondence: gagyor_i@ukw.de
[†]Kambiz Afshar and Nina Fleischmann contributed equally to this work.
[7]Department of General Practice Universitätsklinikum Wurzburg, Josef-Schneider-Str. 2/D7, 97080 Würzburg, Germany
Full list of author information is available at the end of the article

Background

Acute urinary tract infections (UTI) represent a common condition in general practice and are usually treated with antibiotics. Though known to be self-limiting in many cases [1–5], UTI account for a significant number of antibiotic prescriptions [6]. This contributes to increasing resistance rates in UTI uropathogenic bacteria and is being discussed critically [7].

Antibiotic prescriptions can be problematic with regard to resistance rates, side effects and costs [8]. Furthermore, several studies show that women with uncomplicated UTI are often willing to delay or even decline antibiotic treatment because they are aware of possible adverse events [5, 9]. Considering these factors, there is a need for evidence of alternative treatment strategies in women with uncomplicated UTI.

In a recent trial, the strategy of initial symptomatic treatment with ibuprofen was proven to be effective in women with uncomplicated UTI and mild to moderate symptom burden [10]. Currently, another randomized controlled trial is being conducted by Vik and colleagues comparing ibuprofen versus mecillinam for uncomplicated cystitis [11]. Since ibuprofen is not suitable for all women equally, other treatment strategies should be explored alternatively. *Arctostaphylos uva-ursi* (UU, bearberry extract arbutin) has traditionally been used to treat UTI symptoms. Former studies have shown antiseptic and antimicrobial properties of UU which are attributed to hydroquinones and tannins [12]. UU is concentrated in the urine and has shown efficacy against bacteria causing UTI [13]. It is safe, only mild adverse events (AE) have been described previously (i.e. gastrointestinal complaints) and detailed investigation did not reveal any toxicity related to the ingestion of UU [14, 15]. In over the counter use, patients should be advised to respect recommended dosage and duration [16]. Being a herbal preparation, a generally high acceptance of UU by patients may be presumed [17]. Limited clinical data from small studies suggest that UU is effective in preventing UTI even in high risk patients [15, 18]. However, its clinical effectiveness in treating acute uncomplicated UTI and its potential to reduce antibiotic use has not yet been subject of a fully powered randomized controlled trial.

The main research questions of this study are:

1) Does initial treatment with UU in women with uncomplicated UTI (starting treatment with UU and prescribing antibiotics only if symptoms persist) reduce the number of antibiotic courses without significantly increasing symptom burden?
2) Is the suggested strategy safe with regard to complications and recurrences?

Methods

The study protocol of REGATTA is based on the previous trial "Ibuprofen versus fosfomycin for uncomplicated urinary tract infection in women: randomised controlled trial" (ICUTI) [10].

Study design

REGATTA is a double-blind, randomized, controlled comparative effectiveness trial with active control and parallel groups comparing initial herbal treatment of uncomplicated UTI with immediate antibiotic therapy.

Trial objectives

Co-primary endpoints

Two co-primary endpoints are: 1) number of antibiotic courses day 0–28 and 2) symptom burden (AUC) day 0–7, defined as a weighted sum of the daily total symptom scores, measured as the area under the curve (AUC) of the total symptom score. The trial result is considered positive if superiority of initial treatment with UU is demonstrated with reference to the co-primary outcome number of antibiotic courses and non-inferiority of initial treatment with UU with reference to the co-primary outcome symptom burden. We assume non-inferiority if the symptom burden under UU is increased by less than 25% in comparison to the active control.

Key secondary endpoints

With reference to effectiveness: number of early relapses defined as recurrent symptoms until day 14 after initial symptom resolution, number of patients with recurrent UTI day 15–28, defined as recurrent UTI symptoms after initial symptom resolution, number of patients with symptom resolution on day 4 and 7, mean daily symptom sum scores day 0–7, symptom burden (AUC) for individual symptoms (dysuria, urgency, frequency, lower abdominal pain) day 0–7, symptom burden (AUC) day 0–7 of patients with positive and patients with negative urine culture, activity impairment by UTI symptoms days 0–7 (AUC), use of painkillers (defined daily dose, DDD) day 0–7, number of patients taking painkillers, antibiotic use (DDD) day 0–28, number of UTI related visits day 0–28, number of days of UTI related sick leave day 0–28.

With reference to safety: number of patients with temperature > 38 °C day 0–7, number of patients with worsening symptoms, number of patients with prolonged symptoms (> 7 days after inclusion), episodes of pyelonephritis day 0–28 according to general practitioner's (GP) diagnosis, number of AE and SAE by system organ class day 0–28, proportion of patients with at least 1 AE / 2 AE. All patients will be followed up until symptom resolution. Symptom resolution is defined as max. One score point on each symptom scale.

Sample size

Demonstrating non-inferiority regarding co-primary endpoint symptom burden drives the sample size. Based on data of the ICUTI trial [10], it was assumed that the coefficient of variation of symptom burden will be 70%. With this coefficient of variation the sample size required to demonstrate non-inferiority as defined above at a one-sided significance level of 2.5% with a power of 90% will be 170 patients per group, i.e. Three hundred forty patients in total give no difference in symptom burden between the groups. A Wilcoxon rank sum test comparing the two treatment groups with regard to the co-primary endpoint number of antibiotic courses has a power of at least 90% given the sample size of 170 patients per group and a probability of at least 61% that a patient in the intervention group takes fewer antibiotic courses than a patient in the control group. This is a conservative assumption as this probability was estimated to be in excess of 80% from data in the ICUTI study [10]. Adjusting for a drop-out rate of 20%, 430 patients have to be randomized. The sample sizes were calculated using nQuery Advisor® Version 7.0.

Trial population

Setting and recruitment

General practices in Germany (Lower Saxony, Hesse, North-Rhine Westphalia, Thuringia and Bremen) will participate in the trial and recruit 430 patients during a 16 months recruitment period. The academic study centers in Göttingen and Hannover will provide structured practice support to optimize patient recruitment with newsletters, telephone calls and incentives.

On site monitoring visits are planned at the beginning and during the study for source data verification and to ensure correct procedures and documentation.

Inclusion and exclusion criteria

Women between 18 and 75 years with suspected UTI presenting at general practice with at least two of the following symptoms: dysuria, urgency, frequency and lower abdominal pain will be asked for participation, assessed for eligibility and included after written informed consent.

Key exclusion criteria comprise any signs of complicated UTI (i.e. temperature > 38 °C, loin tenderness), any conditions that may lead to complicated infections (i.e. renal diseases, patients with urinary catheter), pregnancy or breastfeeding, current self-medication with UU preparations, antibiotic use in the last 7 days, previous UTI in the past 2 weeks, history of pyelonephritis, contraindications for trial drugs, severe diseases (i.e. serious infection, multiple sclerosis), inability to understand trial information, and current participation in another clinical trial.

Trial drug and interventions

UU is a dry extract (dry extract ratio 2.5–4.5:1), extraction solvent water, containing 20–28% of hydroquinone derivatives calculated as anhydrous arbutin (spectrophotometry). The dosage for UU will be 3 × 2 105 mg arbutin for 5–6 days until all tablets have been completed. This will give a daily total of 630 mg arbutin, which is below the maximum dose of 840 mg as recommended by the European Medicines Agency (EMA). Haupt Pharma Wülfing GmbH, Member of the Aenova Group, is charged with the production of the UU tablets (Arctuvan®) and with the repacking of the tablets in new blisters. Six tablets will be packed in a blister and 5 blisters will be packed into a box. The blisters will be labeled by the Hospital Pharmacy of the University Hospital of Schleswig-Holstein (UKSH) who will prepare the drug as a clinical trial product. The shelf life is 3 years.

After written informed consent, patients receive either antibiotic therapy with fosfomycin 1 × 3 g or initial treatment with UU tablets (3 × 2 105 mg arbutin) for 5 days. In case of persistent or worsening symptoms, specific antibiotic treatment in line with the results of the urine culture can be initiated at the discretion of the GP. Since fosfomycin is only orally available as granules, a double dummy design is planned. The intervention group takes placebo granule sachets once additional to UU tablets (3 × 2 105 mg arbutin) whereas the control group takes placebo tablets 3 × 2 for 5 days additional to fosfomycin. Patients will be instructed to take preexisting co-medication as usual. Co-medication as well as any analgesics or other additional drugs will be documented in the electronic case report form (eCRF).

Randomization will be performed on patient level. Drug units will be labelled with code numbers from a computer generated random list. At inclusion, patients receive a drug unit, and the code number from the drug unit will be assigned to the patient.

Clinical trial procedures

At inclusion (day 0), patients complete a symptom questionnaire after informed consent. Further, patients provide a urine specimen for dipstick, culture and pregnancy test, and body temperature will be taken in the ear or orally. GPs hand over the drug unit and recommend patients to visit again if symptoms persist or worsen or if fever occurs. If patients return therapy will be changed at the discretion of the GP and according to the German UTI guideline [19], results of the microbiological tests will be available after 4–5 days. Native urine samples will be stored in the refrigerator max. 24 h until collection to the laboratory. All urine cultures will be performed in one central laboratory.

Data collection and management

Participant timeline in REGATTA with information on schedule for enrolment, interventions, assessments, and visits is provided in Table 1.

Inclusion: Symptom questionnaire

Patients will complete a symptom questionnaire which has been used in previous UTI studies but has not been validated yet [4, 10]. Duration and severity of symptoms and activity impairment will be documented. Symptom evaluation will cover the symptoms dysuria, urgency, frequency and lower abdominal pain, each scored from 0 (none) to 4 (very strong). UTI-related activity impairment covers impairment by each single symptom (see above), scored as well from 0 (none) to 4 (very strong) [20]. Data will be transferred to the web-based eCRF by practice staff.

Follow-up

Patients will be asked to record daily symptom severity and activity impairment in the patient diary for at least 7 days. Additionally, pain killer intake and any antibiotic treatment between day 0–7 will be documented. The diaries will be sent back by the patients to the general practice. There will be a follow-up documentation on day 28, where patients will complete the follow-up survey including antibiotic intake, relapses and recurrent UTI, AEs/SAEs, UTI-related consultations and days of sick leave. Study nurses will transfer these data to the web-based eCRF.

Statistical analysis and reporting

The primary analysis will be based on the results of two statistical tests corresponding to two co-primary endpoints. The first test will be on the following two hypotheses H0 (H1): The rate of antibiotic courses per patient within the interval 0–28 days in the UU group is greater or equal (lower) than the rate in the fosfomycin group. The second test will be on the following two hypotheses: H0 (H1): The symptom burden within the interval 0–7 days in the UU group is greater or equal (lower) than 125% of the corresponding symptom burden in the fosfomycin group. Since both criteria have to be fulfilled for the study to be positive, both hypotheses are tested at a one-sided level of 2.5% and the overall type I error rate will still be controlled at the one-sided level of 2.5% (intersection-union method).

The number of antibiotic courses within the interval 0–28 days will be compared between treatment groups using a Wilcoxon rank sum test. The treatment effect will be reported in terms of the so-called relative effect (or also probabilistic index) with 95% confidence interval [21]. As supporting analyses, the number of antibiotic courses will be modelled using suitable parametric models such as negative binomial regressions with treatment group and study center as factors and baseline symptom score as covariate.

An analysis of covariance (ANCOVA) of log symptom burden will be performed with the treatment group as factor and the day-0 (inclusion) log sum of symptom scores as covariate. From this model, a two-sided 95%

Table 1 Participant timeline in REGATTA

Activity	Patient Contact	Baseline	Follow-up							
Day		0	1	2	3	4	5	6	7	28
Visit Number		I								II
Screening		X								
Informed Consent		X								
Inclusion / Exclusion criteria		X								
Medical History, Examination		X								
Urine Tests[a]		X								
Pregnancy Test		X								
Drug Intake[b]		X	X	X	X	X	X			
Symptom Assessment and Activity Impairment (Diary)		X	X	X	X	X	X	X	X	
Additional Antibiotic Courses			X	X	X	X	X	X	X	X
Painkiller Intake			X	X	X	X	X	X	X	X
Adverse Events and Complications			X	X	X	X	X	X	X	X
Recurrent UTI (Questionnaire)										X
Return of Drug Packages										X
Phone Calls to Remind Patients (Diary, Drug Return, Questionnaire)			X						X	X

[a]Midstream urine for on-site dipstick test (leukocytes, nitrite, red blood cells) and for urine culture (pathogens and resistances)
[b]Drug intake until all 30 tablets are finished (= 3 × 2 tablets uva-ursi daily for 5 days)

confidence interval for the ratio of the expected total symptom burden of conditional antibiotic use vs. immediate use will be derived and compared to the non-inferiority margin of 125%.

Secondary endpoints will be explored using regression models appropriate for type of scale, without adjustment for multiplicity.

Patient safety

At inclusion, patients will be advised to consult their GPs at any time in case of ongoing or worsening symptoms. In this case, specific antibiotic therapy can be provided as soon as the resistogram of the urine culture taken at inclusion is available. Adverse events (AE) leading to consultation will be documented in the eCRF by the GP. Serious AE (SAE) will have to be reported by fax within 24 h after becoming aware of it. An independent Data and Safety Monitoring Board (DSMB) will be established to assess safety risks based on the safety related data regularly. In case of cumulative occurrence of SAE or pyelonephritis, the DSMB will decide whether to continue or discontinue the trial.

Ethical considerations

Ethical approval has been obtained by the Independent Ethics Committee of the University Medical Center Göttingen (No. 16/11/16). The study will be conducted according to the principles of Good Clinical Practice (GCP). The patient information sheet has been developed according to current ethic committee's standards. At inclusion, GPs ensure complete orally information about risks, benefits, and study procedures, and take patients' informed consent. Patients declare their agreement to disclosure of pseudonymized data based on current data protection regulations. All patient related data will be treated confidentially. Patients can withdraw their consent for the trial at any time.

This trial is ethically justifiable since harm is unlikely due to the good prognosis of the condition and the use of known and authorized medicines for a period of only 5 days. Additionally, patients will be informed that if their symptoms persist or reoccur they can return to the practice at any time and that, if needed, specific antibiotic treatment can be initiated.

The benefit for individuals comprises saving patients from unnecessary antibiotic treatment and possible antibiotic side effects. In general, the reduction of unnecessary antibiotic prescriptions helps to decrease resistance development.

Patient involvement

We use different approaches to include the patients' perspectives into the design and conduction of this trial.

Patient board

A patient board involving 10 patients with previous UTI will accompany all study procedures, some board members have already participated in the previous trial on UTI [10]. The patient board meets on a regular basis and is involved in the discussion on study documents and material. They will also contribute their perspectives to assist the recruitment of patients, discuss outcomes and support the implementation of results.

Involvement of patient representatives

The patient representative involved in the update of the German guideline on UTI [19], approved the REGATTA trial, its design, endpoints and patient-related aspects. No further changes in the protocol were requested.

Previous experiences

Patients of the previous ICUTI trial have been interviewed after study participation [22]. They pointed out the importance of feeling "safe" in the trial with regard to reliable symptom relief. These results were considered in the planning of REGATTA. Consequently, we do not have a placebo arm but remain with a two-active-treatments design. Furthermore, as patients appreciated in ICUTI, GPs will recommend consultation in cases of persistent symptoms.

The concept to delay antibiotic therapy is supported by different international studies [5, 23]. In a Dutch cohort study for instance [5] one third of women with suspected UTI were willing to delay antibiotic therapy – although in this study no alternative therapy besides watchful waiting was provided.

Registration

This study is registered at clinical trials.gov (NCT03151603) with the acronym REGATTA.

Discussion

This study will show if the use of antibiotics for uncomplicated UTI can be reduced by this alternative treatment. We want to investigate whether the initial treatment with UU is a safe and effective alternative treatment strategy in women with uncomplicated UTI. By choosing a comparative effectiveness design, we will be able to prove the effectiveness of two therapeutic strategies and not only the drug efficacy.

REGATTA is designed to create evidence for an alternative treatment option in UTI and to provide information about the clinical effectiveness and potential to reduce antibiotic use. The study results can indicate an alternative treatment for women who are willing to avoid antibiotic treatment, and may possibly change the management of UTI by this approach that fits perfectly in the daily routines of primary care. In contrast to many UTI trials focusing on patients with microbiologically proven UTI, this study, similarly to the previous study ICUTI, follows a more pragmatic approach by including patients presenting with typical symptoms. The study sample of patients with uncomplicated UTI who are otherwise healthy represent a typical practice population. Thus, external validity is high and results can easily be transferred to routine in general practice.

To assess bacterial count and species, urine cultures will be provided at inclusion for trial reasons only. The results will allow a distinction between patients with and without bacterial infections in the analysis and provide data on resistance in case a secondary antibiotic treatment is needed. Again, this represents a pragmatic approach since treatment decisions for uncomplicated UTI are usually made without microbiological specification in general practice.

Trial objectives

In this study, we aim to investigate benefits and potential risks of two different treatment strategies in UTI. The benefit will consist of a reduced number of antibiotic prescriptions which implies a decrease of resistance rates, side effects and costs. Simultaneously, a potential risk of higher symptom burden will be considered very carefully. Therefore, two co-primary endpoints were chosen to reflect both aspects. Additionally, safety criteria will be assessed by several safety endpoints such as patients with poor outcomes, UTI recurrences and complications, pyelonephritis and number of AE and SAE up to day 28.

Trial drug

UU has antiseptic and antimicrobial properties which are attributed to hydroquinones and tannins [12]. UU is concentrated in the urine and has shown efficacy against bacteria causing UTI [13]. Since there is only few data about the safety and efficacy of UU in uncomplicated UTI there is a need for further investigation. A similar trial investigates whether UU compared to placebo and the advice to take ibuprofen compared to no advice provides relief from urinary symptoms in women with uncomplicated UTI. Results of this study and of REGATT A will provide evidence of strategies to reduce antibiotic use [24].

The control group in REGATTA will be treated with fosfomycin as recommended by the German UTI guideline as one of the first line treatment options in uncomplicated UTI [19]. The resistance rates of fosfomycin with respect to *E. coli* are low [5] and the treatment of symptoms is effective. According to product information and guideline recommendations a single dose treatment is sufficient in UTI [25–27].

As UTI may resolve spontaneously, a third group with observation only could generate further data on the effects of a watch and wait treatment strategy. However, this might also lead to a less participation rate. Patients in this study will receive an active substance irrespective of which group they are randomized to.

Trial procedures

Uncomplicated UTIs have a good prognosis and usually do not require follow-up consultations. To follow this pragmatic approach and to influence the course of the symptoms as little as possible, only one final visit at day 28 without a GP contact is planned in this study. Return visits are possible at any time if symptoms persist or reoccur.

Study-related changes of usual GP procedures are minimized in order to optimize external validity. Nevertheless, GPs can decide whether further diagnostic procedures or an alteration of the initial treatment strategy is necessary in patients with i.e. persistent or worsening symptoms. In this study we tried to keep GPs' and patients' effort as simple and reasonable as possible. Results of a qualitative study of physicians' experiences with a clinical trial confirm that trial procedures should be as simple as possible to successfully implement a clinical trial in family medicine [28]. Therefore, additional procedures (i.e. measurement of the fluid intake or ultrasound for residual urine or renal calculi) were not assessed.

Patient safety

No trial-related invasive procedures are planned. A urine culture will be performed at inclusion so that specific antibiotic therapy can be initiated if necessary in case of persistent or recurrent symptoms.

We estimate that adverse drug events will occur less frequently with UU than with antibiotic therapy and we do not expect complicated disease courses, since UTI is a benign condition. Besides, in both groups the treatment courses are very short.

Although only few data exist, the risk of pyelonephritis after non-antibiotic treatment of UTI is mentioned frequently [3, 29]. In ICUTI comparing ibuprofen versus fosfomycin for uncomplicated UTI, only 5 of 241 patients treated with ibuprofen were suspected to have a pyelonephritis [10]. We expect that some patients will require antibiotic treatment after failure of non-antibiotic treatment, but this will be predominated by the benefits of patients with symptom resolution without antibiotics. Eventually, the rate of relapses might increase – this will be assessed within the trial. The incidence of pyelonephritis/ febrile UTI and poor outcomes in both groups will be monitored. In a follow-up study, we will assess the number of patients with recurrent UTI or pyelonephritis after 3 months.

Conclusions

A confirmation of the trial hypothesis could lead to a revision of the recommended treatment for uncomplicated UTI. Using UU as a first line treatment option may be proven as effective in resolution of UTI symptoms and reduction of antibiotic use. It may also provide favorable effect on resistance rates.

Acknowledgements

The authors thank all GPs and practice staff for participating in this study. We thank the Clinical Study Management (KSM), Göttingen, for preparing the trial (regulatory affairs and project management), the Hospital Pharmacy of the University Hospital of Schleswig-Holstein (UKSH), Haupt Pharma Wülfing GmbH, Member of Aenova Group, Gronau, and the Laboratory Amedes Medizinische Dienstleistungen GmbH, Göttingen for their cooperation.

Funding

The German Federal Ministry of Education and Research fund the study (No. 01KG1601). The funder had no role in the trial design and will have no influence on data collection, analysis, or reporting.

Authors' contributions

IG, EHP, GS, JB and MM had the original idea for the study. All authors substantially contributed to the implementation of the study and have given relevant intellectual input. IG, JB and GS will supervise the practices and manage the trial on a day-to- day basis. KA, NF, IG, JB and EHP wrote the manuscript. TF and KW made substantial contributions to the statistical analysis. All authors read and approved the final manuscript.

Competing interests

The authors have no conflicts of interest to declare. Haupt Pharma Wulfing GmbH was contracted to produce and repack the trial medication (Arctuvan®). The company did not have influence on the study design and will participate neither in the clinical project management nor in the collection, analysis, and interpretation of data.

Author details

[1]Institute for General Practice, Hannover Medical School, Carl-Neuberg-Str. 1, 30625 Hannover, Germany. [2]Department of General Practice, University Medical Center Göttingen, Humboldtallee 38, 37073 Göttingen, Germany. [3]Department for Health Services Research, Institute for Public Health and Nursing Research, University of Bremen, Bremen, Germany. [4]Department of Medical Statistics, University Medical Center Göttingen, Humboldtallee 32, 37073 Göttingen, Germany. [5]Department of Medical Biometry and Epidemiology, University Medical Center Hamburg-Eppendorf, Martinistr, 52, 20246 Hamburg, Germany. [6]Primary Care and Population Science, University of Southampton Faculty of Medicine, Aldermoor Health Centre, Southampton SO16 5ST, UK. [7]Department of General Practice Universitätsklinikum Wurzburg, Josef-Schneider-Str. 2/D7, 97080 Würzburg, Germany.

References

1. Little P, Merriman R, Turner S, Rumsby K, Warner G, Lowes JA, et al. Presentation, pattern, and natural course of severe symptoms, and role of antibiotics and antibiotic resistance among patients presenting with suspected uncomplicated urinary tract infection in primary care: observational study. BMJ. 2010;340:b5633. https://doi.org/10.1136/bmj.b5633.
2. Little P, Moore MV, Turner S, Rumsby K, Warner G, Lowes JA, et al. Effectiveness of five different approaches in management of urinary tract infection: randomised controlled trial. BMJ. 2010;340:c199. https://doi.org/10.1136/bmj.c199
3. Christiaens TCM, De Meyere M, Verschraegen G, Peersman W, Heytens S, De Maeseneer JM. Randomised controlled trial of nitrofurantoin versus placebo in the treatment of uncomplicated urinary tract infection in adult women. Br J Gen Pract. 2002;52:729–34.
4. Bleidorn J, Gagyor I, Kochen MM, Wegscheider K, Hummers-Pradier E. Symptomatic treatment (ibuprofen) or antibiotics (ciprofloxacin) for uncomplicated urinary tract infection?–results of a randomized controlled pilot trial. BMC Med. 2010;8:30. https://doi.org/10.1186/1741-7015-8-30.
5. Knottnerus BJ, Geerlings SE, van Charante EP, ter Riet G. Women with symptoms of uncomplicated urinary tract infection are often willing to delay antibiotic treatment: a prospective cohort study. BMC Fam Pract. 2013;14:71. https://doi.org/10.1186/1471-2296-14-71.
6. Ong DSY, Kuyvenhoven MM, van Dijk L, Verheij TJM. Antibiotics for respiratory, ear and urinary tract disorders and consistency among GPs. J Antimicrob Chemother. 2008;62:587–92. https://doi.org/10.1093/jac/dkn230.
7. Hollis A, Ahmed Z. Preserving antibiotics, rationally. N Engl J Med. 2013;369: 2474–6. https://doi.org/10.1056/NEJMp1311479.
8. Foxman B, Barlow R, D'Arcy H, Gillespie B, Sobel JD. Urinary tract infection: self-reported incidence and associated costs. Ann Epidemiol. 2000;10:509–15.
9. Leydon GM, Turner S, Smith H, Little P. Women's views about management and cause of urinary tract infection: qualitative interview study. BMJ. 2010; 340:c279. https://doi.org/10.1136/bmj.c279.
10. Gágyor I, Bleidorn J, Kochen MM, Schmiemann G, Wegscheider K, Hummers-Pradier E. Ibuprofen versus fosfomycin for uncomplicated urinary tract infection in women: randomised controlled trial. BMJ. 2015;351:h6544. https://doi.org/10.1136/bmj.h6544.
11. Vik I, Bollestad M, Grude N, Baerheim A, Molstad S, Bjerrum L, Lindbaek M. Ibuprofen versus mecillinam for uncomplicated cystitis–a randomized controlled trial study protocol. BMC Infect Dis. 2014;14:693. https://doi.org/10.1186/s12879-014-0693-y.
12. Gruenwald J, Brendler T, Jaenicke C. PDR for herbal medicine. 4th ed. Montvale, NJ: Thompson Healthcare Inc.; 2007.
13. Kedzia B, Wrociński T, Mrugasiewicz K, Gorecki P, Grzewińska H. Przeciwbakteryjne działanie moczu zawierajacego produkty metabolizmu arbutyny. Med Dosw Mikrobiol. 1975;27:305–14.
14. European Medicines Agency, Committee on Herbal Medicinal Products (HMPC). Community herbal monograph on Arctostaphylos uva-ursi (L.) Spreng, folium; 2012. p. 1–6.
15. Albrecht J, Kreyes G. Langzeitbehandlung von Dauerkatheterpatienten: Chemoprophylaxe oder Phytotherapie? Extr urol. 1988;11(5):277–80.
16. Flower A, Wang L, Lewith G, Liu JP, Li Q. Chinese herbal medicine for treating recurrent urinary tract infections in women. Cochrane Database Syst Rev. 2015;(6):CD010446. https://doi.org/10.1002/14651858.CD010446.pub2.
17. Joos S, Glassen K, Musselmann B. Herbal medicine in primary healthcare in Germany: the Patient's perspective. Evid Based Complement Alternat Med. 2012;2012:294638. https://doi.org/10.1155/2012/294638.
18. Larsson B, Jonasson A, Fianu S. Prophylactic effect of UVA-E in women with recurrent cystitis: a preliminary report. Curr Ther Res. 1993;53:441–3. https://doi.org/10.1016/S0011-393X(05)80204-8.
19. Kranz J, Schmidt S, Lebert C, et al. Epidemiology, diagnostics, therapy, prevention and management of uncomplicated bacterial outpatient acquired urinary tract infections in adult patients: update 2017 of the interdisciplinary AWMF S3 guideline (article in German). Urologe A. 2017; 56(6):746–58. https://doi.org/10.1007/s00120-017-0389-1.
20. Wild DJ, Clayson DJ, Keating K, Gondek K. Validation of a patient-administered questionnaire to measure the activity impairment experienced by women with uncomplicated urinary tract infection: the activity impairment assessment (AIA). Health Qual Life Outcomes. 2005;3:42.
21. Kieser M, Friede T, Gondan M. Assessment of statistical significance and clinical relevance. Stat Med. 2013;32:1707–19.
22. Bleidorn J, Bucak S, Gágyor I, Hummers-Pradier E, Dierks M. Why do - or don't - patients with urinary tract infection participate in a clinical trial? A qualitative study in German family medicine. Ger Med Sci. 2015;13:Doc17.
23. Butler CC, Hawking MK, Quigley A, McNulty CA. Incidence, severity, help seeking, and management of uncomplicated urinary tract infection: a population-based survey. Br J Gen Pract. 2015;65(639):e702–7.
24. Trill J, Simpson C, Webley F, et al. Uva-ursi extract and ibuprofen as alternative treatments of adult female urinary tract infection (ATAFUTI): study protocol for a randomised controlled trial. Trials. 2017;18:421. https://doi.org/10.1186/s13063-017-2145-7.

25. Minassian MA, Lewis DA, Chattopadhyay D, Bovill B, Duckworth GJ, Williams JD. A comparison between single-dose fosfomycin trometamol (Monuril) and a 5-day course of trimethoprim in the treatment of uncomplicated lower urinary tract infection in women. Int J Antimicrob Agents. 1998;10:39–47.
26. Lobel B. Short term therapy for uncomplicated urinary tract infection today. Clinical outcome upholds the theories. Int J Antimicrob Agents. 2003; 22(Suppl 2):85–7.
27. Stein GE. Comparison of single-dose fosfomycin and a 7-day course of nitrofurantoin in female patients with uncomplicated urinary tract infection. Clin Ther. 1999;21:1864–72. https://doi.org/10.1016/S0149-2918(00)86734-X.
28. Bleidorn J, Költzsch C, Hummers-Pradier E, Gágyor I, Theile G. Family physicians as clinical trial investigators? - a qualitative study of physicians' experiences with a double-blind clinical trial. Fam Med Med Sci Res. 2014;3: 122. https://doi.org/10.4172/2327-4972.1000122.
29. Richards D, Toop L, Chambers S, Fletcher L. Response to antibiotics of women with symptoms of urinary tract infection but negative dipstick urine test results: double blind randomised controlled trial. BMJ. 2005;331(7509): 143. Epub 2005 Jun 22

Dietary supplement use among undergraduate male students in health and non-health cluster colleges of a public-sector university in Dammam, Saudi Arabia

Atta Abbas Naqvi[1*], Rizwan Ahmad[2], Abdullah Abdul Wahid Elewi[3], Ayman Hussain AlAwa[3] and Moayed Jafar Alasiri[3]

Abstract

Background: Dietary supplements (DS) are nutraceuticals that improve overall health and well-being of an individual as well as reduce the risk of diseases. Evidence indicates a rising prevalence of these products worldwide especially among college students. Studies have reported an increasing use of supplements among Saudi students. However, the scope of those researches was limited to prevalence data. Hence, the aim of our study was to document the prevalence, opinions, attitudes, reasons for use and monthly cost attributed to dietary supplement use.

Methods: A 3-month cross-sectional study was conducted to evaluate use of dietary supplement among health and non-health college students at a public-sector university in Dammam city, Saudi Arabia. It was conducted using Arabic version of the Dietary supplement questionnaire (DSQ-A). A total of 469 male students responded to the survey giving a response rate of 93.8%. The students were from ten colleges of the university. The data was analyzed by SPSS version 22. The study was approved by Institutional Review Board of Imam Abdulrahman Bin Faisal University, Dammam, Saudi Arabia (IRB-UGS-2018-05-074).

Results: The overall prevalence of dietary supplement use in the university was 29.42%. In health cluster colleges, it was reported at 35.91% while in non-health cluster college it was 23.69%. Maintaining general health and well-being was the most common reason for use. Prevalence of multivitamins and whey proteins was approximately 23%. Average monthly cost of supplement was SAR 278.92 (USD 74.39). Cost was positively correlated ($\rho = 0.305$) with satisfaction score. Students preferred brand products (16.4%). 41.4% students opined that DS may prevent chronic illness if used regularly and agreed that they are good for health. Majority of students (65%) recommended DS use only upon physician's recommendation. College clusters and study-year was associated (p-value< 0.01) with students' opinion. Students in health cluster colleges were more likely to recommend supplements (OR 3.715, p-value< 0.0001).

Conclusion: Prevalence of dietary supplement use was lower than other local and international university students. Health cluster colleges had higher prevalence as compared to non-health cluster colleges. Multivitamins and whey protein were the most commonly used types of DS. Students preferred brand products, had positive opinions and attitudes towards dietary supplement. However, they recommended supplements use to others only upon a physician's recommendation.

Keywords: Dietary supplement, Undergraduate students, Prevalence, Opinions, Attitudes, Cost, Saudi Arabia

* Correspondence: naqviattaabbas@gmail.com; aaghulam@iau.edu.sa
[1]Department of Pharmacy Practice, College of Clinical Pharmacy, Imam Abdulrahman Bin Faisal University, Dammam 31441, Saudi Arabia
Full list of author information is available at the end of the article

Background

Appropriate nutrition is essential for proper development and maintenance of the human body. Dietary supplement (DS) improves general health and well-being when used as recommended [1]. It includes multivitamins, minerals and, natural products extracts [2]. The use of DS is quite common in the developed world [3]. According to the 3rd National Health and Nutrition Examination Survey (NHANES), the overall prevalence of dietary supplement use in the United States (US) was 40% [3]. Evidence indicates that individuals may use a single or a combination of different dietary supplements as means to improve their nutrition intake, maintaining general health and well-being, as well as reduce risk of diseases [3]. Conversely, studies have reported adverse drug events and mortalities because of over dose, drug-drug and drug-disease interactions associated with supplement use [4]. For instance, excessive use of cholecalciferol, i.e., vitamin D, may adversely affect soft tissues and kidney functions [5]. Supplements may also interact with drugs for managing cardiovascular illnesses [6, 7].

Studies have reported a higher consumption of supplements in subgroups as compared to overall population and, several demographic determinants such as higher education, attitudes, etc., have been reported to be associated with a greater likelihood of dietary use [3, 8, 9]. Literature highlights that more than half (66%) of college students in the US used dietary supplements and students with a health study background used DS more regularly than students belonging to non-health study field [1, 10, 11].

The monetary value of dietary supplements in 2014 amounted to United States dollar (USD) 165.62 billion and was rising with a compound annual growth rate (CAGR) of 7.3%. The projected market worth is expected to touch USD 278.96 billion by 2021. Asia Pacific region has emerged as the second largest market for dietary supplements after US and Canada [12]. Saudi Arabia is the biggest market for dietary supplements in the Middle East region as DS accounts for 4% of total pharmaceuticals sold in the country with an estimated worth of USD 2 billion [13, 14].

Dietary supplements may be marketed as brand or generic products. A brand is a pharmaceutical product that is developed by a pharmaceutical company after years of research and financial investment. These pharmaceutical products are legally protected by patents granted from health regulatory agencies for several years. The patent gives the manufacturer the sole legal right to sell the product for the stated period of patent. After the expiry of the patent, other pharmaceutical firms may manufacture the product after approval from the health regulatory agency. These products are termed as generic. Since generic products utilize the research of the parent brand drug, they do not require investment of huge finances in research and therefore, are cheaper than their brand counterparts. However, studies have reported that despite same product quality, brands may be preferred over generics due to a positive patient perception [15].

College students studying in Saudi Arabia were more likely to use DS as compared to general population [10]. Although, a few studies reported that the use of supplements had increased in general population as well as undergraduate students of Saudi Arabia. However, the findings were limited to prevalence data [14, 16]. There is a scarcity of data that reports common supplements used by Saudi students. Moreover, the reasons as well as attitudes towards DS use have not been studied before. A study by Albusalih et al., conducted at this venue reported an increasing use of dietary supplement among students [16]. However, it established a mere prevalence of multivitamins. Hence, the aim of this study was to report the use of dietary supplements in students including its prevalence data, i.e., overall, college-wise and study year-wise prevalence as well as individual prevalence of each supplement. In addition, students' opinion, attitudes, reasons for use as well as monthly cost attributed to dietary supplement use, was documented.

Methods

A cross-sectional study was conducted in undergraduate students studying in health and non-health cluster colleges at Imam Abdulrahman Bin Faisal University located in Dammam, Saudi Arabia.

Operational definitions

Dietary supplements

Dietary supplements are nutraceuticals and natural products extracts, that are available without prescription and are used by individuals in recommended dose for improving performance, general health and well-being as well as reducing the risk of diseases [1].

Dietary supplement prevalence (point prevalence)

The regular use of dietary supplements in a population over a defined time-period [1].

Brand and generic pharmaceutical products

A brand is a pharmaceutical product that is developed by a pharmaceutical company after years of research and financial investment. They are legally protected by patents granted from health regulatory agencies for several years that gives the manufacturer the sole legal right to sell the product for the stated period of patent. After the expiry of the patent, other pharmaceutical firms may manufacture the product after approval from the health regulatory agency. These products are termed as generics and are cheaper than brands because they utilize the research of the parent brand drug and do not require investment of huge finances in research [15].

Target population and inclusion criteria

The study included male students studying in health and non-health colleges affiliated to IAU who were willing to participate. Health cluster included four colleges namely clinical pharmacy, medicine, nursing and applied medical science. Non-health cluster included six colleges namely sharia and law, architecture and planning, engineering, applied studies and community service, business and, science. Female students, students who had graduated from the university and non-consenting students were excluded. Female students could not be included as male and female students were segregated and studied in different campuses with separate and independent administration. The study included only male investigators and it was not possible to conduct the study in female campuses. This is mentioned as a limitation of our study.

Sample size and procedure

We employed purposive sampling methodology and selected most convenient time such as prayer and lunch breaks to approach students. Students from different health and non-health cluster colleges of university were invited to participate. Sample size was calculated based on number of undergraduate students studying in Saudi universities. According to official figures, there were 1597 students enrolled at IAU [17]. This figure was identified as target population. Sample size was calculated from online calculator [18]. The sample size calculated was 310. Our study gathered data from 469 students which was more than the required sample size.

Research instrument and translation process

A survey questionnaire developed by Naqvi and colleagues, known as the Dietary supplement questionnaire (DSQ) [1], was used after its translation into Arabic language that is the native language of Saudi students. The questionnaire contained multiple choice questions, few open-ended questions and a numeric rating scale.

The DSQ includes questions related to the demographic information of respondents such as age, college, year of study, residence status, number of siblings, presence of any major illnesses and if they had used a dietary supplement in the last month. Furthermore, the respondents were asked about the type of dietary supplement they used, what commercial product did they use, i.e., imported brand from foreign countries or a locally produced generic product, the reason for taking supplements and monthly cost attributed to its use. The respondents were also asked if they suffered from any adverse drug event that was related to their supplement use. The respondents were also inquired about their source of information and opinions about supplements. They were asked if they believed that dietary supplements were good for health and whether they would personally recommend supplements to others. Finally, they were asked to rate their satisfaction with supplement use on a rating scale [1].

The translation was carried out considering standard guidelines [19, 20]. The translation process included three Arabic speaking pharmacists whose second language was English. The initial translation was conducted in supervision of the inventors of DSQ to elaborate and clarify meaning in any DSQ item. The initial draft was reviewed by four academic professors specialized in medicine, pharmacy and physics whose first language was Arabic and second language was English. This was done to check for adaptability of the Arabic version (DSQ-A) for respondents belonging to health and non-health background. The three reviewers were kept unaware of the purpose of study to have a balanced review of the tool. DSQ-A was back translated by an academic professor of ethics with same language expertise in collaboration with tool inventors. The face validity and content validity were established and the Arabic version of DSQ was deemed fit to use at this point. The questionnaire is available as an Additional file 1.

Pilot study and acceptability of the DSQ-A

DSQ-A was subjected to pilot study in 100 students belonging to different colleges of the university. A total of 92 responses were received giving a response rate of 92%. No difficulty in understanding of the questionnaire was observed. The DSQ-A was deemed fit to use at this point.

Data analysis

The data was entered and analyzed using statistical software IBM SPSS version 22. Prevalence was calculated using Medcalc. Frequency counts (N), percentages (%) and descriptive statistics such as mean (X) and standard deviation (SD) were used. Prevalence was expressed in percentage (%) and 95% confidence intervals. Inferential statistics such as chi square ($\chi 2$) test to observe associations between student characteristics, i.e., independent variables (IV) and DS study variables, i.e., dependent variables (DV) were performed. Spearman's rank correlations (ρ) was employed to document any correlation among IV and DV. Regression analysis was conducted to report any predictors of DS use.

Ethics approval and consent

The study was approved by the Institutional Review Board of Imam Abdulrahman Bin Faisal University (IRB-UGS-2018-05-074). Students were informed about the study and its objectives. Students who consented to participate in the study were included. The participation was voluntary without any incentive. An informed written consent was sought from students before handing them the questionnaire. Those who consented to participate in the study were handed DSQ-A.

Results

Of total 500 students who were approached, 469 students responded to the survey giving a response rate of 93.8%. The study included students from all study years. The mean age of the students was 21 years (X = 20.96, SD = 1.66). Majority of the students (*N* = 395, 84.2%) lived with their families and had 3–5 siblings (*N* = 262, 55.9%). Few students (*N* = 49, 10.4%) suffered from major illnesses. Of total 49 patients considered as 100% who suffered from illnesses, the proportions of patients were; hypertension (*N* = 3, 6.1%), diabetes mellitus (*N* = 6, 12.2%), sickle cell anemia (*N* = 7, 14.3%), thalassemia (*N* = 1, 2%), glucose 6 – phosphate dehydrogenase (G6PD) (*N* = 17, 34.7%), asthma (*N* = 6, 12.2%), rheumatoid arthritis (*N* = 1, 2%), psoriasis (*N* = 2, 4%), gastro esophageal reflux disorder (GERD) (*N* = 1, 2%), migraine (*N* = 2, 4%), obesity (*N* = 2, 4%) and epilepsy (*N* = 1, 2%). The summary of student information is presented in Table 1.

Table 1 Student characteristics

	N	%
College		
Pharmacy	70	14.9
Medicine	92	19.6
Nursing	22	4.7
Sharia and law	39	8.3
Applied medical sciences	36	7.7
Architecture and planning	57	12.2
Engineering	36	7.7
Applied studies and community service	27	5.8
Business	43	9.2
Science	47	10
Study year		
Prep year	84	17.9
2nd year	138	29.4
3rd year	92	19.6
4th year	59	12.6
5th year	89	19
6th year	7	1.5
Residence		
Living with family	395	84.2
Living alone (University accommodation)	74	15.8
Siblings		
Between 1 and 2 siblings	49	10.4
Between 3 and 5 siblings	262	55.9
Between 6 and 8 siblings	102	21.7
More than 8 siblings	50	10.7
No siblings	6	1.3
Any major illness		
Do not suffer from any illness	420	89.6
Suffer from a major illness	49	10.4
DS use in the last month		
Daily	62	13.2
Weekly	24	5.1
Once a month	20	4.3
Never	300	64
Not sure	63	13.4

Table 2 Types and prevalence of dietary supplement used

Types of dietary supplements used	Alone	As combination
Multivitamins	44 (9.4)	42 (9)
Gingko biloba	1 (0.2)	–
Ginseng	–	3 (0.6)
Glucosamine/omega 3 FA	3 (0.6)	32 (6.8)
Whey protein	38 (8.1)	38 (8.1)
Calcium	1 (0.2)	–
Creatine phosphate	–	1 (0.2)
More than one supplement	64 (13.6)	–
Not applicable	318 (67.8)	–
Cluster-wise prevalence	Prevalence (%)	95% confidence interval
All colleges	29.4	25.3–33.8%
Health cluster colleges	35.9	29.6–42.6%
Non-health cluster colleges	23.7	18.5–29.5%
College-wise prevalence		
Pharmacy	34.3	23.4–46.6%
Medicine	39.1	29.1–49.9%
Nursing	18.2	5.2–40.3%
Applied Medical Science	40	23.9–57.9%
Sharia and law	12.8	4.3–27.4%
Architecture and planning	14	6.6–25.8%
Engineering	41.7	25.5–59.2%
Applied studies and community service	18.5	6.3–38.1%
Business	37.2	23–53.3%
Science	19.2	9.2–33.3%
Study year-wise prevalence		
Prep year	16.7	9.4–26.4%
2nd year	24.5	17.6–32.5%
3rd year	29.4	20.3–39.8%
4th year	37.3	25–50.6%
5th year	42.7	32.3–53.6%
6th year	42.9	9.9–81.6%

Types and prevalence of dietary supplement use

Multivitamins were used alone or in combination by a tenth proportion of students, i.e., 9–9.4%. The overall prevalence of dietary supplement use was 29.4%. Health cluster colleges had an overall prevalence of 35.9% while non-health cluster college reported a prevalence of 23.7%. The summary of prevalence by group and individual colleges as well as study year is presented in Table 2.

The college-wise and study year-wise prevalence of multivitamins, glucosamine/omega 3 Fatty Acids (FA), whey protein, ginseng and gingko biloba was documented. The prevalence of ginseng was reported at 2.9% (0.4–9.9 for 95% CI) from pharmacy college. It was also reported at 1.1% (0.03–5.6 for 95% CI) and 1.7% (0.04–8.9 for 95% CI) in 3rd and 4th year students respectively. The prevalence of gingko biloba was reported in pharmacy college at 1.4 (0.04–7.7 for 95% CI) and at 1.7% (0.04–8.9 for 95% CI) in 4th year students respectively. The college and study year-wise prevalence are tabulated in Table 3.

Cost of dietary supplement per month

The average monthly cost attributed to dietary supplement use was reported at SAR 278.92 (USD 74.39) however, the median cost reported was SAR 220 (USD 58.67). Minimum cost incurred was reported at SAR 5 (USD 1.33) and maximum cost incurred on DS use per month was SAR 2170 (USD 578.74).

Reasons and types of dietary supplements used

Most students did not use DS (318, 67.8%). Almost a fifth proportion of students ($N = 82$, 17.5%) selected more than one reason for using dietary supplement.

Students' experience from DS use

Some students ($N = 77$, 16.4%) used a brand product and a few ($N = 51$, 10.9%) did not know if it was a brand or generic product. A third of students ($N = 142$, 30.2%) did not suffer from an adverse reaction to dietary supplement.

Opinion and attitudes towards DS

More than 40% of students ($N = 194$, 41.4%) opined that DS may prevent chronic illness if used regularly followed by similar number of students ($N = 185$, 39.4%) who considered DS as harmless. Slightly less than half of students ($N = 224$, 47.8%) agreed to the notion that DS are good for health and more than half ($N = 305$, 65%) recommended use of DS to others, only upon doctor's recommendation. Student rated their satisfaction with DS use on a scale of 0 (worst) to 5 (best). The average satisfaction score was reported to be almost 3 (X = 2.89, SD = 1.25). The details are presented in Table 4.

Association and correlation of independent and dependent variables

The dependent variable (DV) of student opinion towards dietary supplements, was significantly associated with;

Table 3 College and study year-wise prevalence of multivitamins, glucosamine/Omega 3 FA and whey protein

	Prevalence % (95% CI)		
	Multivitamins	Glucosamine/Omega 3 FA	Whey protein
Colleges			
Pharmacy	18.6 (10.3–29.7)	10 (4.1–19.5)	22.9 (13.7–34.5)
Medicine	21.7 (13.8–31.6)	6.5 (2.4–13.7)	25 (16.6–35.1)
Nursing	9.1 (1.1–29.2)	9.1 (1.1–29.2)	12.5 (2.7–32.4)
Applied Medical Science	18.2 (8.2–32.8)	10 (2.8–23.7)	16.3 (6.8–30.7)
Sharia and law	9.3 (2.6–22.2)	2.5 (0.1–13.2)	4.9 (0.6–16.5)
Architecture and planning	10.9 (4.5–21.3)	9.5 (3.6–19.6)	13.6 (6.4–24.3)
Engineering	18.2 (8.2–32.7)	12.2 (4.1–26.2)	12.2 (4.1–26.2)
Applied studies and community service	10 (2.1–26.5)	–	12.9 (3.6–29.8)
Business	23.2 (3–36.4)	2.3 (0.1–12)	17.3 (8.2–3.3)
Science	16.1 (7.6–28.3)	6 (1.3–16.6)	9.6 (3.2–21)
Study year			
Prep year	15.2 (8.7–23.8)	3.5 (0.7–9.8)	6.7 (2.5–14)
2nd year	9.8 (5.6–15.7)	7.4 (3.7–12.8)	10.4 (6.1–16.3)
3rd year	17.8 (11.3–26.2)	8.9 (4.2–16.2)	13.2 (7.4–21.2)
4th year	21.3 (12.7–32.3)	6.4 (1.8–15.5)	19.2 (10.9–30.1)
5th year	16.8 (10.3–25.3)	6.3 (2.4–13.2)	23.4 (16.5–32.7)
6th year	30 (6.7–65.2)	22.2 (2.8–60.1)	22.2 (2.8–60.1)

Table 4 Reasons for use, experience with DS, opinions and attitudes towards dietary supplements

Reasons for use	Sample (N)	Percentage (%)
General Health and Well Being	22, 31[a]	4.7, 6.6[a]
Boost immunity	2, 27[a]	0.4, 5.8[a]
Weight gain	2, 18[a]	0.4, 3.8[a]
Doctor's recommendation	7, 17[a]	1.5, 3.6[a]
Enhance memory	3, 16[a]	3.4, 0.6[a]
Increase performance/sports	5, 24[a]	1.1, 5.1[a]
Increase endurance/body building	12, 47[a]	2.6, 10[a]
Malnutrition	9. 35[a]	1.9, 7.5[a]
Energy source	7, 29[a]	1.5, 6.2[a]
More than one reason	82	17.5
Not applicable	318	67.8
Experience with DS use in last month		
Pharmaceutical category used		
Generic	12	2.6
Brand	77	16.4
Both	11	2.3
I do not know	51	10.9
Not applicable	318	67.8
Adverse reactions to dietary supplements		
I suffered from an adverse reaction	1	0.2
I suffered from an adverse reaction but sure if it was related to DS use	8	1.7
No, I did not suffer from any adverse effect	142	30.2
Not applicable to me as I did not use any supplements	318	67.8
Opinion and attitudes		
Opinion about dietary supplements		
Necessary for all ages	49	10.4
They are harmless	185	39.4
Regular use of dietary supplement prevents chronic disease	194	41.4
Dietary supplements may prevent cancer	26	5.5
No opinion	15	3.2
Dietary supplements are good for health		
Agree	224	47.8
I don't know	173	36.9
Disagree	72	15.4
Do you personally recommend use of dietary supplements to others		
Yes, I always recommend	66	14.1
Yes, only when doctors recommend	305	65
Not at all	98	20.9

Legend ([a]) = selected in combination with others

college (p-value< 0.01), college type (p-value< 0.01) and study year (p-value< 0.001). However, there was no statistical significance between the variable of student opinion and demographic information, i.e., siblings (p-value> 0.05). Moreover, the association between student opinion and illness profile was insignificant (p-value> 0.05). The cross tabulation is presented in Table 5. The values presented in brackets are expected counts.

The IV of age and dietary supplement cost were positively correlated with satisfaction score ($\rho = 0.12$ and $\rho = 0.305$ respectively) and the correlation was significant at p-value< 0.01 (Figs. 1 and 2).

Multinomial logistic regression (MLR) was used to interpret the odds ratio for dependent variable (DV) of, 'encouraging dietary supplement use'. The discrete independent variable (IV) of, 'age' was considered as covariate and categorical IV of, 'college type' was fixed. Student attitudes towards encouraging DS use was taken as DV. The parameter of IV, i.e., 'non-health cluster college,' was redundant and therefore, set to zero (0). Parameter of DV, i.e., 'not at all,' was considered as reference category. The regression analysis reported that keeping the categorical IV of 'college type' as constant, the odds of, 'always recommending DS use,' increases with every year-wise increase in age (OR 1.303, p-value< 0.01). Similarly, keeping the IV of 'age' as constant, students studying in 'health cluster colleges' were more likely to, 'recommend DS use' as compared to students studying in 'non-health cluster colleges' (OR 3.715, p-value< 0.0001). The regression analysis is tabulated in Table 6.

Discussion

Dietary supplement use has been previously reported from this university by Albusalih et al., that highlighted the need to conduct a full-scale study to investigate their use including prevalence, cost attributed to DS use and students' attitude and opinion towards it [16]. This study was conducted in ten colleges of the university. The sample size was 310 for 95% confidence interval (CI) however, we focused on gathering sample to satisfy 99% CI. The extensiveness of data collection in ten colleges, large sample size and a high response rate are major strengths of this study.

The average age of students was 21 years and most students lived with their families. Few students had major illnesses, i.e., cardiovascular diseases, endocrine and blood disorders, musculoskeletal diseases, gastrointestinal and central nervous system disorders. Previous studies conducted in this population have also reported similar student health profile [16, 21–23].

The overall prevalence of DS use at the university was 29.42%. This reiterates the findings of Albusalih et al.,

Table 5 Cross tabulation between students' demographic characteristics and opinion

Independent Variable	Dietary supplements are good for health			*P*-value
	Agree	Do not know	Disagree	
College				*< 0.01*
Clinical pharmacy	49 (33.4)	17 (25.8)	4 (10.7)	
Medicine	62 (43.9)	23 (33.9)	7 (14.1)	
Nursing	7 (10.5)	9 (8.1)	6 (3.4)	
Applied medical sciences	12 (17.2)	14 (13.3)	10 (5.5)	
Sharia and law	10 (18.6)	23 (14.4)	6 (6)	
Architecture and planning	15 (27.2)	32 (21)	10 (8.8)	
Engineering	21 (17.2)	9 (13.3)	6 (5.5)	
Applied studies and community service	7 (12.9)	13 (10)	7 (4.1)	
Business	27 (20.5)	11 (15.9)	5 (6.6)	
Science	14 (22.4)	22 (17.3)	11 (7.2)	
College cluster				*< 0.001*
Health	130 (105.1)	63 (81.2)	27 (33.8)	
Non-health	94 (118.9)	110 (91.8)	45 (38.2)	
Study year				*< 0.001*
Prep Year	26 (40.1)	39 (31)	19 (12.9)	
2nd Year	52 (65.9)	63 (50.9)	23 (21.2)	
3rd Year	47 (43.9)	32 (33.9)	13 (14.1)	
4th Year	35 (28.2)	17 (21.8)	7 (9.1)	
5th Year	61 (42.5)	19 (32.8)	9 (13.7)	
6th Year	3 (3.3)	3 (2.6)	1 (1.1)	
Siblings				*> 0.05*
Between 1 and 2 siblings	28 (23.4)	14 (18.1)	7 (7.5)	
Between 3 and 5 siblings	120 (125.1)	103 (96.6)	39 (40.2)	
Between 6 and 8 siblings	54 (48.7)	35 (37.6)	13 (15.7)	
More than 8 siblings	22 (23.9)	17 (18.4)	11 (7.7)	
No siblings	0 (2.9)	4 (2.2)	2 (0.9)	
Any major illness				*> 0.05*
Do not suffer from any illness	198 (200.6)	156 (154.9)	66 (64.5)	
Suffer from a major illness	26 (23.4)	17 (18.1)	6 (7.5)	

that reported a 30% prevalence of the same [16]. Though, that figure was reported in male and female students cumulatively. Our results are in the range of 26.31–35% as reported by Albusalih et al., [16]. Naqvi and colleagues reported a prevalence of dietary supplement use at 51% in male undergraduate pharmacy students of Pakistani universities [1]. Our finding was much lower than figures reported from American, Nigerian and South African university students [1, 14, 24, 25]. However, it was higher than that reported in Japanese students [26]. Our study further documented college-wise and study-year wise prevalence data as well. We tested the hypothesis that health students use such products more than non-health students. Studies have reported that students with a health background tend to use supplements more than their counterparts which could be due to better awareness and education that may shape their opinions in favour of using supplements [26, 27]. The prevalence of DS use in health cluster colleges was reported at 35.91% while it was 23.69% in non-health cluster. Similarly, highest prevalence of DS use was reported from applied medical science, medicine and pharmacy colleges. Students of engineering college, i.e., a non-health college, reported prevalence similar to that reported in students of applied medical science college. This reiterates the findings of Kobayashi et al., that prevalence was higher in students with health background compared to those with a non-health background [11, 26]. An inclining trend was evident while

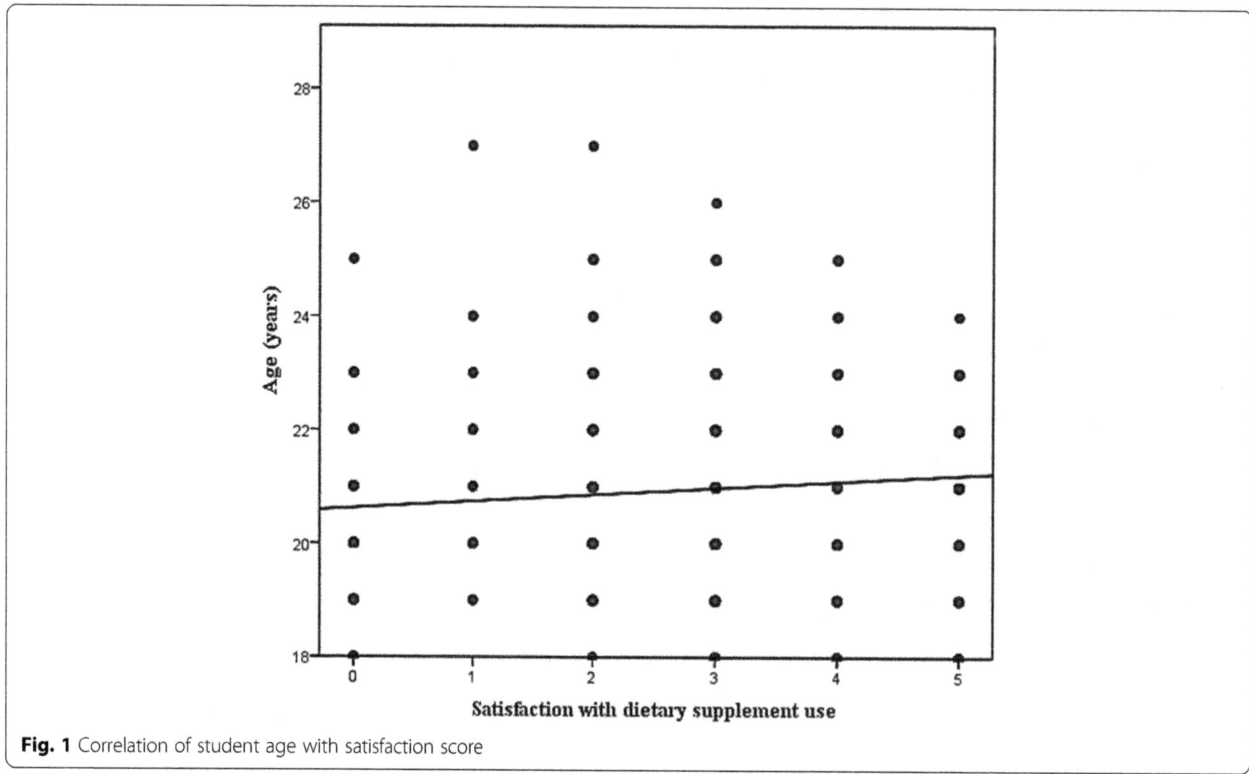

Fig. 1 Correlation of student age with satisfaction score

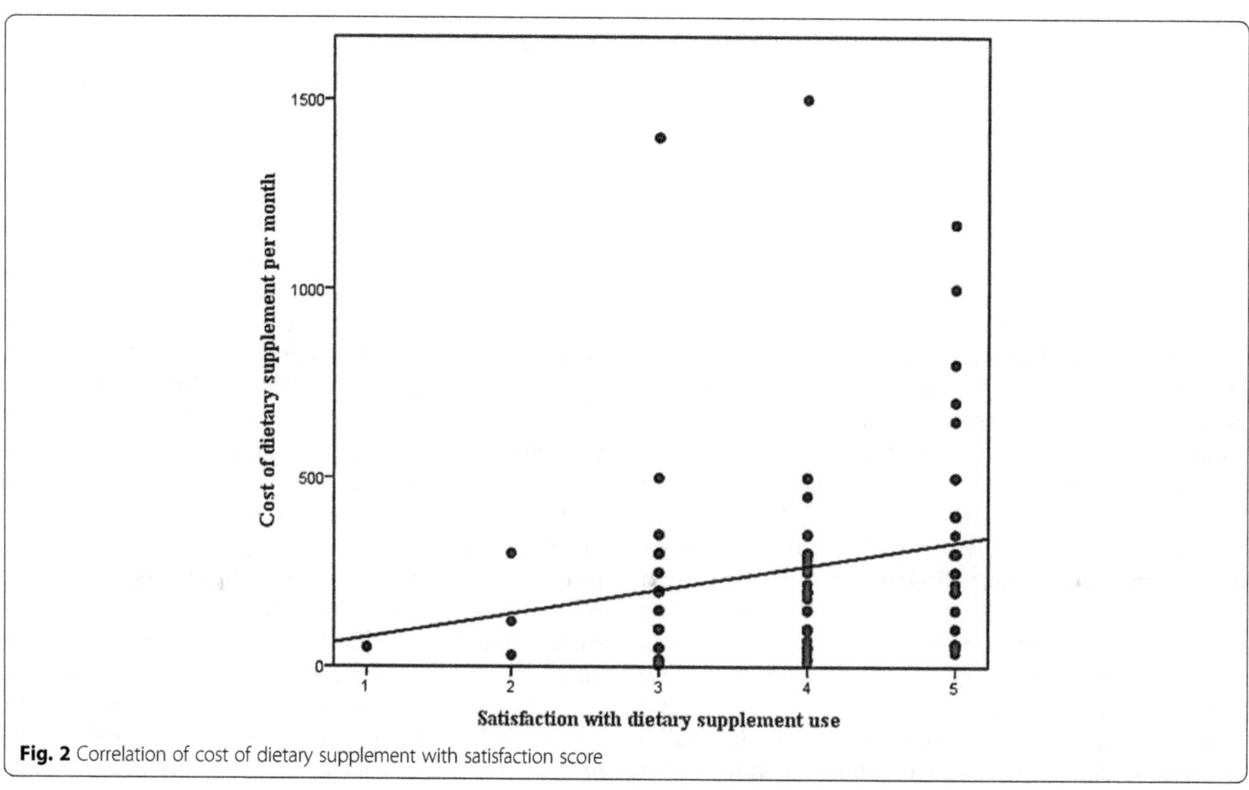

Fig. 2 Correlation of cost of dietary supplement with satisfaction score

Table 6 Multinomial logistic regression analysis

Encourage dietary supplement use?		Coefficient	Odds ratio	95% Confidence interval	
				Lower bound	Upper bound
Yes, I always recommend	Age	0.265	1.303	1.080	1.572
	Health cluster college	1.312	3.715	1.899	7.266
	Non-health cluster college	0[a]	–	–	–
Yes, only when doctor recommends	Age	0.068	1.07	0.93	1.231
	Health cluster college	1.133	3.104	1.868	5.156
	Non-health cluster college	0[a]	–	–	–

[a]Reference category

investigating prevalence data based on study year. This occurrence has been reported previously among university student in Japan. Hence, our findings are consistent with Kobayashi and colleagues [26].

Prevalence of some dietary supplements that were observed to be common amongst students in all colleges was also determined. These included multivitamins, glucosamine/Omega 3 fatty acids, whey protein, ginseng and gingko biloba extracts. Most notable figures were documented for whey protein use. The prevalence remained consistent throughout all colleges. Evidence indicates that protein supplementation is quite common among male university students as it improves physical performance [28, 29]. Multivitamin use prevailed in all colleges with highest prevalence in business college, i.e., around 23% and lowest in nursing college, i.e., 9.1%.

The use of glucosamine/Omega 3 fatty acids (FA) was more widespread in health cluster as compared to non-health cluster. Omega 3 FA may improve sleep quality, reduce depression and anxiety among students [30, 31]. Abbas et al., have reported that anxiety and depression due to academic studies may prevail in undergraduate students [32–34]. Prohaska reported improvement in sleep efficiency by omega 3 FA supplementation in clinically depressed undergraduate students [31]. Studies by Al Rasheed et al., and Al-Shagawi et al., have reported high academic stress and anxiety in Saudi undergraduate students studying medicine and allied health subjects [21, 22]. Hence, its prevalent use could be due to the stress and anxiety among health track students. Use of omega 3 fatty acids has been reported from other colleges in Saudi Arabia as well [14]. However, we could not conclude that high academic stress, depression and anxiety was the reason behind prevalent use of omega 3 FA in our sample.

The use of ginseng and gingko biloba was reported in very low percentages mainly from 3rd and 4th year pharmacy students. This is relevant as pharmacy students study natural products and alternative medicines as well as pharmacognosy courses that may increase their knowledge and awareness of natural products [23]. Use of ginseng and gingko biloba has also been reported from other Saudi universities [14].

Most common reason mentioned for using DS was maintenance of general health and well-being. Students in Pakistani universities mentioned physician's advice as most common reason to use dietary supplement [1]. Furthermore, multivitamins were the most common type of DS used alone, as well as in combination. This occurrence has been reported by studies conducted in local and international academia [8, 14, 16, 26].

The average monthly cost attributed to dietary supplement use was reported at SAR 278.92, i.e., USD 74.39. No studies have been conducted in Saudi universities till date, that document cost attributed to DS use among students. A novel study conducted by Naqvi et al., in Pakistani universities reported average DS cost at USD 13.5 [1]. Hence, our findings highlight a relatively high spending trend among Saudi students. However, this may not be definite as there may be other determinants such as socio-economic status that may affect spending on supplements. We found that students preferred a brand over generic dietary supplement. This may be based on individual buying preference. Studies have demonstrated that an individual may prefer brands as brand products are believed to have better quality as compared to generics [15, 28]. Dwyer and colleagues have reported that poor quality of dietary supplements have resulted in adverse drug events (ADEs) and mortality [6]. Moreover, pharmaceutical packaging may also affect consumers' preferences. Sabah and colleagues mentioned un-attractive packaging as a reason for low preference of generic products in Pakistan [35]. The occurrence of a significantly strong correlation between cost of DS and satisfaction score may explain the buying preference from another dimension. This correlation implied that students appeared more satisfied with expensive supplements. This occurrence has been reported by Jamshed and colleagues from Pakistan's health sector as well [36]. Studies report that brands are generally expensive than generics [15, 36].

Majority of the students opined that regular use of supplements prevented chronic diseases and agreed to the idea that DS were good for health. This was significantly associated with demographic variables of college, college cluster and study year. Students belonging to health cluster colleges agreed that DS were good for health however, responses from non-health track students swayed between uncertainty and disagreement. Similarly, students in advance study years agreed with the notion. These findings agree with Kobayashi and colleagues [26]. Another confirmation of this phenomenon was the occurrence of significant positive correlation between age of students and DS satisfaction score. Most students mentioned that they would recommend DS only upon a physician's recommendation. This finding contradicts the results of El Khoury et al., i.e., Lebanese students recommended use of supplements on relatives, friends and peers' advice [37]. However, there is a plethora of evidence that indicates that dietary supplements may be harmful if not taken in recommended dose [4]. In some cases, over usage of multivitamins may exceed the permissible limits of certain vitamins such as cholecalciferol that may result in adverse effects [5, 6, 38].

Conclusion

The prevalence of dietary supplement was lower than other local and international academic institutions. Prevalence was higher in health cluster colleges as compared to non-health cluster colleges. Multivitamins were most commonly used dietary supplements among university students. Students were more inclined towards expensive brand supplements and had favourable opinion about them. Students had a positive attitude towards dietary supplement use however, they recommended it only upon physician's recommendation. These findings were in line with previously reported literature.

This study used a validated questionnaire after its translation in Arabic language. The translated tool was piloted in students that enhanced understanding of the topic and improved its acceptability. This aspect was lacking in all previous researches.

The prevalence data derived from the study was very extensive. Predictive modelling applied to the data provided novel insights, i.e., prevalence, students' attitudes and, monthly cost incurred on DS. Non-inclusion of female students could be a limitation in our study. Male and female students were segregated in different campuses with independent administration. Inclusion of female students would have helped the researchers to understand how DS use and its opinions differ gender-wise in the same population. The researchers recommend conducting the study in female population.

Abbreviations

CAGR: Compound annual growth rate; DS: Dietary supplement; DSA-A: Dietary supplement questionnaire – Arabic version; DSQ: Dietary supplement questionnaire; DV: Dependent variable; FA: Fatty acids; G6PD: Glucose 6 – phosphate dehydrogenase; IAU: Imam Abdulrahman Bin Faisal University; IV: Independent variable; KSA: Kingdom of Saudi Arabia; NHANES: National Health and Nutrition Examination Survey; SAR: Saudi Arabian riyal; SD: Standard deviation; USA: United States of America; USD: United States dollar

Acknowledgements

We extend our gratitude to all students for their participation in the study. We acknowledge the support of Naqvi and colleagues from Pakistan in providing questionnaire. This arrangement was made under the Evidence Based Improvement initiative [39–41].

Authors' contributions

AAN conceived the idea, designed the study with RA, AWE, AHA and MJA. AAN wrote the introduction with RA, AWE, AHA and MJA. AWE, AHA and MJA conducted literature review. RA and AAN designed the data collection tool and wrote the abstract and methodology. The data was collected and entered in SPSS by AWE, AHA and MJA. AAN conducted statistical tests and wrote the results section. RA and AAN wrote the discussion and conclusion with assistance from AWE, AHA and MJA. AAN edited the final draft of the manuscript. The authors AWE, AHA and MJA contributed equally. All authors read and approved the manuscript.

Competing interests

The authors declare that they have no competing interests.

Author details

[1]Department of Pharmacy Practice, College of Clinical Pharmacy, Imam Abdulrahman Bin Faisal University, Dammam 31441, Saudi Arabia. [2]Natural Products and Alternative Medicines, College of Clinical Pharmacy, Imam Abdulrahman Bin Faisal University, Dammam 31441, Saudi Arabia. [3]College of Clinical Pharmacy, Imam Abdulrahman Bin Faisal University, Dammam 31441, Saudi Arabia.

References

1. Naqvi AA, Ahmad R, Zehra F, Yousuf R, Kachela B, Nadir MN. Dietary supplement use among students of pharmacy colleges in the City of Karachi, Pakistan: prevalence, opinions, and attitudes. Journal of Dietary Supplements. https://doi.org/10.1080/19390211.2018.1443191.
2. Bailey RL, Gahche JJ, Miller PE, Thomas PR, Dwyer JT. JAMA Intern Med. 2013;173(5):355–61.
3. Radimer K, Bindewald B, Hughes J, Ervin B, Swanson C, Picciano MF. Dietary supplement use by US adults: data from the National Health and nutrition examination survey, 1999–2000. Am J Epidemiol. 2004;160:339–49.
4. Maughan RJ, King DS, Lea T. Dietary supplements. J Sports Sci. 2004;22(1): 95–113.
5. Drüeke TB, Massy ZA. Role of vitamin D in vascular calcification: bad guy or good guy? Nephrol Dial Transplant. 2012;27(5):1704–7.
6. Dwyer JT, Coates PM, Smith MJ. Dietary supplements: regulatory challenges and research resources. Nutrients. 2018;10(1):41.
7. Gardiner P, Phillips R, Shaughnessy AF. Herbal and dietary supplement--drug interactions in patients with chronic illnesses. Am Fam Physician. 2008;77(1): 73–8.
8. Rock CL. Multivitamin-multimineral supplements: who uses them? Am J Clin Nutr. 2007;85(1):277S–9S.
9. Foote JA, Murphy SP, Wilkens LR, Hankin JH, Henderson BE, Kolonel LN. Factors associated with dietary supplement use among healthy adults of five ethnicities. Am J Epidemiol. 2003;157:888–97.
10. Lieberman HR, Marriott BP, Williams C, Judelson DA, Glickman EL, Geiselman PJ, Dotson L, Mahoney CR. Patterns of dietary supplement use among college students. Clin Nutr. 2015;34:976–85. https://doi.org/10.1016/j.clnu.2014.10.010 PMID:25466950.
11. Moore KL, Saddam AM. Dietary supplement use among undergraduate college students. J Acad Nutr Dietet. 1999;99:SA96.
12. Transparency Market Research. Nutraceuticals market—global industry analysis, size, share, growth, trends, and forecast 2015–2021. 2015. https://www.transparencymarketresearch.com/pressrelease/global-nutraceuticals-product-industry.htm. Accessed 24 Sept.

13. NHP Consulting. Saudi Arabia. http://www.nhpconsulting.ca/services/world/middle-east/saudi-arabia/. Accessed 24 July 2018.
14. Alfawaz HA, Khan N, AlOteabi N, Hussain SD, Al-Daghri NM. Factors associated with dietary supplement use in Saudi pregnant women. Reprod Health. 2017;14:104.
15. Zehra F, Naqvi AA, Tasneem S, Ahmad R, Ahmad N, Shamsi AZ, Asghar NA, Khan GU. Brand versus generic dispensing trend for ciprofloxacin 500 mg, levofloxacin 500 mg, and moxifloxacin 400 mg (oral dosage forms) among pharmacies of Karachi, Pakistan. Int J Pharma Investig. 2017;7(2):70–6.
16. Albusalih FA, Naqvi AA, Ahmad R, Ahmad N. Prevalence of self-medication among students of pharmacy and medicine colleges of a public Sector University in Dammam city, Saudi Arabia. Pharmacy (Basel). 2017;5(3):E51.
17. Ministry of Education. Educational statistics in detail. 2015–16. Available from: https://departments.moe.gov.sa/PLANNINGINFORMATION/RELATEDDEPARTMENTS/EDUCATIONSTATISTICSCENTER/EDUCATIONDETAILEDREPORTS/Pages/default.aspx. Accessed 24 Sept.
18. Raosoft. Sample size calculator. Available from: http://www.raosoft.com/samplesize.html. Accessed 23 March
19. Beaton DE, Bombardier C, Guillemin F, et al. Guidelines for the process of cross-cultural adaptation of self-report measures. Spine. 2000;25:3186–91.
20. Wild D, Grove A, Martin M, Eremenco S, McElroy S, Verjee-Lorenz A, Erikson P, Mar-Apr, ISPOR Task Force for Translation and Cultural Adaptation. Principles of Good Practice for the Translation and Cultural Adaptation Process for Patient-Reported Outcomes (PRO) Measures: report of the ISPOR Task Force for Translation and Cultural Adaptation. Value Health. 2005;8(2):94–104.
21. Al Rasheed F, Naqvi AA, Ahmad R, Ahmad N. Academic stress and prevalence of stress-related self-medication among undergraduate female students of health and non-health cluster colleges of a public Sector University in Dammam. Saudi Arabia J Pharm Bioallied Sci. 2017;9(4):251–8.
22. Al-Shagawi MA, Ahmad R, Naqvi AA, Ahmad N. Determinants of academic stress and stress-related self-medication practice among undergraduate male pharmacy and medical students of a tertiary educational institution in Saudi Arabia. Trop J Pharm Res. 2017;16(12):2997–3003.
23. Ahmad R, Naqvi AA, Ahmad N, Baraka M, Mastour M, Al Sharedah S, Al Ghamdi S, Al Rabea G, Al Ghamdi MS. Awareness, perception, attitude, and knowledge regarding complementary and alternative medicines (CAMs) among the pharmacy and medical students Public University in Saudi Arabia. Arch Pharm Pract. 2017;8:51–63.
24. Aina BA, Ojedokun OA. Knowledge and use of dietary supplements by students of College of Medicine, University of Lagos, Idi-araba, Lagos, Nigeria. J Basic Clin Pharm. 2014;5:34–9.
25. Steele M, Senekal M. Dietary supplement use and associated factors among university students. SAJCN. 2005;18:17–30.
26. Kobayashi E, Sato Y, Umegaki K, Chiba T. The prevalence of dietary supplement use among college students: a Nationwide survey in Japan. Nutrients. 2017;9(11):1250.
27. Pouchieu C, Andreeva VA, Péneau S, Kesse-Guyot E, Lassale C, Hercberg S, Touvier M. Sociodemographic, lifestyle and dietary correlates of dietary supplement use in a large sample of French adults: results from the NutriNet-Santé cohort study. Br J Nutr. 2013;110(8):1480–91.
28. Sung Y, Choi J. Protein supplement usage among Male University students: comparisons between current and previous users. J Am Coll Nutr. 2018; 37(2):127–32.
29. Solak BB, Akin N. Health benefits of whey protein: a review. J Food Sci Eng. 2012;2(3):129–37.
30. Kiecolt-Glaser JK, Belury MA, Andridge R, Malarkey WB, Glaser R. Omega-3 supplementation lowers inflammation and anxiety in medical students: a randomized controlled trial. Brain Behav Immun. 2011;25(8):1725–34.
31. Prohaska J. Omega-3 Fatty acid supplementation and sleep. University of Kansas. 2008. [Master's thesis]. Available from: https://pdfs.semanticscholar.org/123e/5d79a8f2ab9e61e23d81cb602cb3954e2176.pdf.
32. Abbas A, Rizvi SA, Hassan R, Aqeel N, Khan M, Bhutto A, Khan Z, Mannan Z. The prevalence of depression and its perceptions among undergraduate pharmacy students. Pharm Educ. 2015;15(1):57–63.
33. Khan M, Aqeel N, Abbas A. An overview of depression and its pharmacotherapy. Int J of Res Pharmacol Pharmacotherapeutics. 2014;3(1):1–6.
34. Abbas A, Ahmed FR, Yousuf R, Khan N, Nisa ZU, Ali SI, Rizvi M, Sabah A, Tanwir S. Prevalence of self-medication of psychoactive stimulants and antidepressants among undergraduate pharmacy students in twelve Pakistani cities. Trop J Pharm Res. 2015;14(3):527–32.
35. Sabah A, Abbas A, Tanwir S, Ahmed FR, Arsalan A, Arif A, Ali SI, Adnan S, Haroon S, Rizvi SA. Consumer's perception regarding pharmaceutical product packaging: a survey of Pakistan. Int J Pharm Analytical Res. 2014; 3(1):118–25.
36. Jamshed SQ, Ahmad Hassali MA, Mohamed Ibrahim MI, Babar ZUD. Knowledge attitude and perception of dispensing doctors regarding generic medicines in Karachi, Pakistan: a qualitative study. J Pak Med Assoc. 2011;61(1):80–3.
37. El Khoury G, Ramadan W, Zeeni N. Herbal products and dietary supplements: a cross-sectional survey of use, attitudes, and knowledge among the Lebanese population. J Commun Health. 2016;41(3):566–73.
38. Rooney MR, Harnack L, Michos ED, Ogilvie RP, Sempos CT, Lutsey PL. Trends in use of high-dose vitamin D supplements exceeding 1000 or 4000 international units daily, 1999-2014. JAMA. 2017;317(23):2448–50.
39. Abbas A. Evidence based improvements in clinical pharmacy clerkship program in undergraduate pharmacy education: the evidence based improvement (EBI) initiative. Pharmacy. 2014;2(4):270–5.
40. Khan N, Abbas A. The need to modernize clinical pharmacy curriculum in undergraduate pharmacy teaching institutes of Pakistan. Med Sci. 2014; 10(36):12–3.
41. Naqvi AA. Evolution of clinical pharmacy teaching practices in Pakistan. Arch Pharma Pract. 2016;7:26–7.

16

Mechanical and aesthetics compatibility of Brazilian red propolis micellar nanocomposite as a cavity cleaning agent

Isabel Cristina Celerino de Moraes Porto[1,2,3*†], Dayse Chaves Cardoso de Almeida[1†], Gabriela Vasconcelos Calheiros de Oliveira Costa[1†], Tayná Stéphanie Sampaio Donato[1†], Letícia Moreira Nunes[1†], Ticiano Gomes do Nascimento[3†], José Marcos dos Santos Oliveira[3†], Carolina Batista da Silva[4†], Natanael Barbosa dos Santos[5†], Maria Luísa de Alencar e Silva Leite[6†], Irinaldo Diniz Basílio-Júnior[3†], Camila Braga Dornelas[3†], Pierre Barnabé Escodro[7†], Eduardo Jorge da Silva Fonseca[3†] and Regianne Umeko Kamiya[8]

Abstract

Background: Propolis is a natural substance produced by bees and is known to have antimicrobial activity. Our aim was to evaluate the antimicrobial effect of micellar nanocomposites loaded with an ethyl acetate extract of Brazilian red propolis as a cavity cleaning agent and its influence on the color and microtensile bond strength (μTBS) of the dentin/resin interface.

Methods: An ultra-performance liquid chromatography coupled with a diode array detector (UPLC-DAD) assay was used to determine the flavonoids and isoflavones present in an ethyl acetate extract of Brazilian red propolis (EARP) and micellar nanocomposites loaded with EARP (MNRP). The antimicrobial activity of EARP and MNRP was tested against *Streptococcus mutans*, *Lactobacillus acidophilus*, and *Candida albicans*. One of the following experimental treatments was applied to etched dentin (phosphoric acid, 15 s): 5 μL of MNRP (RP3, 0.3%; RP6, 0.6%; or RP1, 1.0% *w/v*), placebo, and 2% chlorhexidine digluconate. Single Bond adhesive (3 M/ESPE) was applied and a 4-mm-thick resin crown (Z350XT, 3 M/ESPE) was built up. After 24 h, the teeth were sectioned into sticks for the μTBS test and scanning electron microscopy. Spectrophotometry according to the CIE L*a*b* chromatic space was used to evaluate the color. Data were analyzed using one-way ANOVA and the Tukey test or Kruskal-Wallis test and the same test for pairwise comparisons between the means ($P < 0.05$).

(Continued on next page)

* Correspondence: isabel.porto@foufal.ufal.br
†Isabel Cristina Celerino de Moraes Porto, Dayse Chaves Cardoso de Almeida, Gabriela Vasconcelos Calheiros de Oliveira Costa, Tayná Stéphanie Sampaio Donato, Letícia Moreira Nunes, Ticiano Gomes do Nascimento, José Marcos dos Santos Oliveira, Carolina Batista da Silva, Natanael Barbosa dos Santos, Maria Luísa de Alencar e Silva Leite, Irinaldo Diniz Basílio Júnior, Camila Braga Dornelas, Pierre Barnabé Escodro and Eduardo Jorge da Silva Fonseca contributed equally to this work.
[1]Postgraduate Program in Health Research, Cesmac University Center, Rua Cônego Machado, 825, Farol, Maceió, Alagoas, Brazil
[2]Department of Restorative Dentistry, Faculty of Dentistry, Federal University of Alagoas, Campus AC Simões, Av. Lourival Melo Mota, S/N, Tabuleiro do Martins, Maceió, Alagoas, Brazil
Full list of author information is available at the end of the article

(Continued from previous page)
Results: The UPLC-DAD assay identified the flavonoids liquiritigenin, pinobanksin, pinocembrin, and isoliquiritigenin and the isoflavonoids daidzein, formononetin, and biochanin A in the EARP and micellar nanocomposites. EARP and MNRP presented antimicrobial activity against the cariogenic bacteria *Streptococcus mutans* and *Lactobacillus acidophilus*, and for *Candida albicans*. Δ*E* values varied from 2.31 to 3.67 ($P = 0.457$). The mean μTBS for RP1 was significantly lower than for the other groups ($P < 0.001$). Dentin treated with RP1 showed the shortest resin tags followed by RP6 and RP3.

Conclusions: The EARP and (MNRP) showed antimicrobial activity for the main agents causing dental caries (*Streptococcus mutans* and *Lactobacillus acidophilus*) and for *Candida albicans*. MNRP at concentrations of 0.3 and 0.6% used as a cavity cleaner do not compromise the aesthetics or μTBS of the dentin/resin interface.

Keywords: Red propolis, Dental caries, Cavity disinfectant, Micellar nanocomposites, Dental fillings, Antibacterial activity, Isoflavonoids, UPLC-DAD assay

Background

Propolis is produced by bees to close small gaps in the hive, prevent entry of insects, and reduce the proliferation of fungi and bacteria. Therefore, it is an important natural antibiotic and plays a promising role in medicine and dentistry [1, 2].

Useful knowledge about propolis has been gathered from research in the fields of medicine, pharmacology, food sciences and chemistry [2, 3]. In dentistry, some work has been published on endodontics [4, 5], preventive dentistry [6, 7], cariology [3, 6], surgery [8], and periodontics [9, 10], but there is a shortage of studies in the field of restorative dentistry.

In Brazil, the biodiversity of the flora favors the emergence of 13 types of propolis. Red propolis (RP), the 13th type of Brazilian propolis with a characteristic intense red color, is produced by bees of the species *Apis mellifera* with the sap of *Dalbergia ecastophyllum*, a leguminous plant that inhabits the northeastern mangroves of Brazil [11]. Brazilian RP has unique components that differentiate it from other propolis produced in Brazil and around the world. Isoflavonoids, propolones/guttiferones, terpenes, chalcones, and phenolic compounds are the principal classes of secondary metabolites present in RP [2, 12, 13].

Alencar et al. [14] reported the presence of at least four isoflavones in Brazilian RP that have never been found before: homopterocarpin, medicarpin, 4′,7-dimethoxy-2′-isoflavonol, and 7,4′-dihydroxyisoflavone. Three other new compounds were identified by Awale et al. [15]: (6a*S*,11a*S*)-6a-ethoxymedicarpan, 2-(2′,4′-dihydroxyphenyl)-3-methyl-6-methoxybenzofuran, and 2,6-dihydroxy-2-[(4-hydroxyphenyl)methyl]-3-benzofuranone. In Brazilian RP from Alagoas state, a newer study [16] identified other unique components, such as 3,4,2′,3′-tetrahydroxychalcone and a flavone C-glycoside, not found before in propolis from other sources.

Brazilian RP has potent antimicrobial activity even at low concentrations (0.1 and 1.0%). Several studies have proved the effective action of Brazilian RP against *Streptococcus mutans* and *Lactobacillus* [3, 7, 17–19] attributed to the high concentration of flavonoids and phenolic compounds in Brazilian RP [20]. The best results were obtained with an acetone fraction of an alcoholic extract of Brazilian propolis, possibly because of its high polarity; the acetone fraction contains a greater amount of active phenolics, which increases the antimicrobial activity [21]. However, propolis is poorly soluble in water, and at higher concentrations (2, 10, 20, 30%) it causes unacceptable color changes [22] and obliteration of the dentinal tubules with possible damage to adhesive procedures [9].

A wide variety of new chemicals are emerging from natural products, and many active components extracted from them are water insoluble, which represents a great challenge for the development of new products. Micellar nanocomposites, which are submicrometer colloidal dispersions of pure drug particles that are stabilized by a small percentage of excipients, could dramatically enhance the solubility and dissolution rate of drug particles. Furthermore, micellar nanocomposites are the most suitable vehicle for drugs that require high doses or limited volume to be administered. Micellar nanocomposites are a promising technique for the development of poorly water-soluble drugs, especially for screening and early evaluation of candidate active pharmaceutical ingredients. In addition, they may provide many advantages for drug delivery, such as increased drug loading, improved drug absorption, and retention for various delivery routes [23].

Dental caries is considered a chronic and multifactorial disease and occurs as a result of the dissolution of tooth mineral by acids derived from bacterial fermentation of dietary carbohydrates, mainly by *Streptococcus mutans* and *Lactobacillus* ssp., which are involved in the initiation and progression of the lesions, respectively [24].

Contemporary dentistry seeks to arrest the evolution of caries and to prevent new lesions, with minimal restorative intervention and trying to preserve tooth vitality. Traditionally, caries treatment involves the removal of carious tissue and replacing it with a restorative material. However, conventional removal of carious tissue and cavity preparation procedures do not guarantee complete elimination of oral cariogenic bacteria that might be entrapped within the dentin tubules or the smear layer [25]. In addition, in deep cavities, the removal of large amounts of dentin can lead to pulp exposure, and consequently bacterial contamination, which may lead to the need for endodontic treatment [26]. Thus, the removal of only the infected carious dentin layer and preservation of the innermost layer, which can be re-mineralized, provides greater protection to the pulp and is therefore applicable when pulp exposure is imminent [26–29]. Greater benefits can be achieved through measures to eliminate the maximum amount of bacteria remaining in the dental tissue, such as disinfection of the cavity before the restorative procedure [30].

Because Brazilian RP contains waxes and resins and is an intense red color, its use as a natural antimicrobial agent in carious cavities is a challenge. Thus, it is important to investigate its influence on the bond strength and aesthetics of the restoration. The aim of this study was to evaluate the antimicrobial effect of micellar nanocomposites loaded with an ethyl acetate extract of Brazilian RP as a cavity disinfection agent and its influence on the color and microtensile bond strength of the dentin/resin interface.

Methods

Fifty-four extracted, human, caries-free third molars were obtained from adult patients of both genders were stored in 0.5% chloramine T solution at 4 °C and used within 2 months of extraction. Written informed consent was obtained from all subjects. All procedures followed in this study were in accordance with the ethical principles of the Declaration of Helsinki.

Preparation of Brazilian red propolis micellar nanocomposite

Brazilian RP raw material was collected from Marechal Deodoro, Alagoas, Brazil. Propolis was collected from the Ilha do Porto apiary (geographic coordinates 9° 44.555′ S, 35° 52.080′ W, and 18.1 m above sea level) during the month of July/2013. To obtain RP extract, raw propolis (250 g) was manually ground and placed in a flask with 600 mL of 80% ethanol, then placed on an agitator (Thornton, Model T14, Thornton Inpec Eletrônica Ltda., Vinhedo, Brazil) for 48 h. The macerate (the liquid portion) was removed using a pipette, and the solid portion (wax) was discarded. The macerate was mixed with 600 mL of 80% ethanol in a glass flask and agitated for 24 h. The resulting macerate was again mixed with 600 mL of 80% ethanol and left for 24 h without agitation. Next, the macerate was removed using a pipette, filtered through filter paper, and subjected to distillation under reduced pressure in a rotary evaporator (model 801/802; Fisatom, São Paulo, Brazil) in a water bath at 80–90 °C (pressure 650 mmHg and speed 80 rpm) to remove the solvent. The extract of Brazilian RP was then placed in a glass container and left for approximately 3 days for the residual solvent to evaporate; a viscous solid mass (162 g) was obtained as a crude extract of RP.

Liquid-liquid extraction of this crude extract was performed to eliminate grease and waxes. The crude extract (8 g) was solubilized with absolute ethanol (35 mL) and 15 mL of distilled water was added in a beaker. This RP crude extract was transferred to a separation funnel and hexane (50 mL) was added to eliminate the grease and wax present in the crude extract. The hexane layer was removed with a separation funnel and then ethyl acetate solvent (200 mL) was added in two liquid-liquid extraction steps to obtain an ethyl acetate extract enriched with the flavonoids and isoflavonoids from the RP, free of grease and wax. The ethyl acetate extract was subjected to distillation under reduced pressure in a rotary evaporator to obtain a solid mass (4.0 g), which was used in all the experiments in this study.

The experimental micellar nanocomposites were prepared as follows. One hundred milligrams of the polymeric nanocomposites of poly-ε-caprolactone (PCL, molecular weight 10,000) and Pluronic F108 copolymer (molecular weight 14,000) in a proportion of 7:3 were weighed and mixed with 100 mg (RP1) or 60 mg (RP6), or 30 mg (RP3) of ethyl acetate extract of Brazilian red propolis (EARP). Then, 8 mL of acetone was enough to solubilize the micellar nanocomposites loaded with EARP under agitation in an ultrasonic bath for 10 min. The final volume was adjusted to 10 mL with acetone to obtain 1.0, 0.6, and 0.3% nanocomposites in a micellar state (≈70 nm).

Determination of Brazilian red propolis markers using the UPLC-DAD method

The identification and quantification of markers in the EARP and 1% micellar nanocomposites loaded with EARP were performed using ultra-performance liquid chromatography coupled with a diode array detector (UPLC-DAD) from Shimadzu (Tokyo, Japan). The equipment consisted of the following modules: a high-pressure pump (model LC-20ADXR), degasser (model DGU-20A3R), auto-injector (model SIL-20AXR), oven chromatographic column, photodiode array detector (model EPDM-20A), a controller (model CBM-20A), and Shimadzu Labsolution software.

The separation of flavonoids occurred using a reversed-phase column (C_{18}, 150 mm 4.6 mm; 5 μm), and a mobile phase that consisted of solvent A (Milli-Q water) and solvent B (acetonitrile), pumped at a flow rate of 0.3 mL/min. The initial elution gradient consisted of 70% water (A) and 30% acetonitrile (B) (*v*/v). The column was eluted by varying the percentage of (B) as follows: 0–2 min 30% B, 2–5 min 36% B, 5–8 min 46% B, 8–11 min 52% B, 11–14 min 52% B, 14–17 min 57% B, 17–20 min 62% B, 20–24 min 62% B, 24–28 min 68% B, 28–32 min 72% B, 32–36 min 90% B, 36–42 min 97% B, 42–50 min 100% B, 50–55 min 100% B, 55–57 min acetonitrile was reduced to 30% and this condition was maintained up to 60 min. This method was based on Nascimento et al. [31]. This long method was developed in order to wash the column during the analysis with 100% acetonitrile, avoid lack of accuracy and loss of precision during the entrapment assay, and avoid column fouling and excessive pressure buildup by irreversible retention of non-polar compounds (terpenes and guttiferones present in Brazilian RP extract). The injection volume was 2 μL. Analytical standards of the flavonoids described as markers (daidzein, liquiritigenin, pinobanskin, isoliquiritigenin, formononetin, pinocembrin, and biochanin A), the EARP, and 1% micellar nanocomposites loaded with EARP were prepared in a stock solution of 10,000 μg/mL, using acetone as solvent and diluted to a concentration of 500 μg/mL. Calibration of the marker quantification method was carried out according to Nascimento et al. [31].

Antimicrobial activity

The EARP, micellar nanocomposite loaded with EARP (MNRP), 0.12% chlorhexidine gluconate (Ao Pharmacêutico, Unidade Maceió, Brazil), and 0.2% triclosan (Ao Pharmacêutico, Unidade Maceió, Brazil) were tested against *Streptococcus mutans* CCT 3440, *Lactobacillus acidophilus* ATCC 4356, and *Candida albicans* ATCC 36801 and 36,802. The strains from Tropical Cultures Collection (CCT) and American Type Culture Collection (ATCC) were provided by Oswaldo Cruz Foundation, Rio de Janeiro, Brazil. All strains were activated in their selective medium, MSB agar (mitis salivarius-bacitracin, 0.2 U/L), Lactobacilli MRS Agar (deMan, Rogosa and Sharpe), and Candida BCG agar (bromocresol green containing cloramphenicol 0.5 g/L), respectively.

The minimal inhibitory concentration (MIC) test or broth microdilution assay was carried out using microplates (96 wells), following the procedure according to the Clinical and Laboratory Standards Institute [32] and Lima et al. [33] for bacteria and EUCAST [34] for yeast, with some modifications. The McFarland Scale 0.5 determined the cell concentration. A standardized inoculum containing about 10^6 bacteria/mL or 10^5 yeast/mL of a pure overnight culture was used in the tests. Serial two-fold dilutions (range from 15.62 μg/mL to 1000 μg/mL) of Ethyl acetate extract of Brazilian RP and MNRP were prepared in 80 μL of Brain Heart Infusion broth (BHI) or Mueller Hinton broth (MHB) in a 96-well microplate. Both ethyl acetate and micellar nanocomposite without Brazilian RP (blank) were also tested for each serial dilution. Microbial cultures were grown in medium without antimicrobial samples (negative control) and with 0.12% chlorhexidine gluconate or 0.2% triclosan (positive controls). Then, 20-μL aliquots of standardized inoculum were added to the wells to give a final volume of 100 μL/well and serial two-fold dilution (15.62, 31.25, 62.50, 125, 250, 500 and 1000 μg/mL). *Candida albicans* were incubated at 37 °C for 24 h in aerobic conditions. *Streptococcus mutans* and *Lactobacillus acidophilus* were incubated in a microaerobic environment at 37 °C for 24 h. The growth of bacterial cells was measured by absorbance at $OD_{550-630}$ nm in an automated microplate reader (Bio-Rad 680, Madison, WI, USA).

The MIC values were defined as the lowest bandwidth concentration of the tested compounds that inhibited 100% of bacterial growth compared with the negative control. All samples were assayed in quadruplicate in three independent experiments. An aliquot (30 μL) of a concentration higher than MIC was cultured on respective selective media for 24 h, at 37 °C to determine the Minimal bactericidal concentration (MBC). MBC was the lowest concentration that allowed no visible bacterial growth on agar.

Color analysis

The teeth were cut perpendicular to the long axis at the level of the enamel–dentin junction with a diamond disc (Extec, Enfield, CT, USA) fitted in a metallographic cutter (Extec Technologies Inc., Enfield, CT, USA) to obtain a flat dentin surface. The exposed dentin surface was wet-abraded with 600-grit silicon carbide paper for 60 s to create a standardized smear layer. Then, the dentin surfaces were examined under a stereomicroscope at 40× magnification for the presence of enamel.

The teeth were randomly divided into three groups ($n = 10$) according to the treatment: micellar nanocomposites loaded with EARP (RP3, 0.3%; RP6, 0.6%; or RP1, 1.0% *w*/*v*). The teeth were sectioned mesiodistally with the same diamond disc under water lubrication to obtain 60 half teeth and then attached to a wax flat base with a thin metal plate between each pair to ensure that only one half tooth half received the experimental treatment. The other half tooth was the negative control (no treatment, baseline).

In this stage of the study, we used two techniques, before and after acid etching of dentin, to apply micellar nanocomposites loaded with EARP: (1) before etching, using propolis micellar nanocomposites as a cavity cleaner; (2) after etching to improve the effect of propolis, which can be totally or partially removed during etching.

The micellar nanocomposites loaded with EARP were applied on the dentin surface for 1 min, which was then etched for 15 s with 37% phosphoric acid (Atack Tec, Caithec Indústria Ltd., Rio do Sul. SC, Brazil) or was applied on etched dentin before application of Adper Single Bond 2 adhesive (3 M do Brasil Ltd., Sumaré, SP, Brazil) followed by a covering of Filtek Z 350XT composite resin (3 M do Brasil Ltda, Sumaré, SP, Brazil). The adhesive and the composite resin were irradiated according to the manufacturer's instructions with an LED device (1150 mW/cm^2; Emitter B; Schuster Com. Equip. Odontológicos Ltda, Santa Maria, RS, Brazil) and stored in distilled water at 37 °C for 24 h.

Color was measured with a spectrophotometer (Minolta CR-321, Konika Minolta, Tokyo, Japan), ensuring that the readings were taken with the half tooth in the same position. The spectrophotometer converted the information obtained from the bonded surface to a digital scale in the CIELAB system (L* a* b*) [35, 36]. In order to limit the area for color readings to the bonded surface, the size of the reading window was reduced to a circumference of approximately 1 mm using black opaque tape. The placebo (micellar nanocomposite without Brazilian red propolis [DL]) and 2% chlorhexidine digluconate (CHX) were not tested because they are colorless.

Microtensile bond strength test

The teeth were divided into groups according to the dentin pretreatment: micellar nanocomposites loaded with EARP 0.3% (RP3); micellar nanocomposites loaded with EARP 0.6% (RP6); micellar nanocomposites loaded with EARP 1.0% (RP1); DL; 2% CHX (FGM, Joinville, Brazil); and no treatment (NT; negative control group). The same restorative procedure was used throughout. The placebo micellar nanocomposite (DL) was used to separate the effect of the micellar nanocomposites loaded with EARP from the effect produced by the EARP.

After storing in distilled water at 37 °C for 24 h, the bonded specimens were serially sectioned using a low-speed diamond saw (Extec Technologies, Inc., Enfield, CT, USA) across the bonded interface in both the x and y directions into beams with a cross-sectional area of ~0.8 mm^2. These specimens were individually attached to a custom-made testing jig with cyanoacrylate glue and were subjected to microtensile testing at a crosshead speed of 0.1 mm/min until failure using a Microtensile OM 100 tester (Odeme, Luzerna, SC, Brazil). Fractured specimens were examined with a stereomicroscope at 40× magnification (Coleman Co. Ltd., Santo André, SP, Brazil) to determine the mode of failure. Selected debonded sticks were observed by scanning electron microscopy (SEM).

Scanning electron microscopy

Two specimens (sticks) from each group were prepared for examination by SEM in order to evaluate the morphology of the dentin/resin interface. The specimens were polished using ascending SiC papers from 600 up to 1200 grit. Further final polishing was performed using 1.00 μm and 0.05 μm alumina suspensions (Buehler, Lake Bluff, IL, USA). The specimens were cleaned in an ultrasonic bath containing distilled water for 15 min at each polishing step. Each specimen was fixed in Karnovsky solution for 12 h, washed in running water for 1 h, etched with 37% phosphoric acid for 1 min to facilitate the observation of the hybrid layer on the dentin/resin interface, then deproteinized with 10% sodium hypochlorite for 5 min, and rinsed with distilled water before being dehydrated in ascending concentrations of ethanol (25, 50, 75, 95, and 100%), followed by soaking in hexamethyldisilazane for 10 min and left to dry for 24 h at room temperature. The specimens were fixed in stubs using adhesive copper-conducting tape and examined at a variety of magnifications in a scanning electron microscope (TM-3000, Hitachi High Technologies, Tokyo, Japan).

Statistical analysis

The color change data were analyzed using one-way factorial analysis of variance (ANOVA) followed by the Tukey test. Microtensile bond strength data were analyzed by Kruskal-Wallis test and the same test was used for pairwise comparisons between the means [37]. The Statistical Package for the Social Sciences, version 21 (SPSS, Chicago, IL, USA) and MEDCALC, version 12.5.0 (MedCalc Software, Acacialaan, Ostend, Belgium) were used for all statistical analyses ($\alpha = 0.05$).

Results

The overlapping chromatograms obtained using the UPLC-DAD technique for the EARP and micellar nanocomposites loaded with EARP are shown in Fig. 1. The corresponding retention times and peak purity at the maximum wavelengths were determined and compared with the analytical standards of flavonoids (Fig. 1a). The markers daidzein (1), liquiritigenin (2), pinobanksin (3), isoliquiritigenin (4), formononetin (5), pinocembrin (6), and biochanin A (7) were identified and quantified using the UPLC-DAD profile of the EARP and the 1% micellar nanocomposites loaded with EARP (Fig. 1b). The values for the corresponding retention times, maximum wavelengths and concentrations of the flavonoids markers in

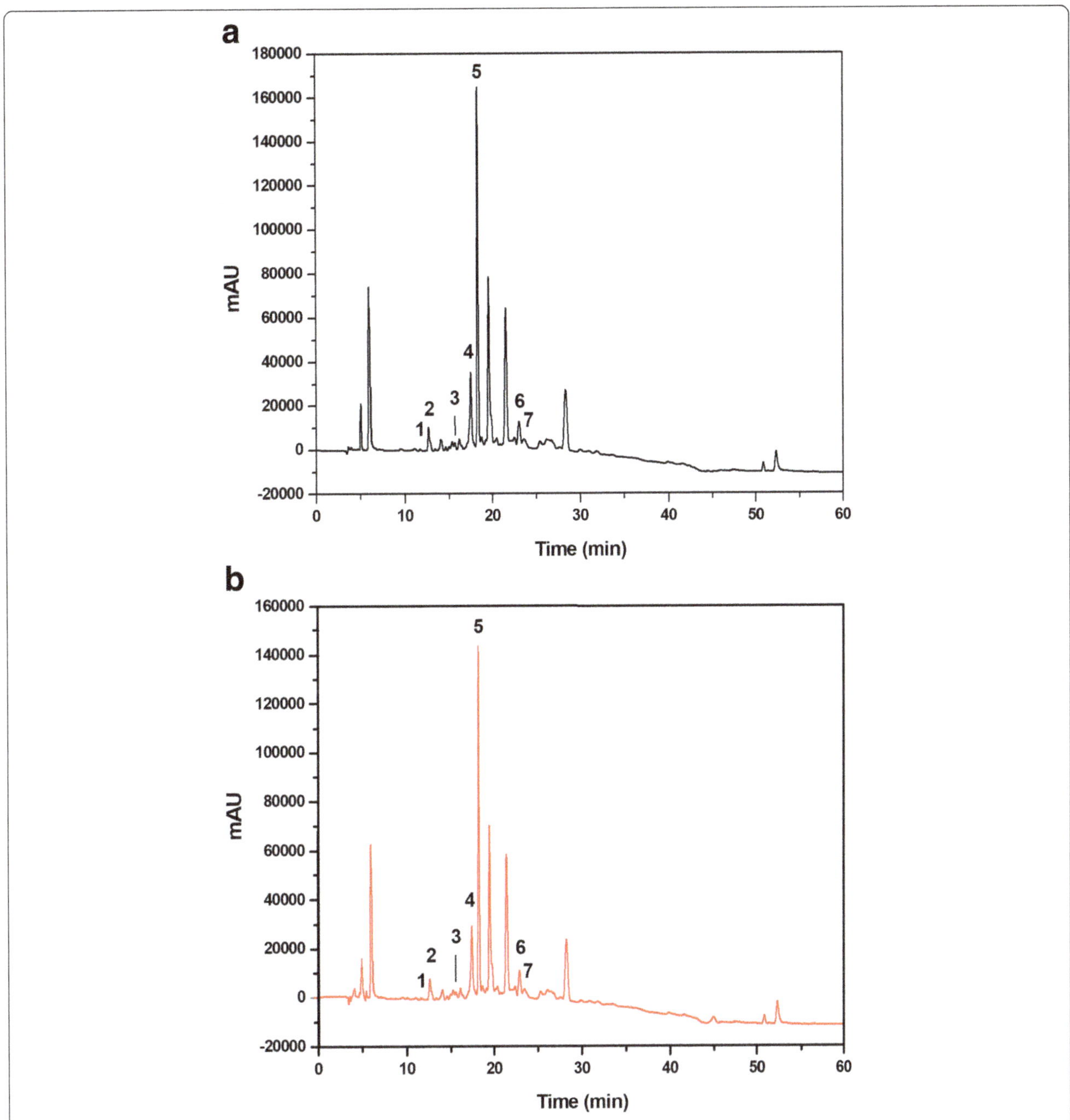

Fig. 1 Markers of Brazilian red propolis extract using UPLC-DAD. Chromatograms of an ethyl acetate extract of Brazilian red propolis (**a**, black line) and 1% micellar nanocomposite loaded with EARP (**b**, red line) at a concentration of 500 μg/mL. Identification of daidzein (1), liquiritigenin (2), pinobanskin (3), isoliquiritigenin (4), formononetin (5), pinocembrin (6), and biochanin A (7) flavonoids in the UPLC-DAD profile at a wavelength of 205 nm

the EARP and 1% micellar nanocomposites loaded with EARP (RP1) are shown in Table 1.

The results of the MIC determination of the EARP and micellar nanocomposite loaded with EARP are presented in Table 2. Both 0.12% chlorhexidine and 0.2% triclosan inhibited the growth of all microorganisms at the concentration range tested. The ethyl acetate solvent without propolis extract and the micellar nanocomposite without EARP (blank) did not inhibit the microorganisms. *Lactobacillus acidophilus* ATCC 4356, *Streptococcus mutans* CCT 3440, *Candida albicans* ATCC 36801, and *Candida albicans* 36,802 were sensitive to the EARP (32–125 μg/mL) and MNRP (15.62–1000 μg/mL) at concentrations below the lowest concentration used in this study (i.e., 3000 μg/mL). The MIC of MNRP against

Table 1 Chromatographic parameters: retention times (RT), maximum wavelength, and concentration of ethyl acetate extract of Brazilian red propolis and 1% of the micellar nanocomposite loaded with EARP using UPLC-DAD

Marker	RT (min)	λ (nm)	Concentration (μg/mL)	Concentration % (*w/w*)
Ethyl acetate extract of Brazilian red propolis: 500 μg/mL				
Daidzein	11.67	249	0.399	0.079
Liquiritigenin	12.68	275	7.131	1.426
Pinobanksin	15.78	289	0.385	0.077
Isoliquiritigenin	17.41	366	5.123	1.024
Formononetin	18.23	249	5.841	1.168
Pinocembrin	22.88	289	1.335	0.267
Biochanin A	23.81	260	0.315	0.063
1% micellar nanocomposite loaded with EARP: 500 μg/mL				
Daidzein	11.67	249	0.179	0.035
Liquiritigenin	12.68	275	6.082	1.216
Pinobanksin	15.78	289	0.299	0.059
Isoliquiritigenin	17.41	366	4.417	0.883
Formononetin	18.23	249	4.990	0.998
Pinocembrin	22.88	289	1.125	0.225
Biochanin A	23.81	260	0.281	0.056

EARP ethyl acetate extract of Brazilian red propolis

Lactobacillus acidophilus ATCC 4356 was found to be < 15.62 μg/mL.

The mean Δ*E* values and standard deviations for all groups are shown in Table 3. The Δ*E* values ranged from 2.31 to 3.67 and showed no significant differences among the groups regarding the propolis protocol, before or after etching ($P = 0.457$). Among all the micellar nanocomposites tested, major color changes were observed in the groups treated with 0.6 and 1.0% micellar nanocomposites loaded with EARP applied after dentin etching.

There was no significant difference in the total color change (Δ*E*) between the processing techniques (before or after etching) or among the micellar nanocomposites loaded with EARP (i.e., RP3, RP6, and RP1) on pairwise comparisons considering the same application technique.

The values of the CIE L*a* b*coordinates (Table 4), regardless of the processing technique, do not show significant differences in the L* coordinate between the RP6 and RP1 groups. There was no significant difference for the a* coordinate (before etching), however, comparing RP3 with RP6 and RP1 (after etching), the difference was statistically significant. For the b* coordinate, the RP6 group before etching and RP1 after etching showed significant differences from all other experimental groups.

Fig. 2 presents the ΔL*, Δa*, and Δb* values according to the processing technique. Except for the group treated with 0.3% micellar nanocomposites loaded with EARP before dentin etching, there was a significant loss of brightness in all groups tested, with greater intensity in the group receiving 0.6% micellar nanocomposites loaded with EARP after dentin etching. There was no

Table 2 Minimal inhibitory concentration (MIC) and minimal bactericidal concentration (MBC) of ethyl acetate extract of Brazilian red propolis and micellar nanocomposite loaded with Brazilian red propolis for *Streptococcus mutans*, *Lactobacillus acidophilus*, and *Candida albicans*

Microorganisms	MIC (μg/mL)		MBC (μg/mL)	
	EARP	MN	EARP	MN
Candida albicans ATCC 36801	31.25–62.50	250–500	500–1000	> 1000
Candida albicans ATCC 36802	31.25–62.50	250–500	250–500	> 1000
Streptococcus mutans CCT 3440	31.25–62.50	250–500	125–250	> 1000
Lactobacillus acidophilus ATCC 4356	31.25–62.50	< 15.62	62.5–125	125–250

EARP ethyl acetate extract of Brazilian red propolis, *MN* micellar nanocomposites loaded with EARP. Mueller Hinton Broth (MHB) was used in the antimicrobial test of *Candida albicans* and Brain Heart Infusion Broth (BHI) was used for *S.mutans* and *L. acidophilus*

Table 3 Mean values of total color variation (Δ*E*) according to treatment and processing technique

Treatment	Color variation (Δ*E*)			
	Micellar nanocomposites loaded with EARP applied before dentin etching		Micellar nanocomposites loaded with EARP applied after dentin etching	
	Mean	Standard deviation	Mean	Standard deviation
Micellar nanocomposites 0.3% (RP3)	2.58	0.99	2.31	1.10
Micellar nanocomposites 0.6% (RP6)	2.67	1.89	3.67	2.67
Micellar nanocomposites 1.0% (RP1)	2.31	1.01	3.30	1.62

EARP ethyl acetate extract of Brazilian red propolis

significant difference in brightness in all groups treated with propolis after dentin acid etching.

Δa* values indicate variations in the red-green axis, with dominance of the reddish color. In the teeth etched before treatment with micellar nanocomposites loaded with EARP, the values corresponding to the yellow-blue axis (Δb*) moved in the direction of the blue axis with a lower to a higher concentration of micellar nanocomposites loaded with EARP (RP1). When propolis was applied before etching, the RP3 and RP6 groups exhibited a more blueish color and the RP1 group showed a more yellowish color. However, Δa* and Δb* values did not differ significantly between the groups ($P > 0.05$).

Data from the bond strength tests are shown in Fig. 3. The RP1 group showed a significant reduction in the interface bond strength compared with the other groups ($P = 0.001$). The mean values for the bond strength for the RP3 and RP6 groups were higher than for the RP1 group and similar to the control group, the DL group, and the CHX group. At 0.3 and 0.6% concentrations, micellar nanocomposites loaded with EARP did not induce any decrease in bond strength. However, micellar nanocomposites loaded with EARP at 1.0% concentration reduced the bond strength by 65%.

The fracture mode distribution according to the experimental groups is shown in Fig. 4. The predominant fracture modes were mixed failure, followed by adhesive failure (cohesive failure in the adhesive and/or in the hybrid layer) regardless of the use of propolis micellar nanocomposite or the processing technique. Few cohesive failures in resin and dentin were recorded for the micellar nanocomposites loaded with EARP tested.

SEM analysis of the dentin and resin surfaces obtained after the bond strength tests revealed the occurrence of mixed fractures (adhesive and cohesive) in almost all the specimens, corroborating the data from the bond strength test. When these specimens were observed under higher magnification, distinct areas of adhesive fractures and cohesive fractures could be observed within the same specimen (Fig. 5).

Fig. 6 shows the micromorphologic aspects of the hybrid layer. The NT and CHX groups show a characteristic image of hybridization of demineralized dentin by adhesive resin with long resin tags deep in the dentinal tubules with lateral branches, which result from the penetration of monomers into the lateral channels that communicate with another dentinal tubule.

In the groups receiving micellar nanocomposites loaded with EARP, the penetration of resin monomers into the dentinal tubules followed by the formation of a zone of interdiffusion dentin/resin (hybrid layer) seems to have been influenced by both the concentration of micellar nanocomposites loaded with EARP and the processing technique (before or after dentin etching). When the propolis micellar nanocomposites were used before dentin etching, application of 0.3% micellar nanocomposites loaded with

Table 4 Means ± standard deviation of the color characteristics in the L*a*b* color space (CIELAB) for each experimental group and the control groups

Treatment	Micellar nanocomposites loaded with EARP applied before dentin etching			Micellar nanocomposites loaded with EARP applied after dentin etching		
	L*	a*	b*	L*	a*	b*
Micellar nanocomposites 0.3% (RP3)	45.46 ± 2.46^{Aa}	-1.08 ± 1.09^{Aa}	3.83 ± 1.67^{Aa}	47.21 ± 2.60^{Aa}	-2.05 ± 0.42^{Ab}	3.66 ± 1.32^{Aa}
RP3 control	45.02 ± 3.04^{Aa}	-1.33 ± 0.53^{Aa}	3.39 ± 1.89^{Aa}	48.90 ± 1.94^{Ab}	-2.25 ± 0.44^{Ab}	3.93 ± 1.23^{Aa}
Micellar nanocomposites 0.6% (RP6)	43.50 ± 1.11^{Ba}	-0.93 ± 0.62^{Aa}	0.98 ± 1.22^{Ba}	43.28 ± 3.75^{Ba}	-0.89 ± 0.88^{Ba}	2.76 ± 0.89^{Aa}
RP6 control	44.85 ± 2.35^{Ba}	-1.61 ± 0.45^{Aa}	1.84 ± 1.63^{Aa}	46.20 ± 1.87^{Aa}	-1.17 ± 0.52^{Aa}	2.84 ± 1.60^{Aa}
Micellar nanocomposites 1.0% (RP1)	44.44 ± 2.41^{Ba}	-1.61 ± 0.53^{Aa}	3.30 ± 1.38^{Aa}	43.33 ± 2.31^{Ba}	-0.94 ± 0.32^{Ba}	1.63 ± 1.74^{Ba}
RP1 control	46.02 ± 2.58^{Aa}	-1.70 ± 0.65^{Aa}	3.04 ± 1.02^{Aa}	45.46 ± 2.92^{Aa}	-1.55 ± 0.48^{Aa}	2.44 ± 1.54^{Aa}

F test (ANOVA) followed by the Tukey test for paired comparisons of L*, a*, and b* CIELAB coordinates. When all the capital letters (columns) are different, there is a significant difference between color changes for each CIELAB coordinate. When all the lower case letters (rows) are different, there is a significant difference between different processing techniques in the same CIELAB coordinate by Tukey's paired comparisons. EARP, ethyl acetate extract of Brazilian red propolis

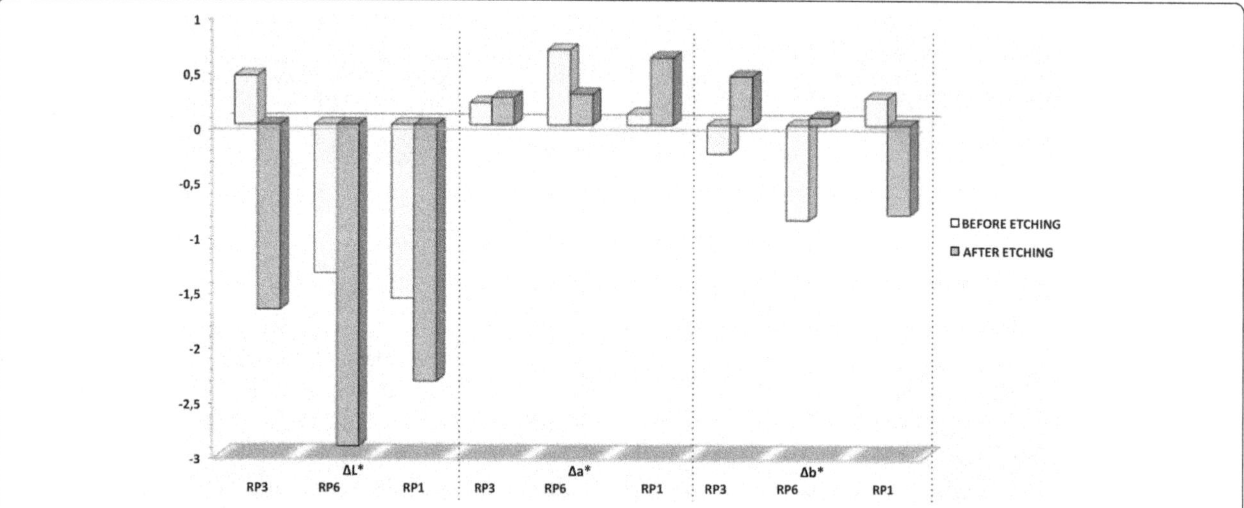

Fig. 2 ΔL*, Δa* e Δb* values per experimental group. F test (ANOVA) has not shown a significant difference in the mean values of Δa* ($P = 0.371$) or Δb* ($P = 0.191$). Comparing different propolis nanosuspensions, ΔL* values are significantly different between RP3 before etching and RP3 after etching ($P = 0.023$). There was also a significant difference between RP3 and RP1 ($P = 0.031$) before etching. There was no statistically significant difference for all other comparisons ($P > 0.05$). RP1, 1% of red propolis micellar nanocomposite; RP6, 0.6% of red propolis micellar nanocomposite; RP3, 0.3% of red propolis micellar nanocomposite

EARP did not affect the formation of the hybrid layer, similar to the NT and CHX groups. When the concentration of micellar nanocomposites loaded with EARP increased to 0.6 and 1.0%, there was a reduction in the size of the resin tags. When micellar nanocomposites loaded with EARP were applied after dentin etching, it seems that there was substance deposition at the entrance and in the dentin tubules, preventing diffusion of adhesive into the tubules and, consequently, shorter tags or tapered structures formed, restricting the entrance to the dentinal tubules (RP1).

Discussion

The flavonoids and isoflavonoids (liquiritigenin, pinobanksin, pinocembrin, isoliquiritigenin, daidzein, formononetin and biochanin A) that were identified by the UPLC-DAD assay in both the ethyl acetate extract and micellar nanocomposites loaded with EARP used in this study, combined with other compounds (quercetin, vestitol, and neo-vestitol) present in the ethyl acetate extract may be responsible for the biological activity against the oral pathogens tested [38]. The antimicrobial

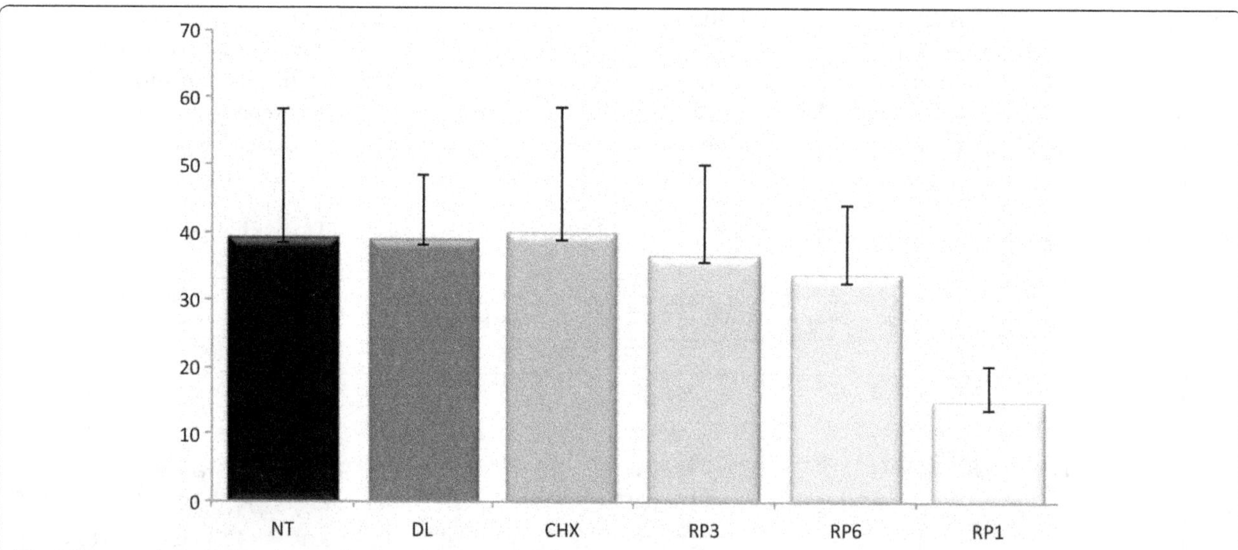

Fig. 3 Microtensile dentin bond strength values in MPa. Kruskal-Wallis test for pairwise comparisons of Brazilian red propolis nanosuspensions showed significantly lower microtensile dentin bond strength values for RP1 ($P = 0.001$). RP1, 1% of red propolis micellar nanocomposite; RP6, 0.6% of red propolis micellar nanocomposite; RP3, 0.3% of red propolis micellar nanocomposite; CHX, 2% digluconate chlorhexidine; DL, placebo (micellar nanocomposites without ethyl acetate extract from Brazilian red propolis); NT, no treatment (negative control)

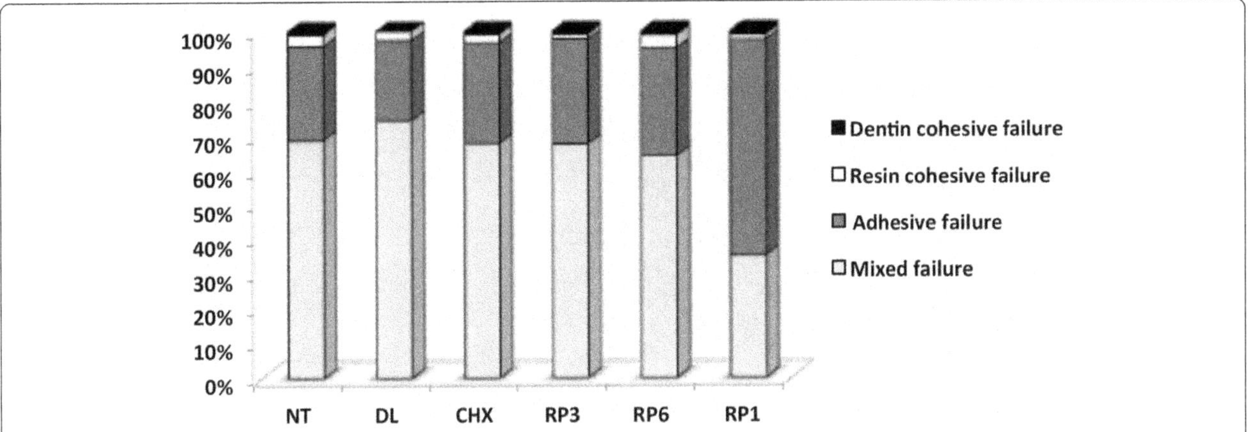

Fig. 4 Percentage of the type of fractures per group. The graph shows the predominance of mixed failures. RP1, 1% red propolis nanosuspension; RP6, 0.6% red propolis nanosuspension; RP3, 0.3% red propolis nanosuspension; CHX, 2% digluconate chlorhexidine; DL, placebo (micellar nanocomposites without ethyl acetate extract from Brazilian red propolis); NT, no treatment (negative control)

activity of propolis is usually credited to the phenolic compounds and diterpenic acids in its composition, such as vestitol, neovestitol, quercetin, pinocembrin, galangin, myricetin, kaempherol, apigenin, caffeic acid, caffeic acid phenethyl ester, cinnamic acids, diterpenic acids, and prenylated benzophenones, which also present antibacterial, anti-plaque, and cariogenic activity against microorganisms involved in oral diseases [38–41].

Our results showed that *Lactobacillus acidophilus* ATCC 4356 strain exhibited higher sensitivity to the MNRP than to EARP, with a very low MIC value (< 15.62 μg/mL), probably due to the effect of charge at its surface. Micellar nanocomposites attach more easily to the surface of bacteria because of their positive surface charge, which facilitates the interaction between micellar nanocomposites and the negatively charged external membrane of gram-positive bacteria.

Although acid-producing microorganisms have been isolated from oral microbiota, *Streptococci* and *Lactobacilli* have been considered to be the most significant bacteria involved in the initiation and progression of dental caries, respectively. Several bacteria can be isolated from deep carious lesions; however, *Lactobacilli* were the most commonly isolated microorganisms on dentin from the floor of a cavity preparation [42].

The high sensitivity of *Lactobacillus acidophilus* to MNRP is not surprising, given that this species grows at low pH (4.0), which is the average pH in deep carious lesions. But the MNRP used in this study could lead to a slight increase in the pH of the environment, disturbing the metabolism of *Lactobacillus acidophilus* and contributing to inhibition of the growth of this species. Nascimento et al. [31] showed that the pH of suspensions of nanoparticles loaded with Brazilian red propolis was weakly acidic (pH 6.00), which can be attributed to PCL-pluronic copolymers.

Independently of growth medium selectivity for *Streptococcus mutans* and *Candida albicans*, EARP performed better than MNRP, which indicates greater adaptation of these microorganisms to the change in pH of the environment, especially from weakly acid to neutral medium. Although higher MIC values have been recorded for *S. mutans* and *Candida albicans* than for *Lactobacillus* strain, they were three times less than the lowest concentration used (3000 μg/mL). Therefore, our MNRP showed a promising effect for the development of dental materials with antimicrobial activity for cleaning cavities.

The antimicrobial activity of *Streptococcus mutans* found in this study was satisfactory and similar to the results of Righi et al.[16] who reported MIC values for *Streptococcus pyogenes* lower than 256 μg/mL using a methanol extract of red propolis. Oldoni et al. [43] found activity against *S. mutans* using vestitol as a chemical marker with MIC and minimum bactericidal concentration (MBC) values of 31–62 μg/mL and 125–250 μg/mL, respectively. Bueno-Silva et al. [18] demonstrated antimicrobial activity against *S. mutans* with MIC values between 25 and 50 μg/mL for neovestitol and between 50 and 100 μg/mL for vestitol. Purified vestitol and neovestitol presented better MIC and MBC values than the crude extract, chloroform extract, or hexane extracts [18, 43].

Ghasempour et al. [44] isolated *Candida albicans* from dental plaque and caries lesions. The authors suggested that *C. albicans* could lead to caries. The contribution of *C. albicans* to total microbial acid formation appears to be relevant for caries progression; this yeast produces 5-fold more acid per colony-forming unit than lactobacilli at pH 7.0 [45]. *Candida albicans* possesses the capacity to dissolve hydroxyapatite approximately 20-fold when compared with *S. mutans* [46]. Moreover,

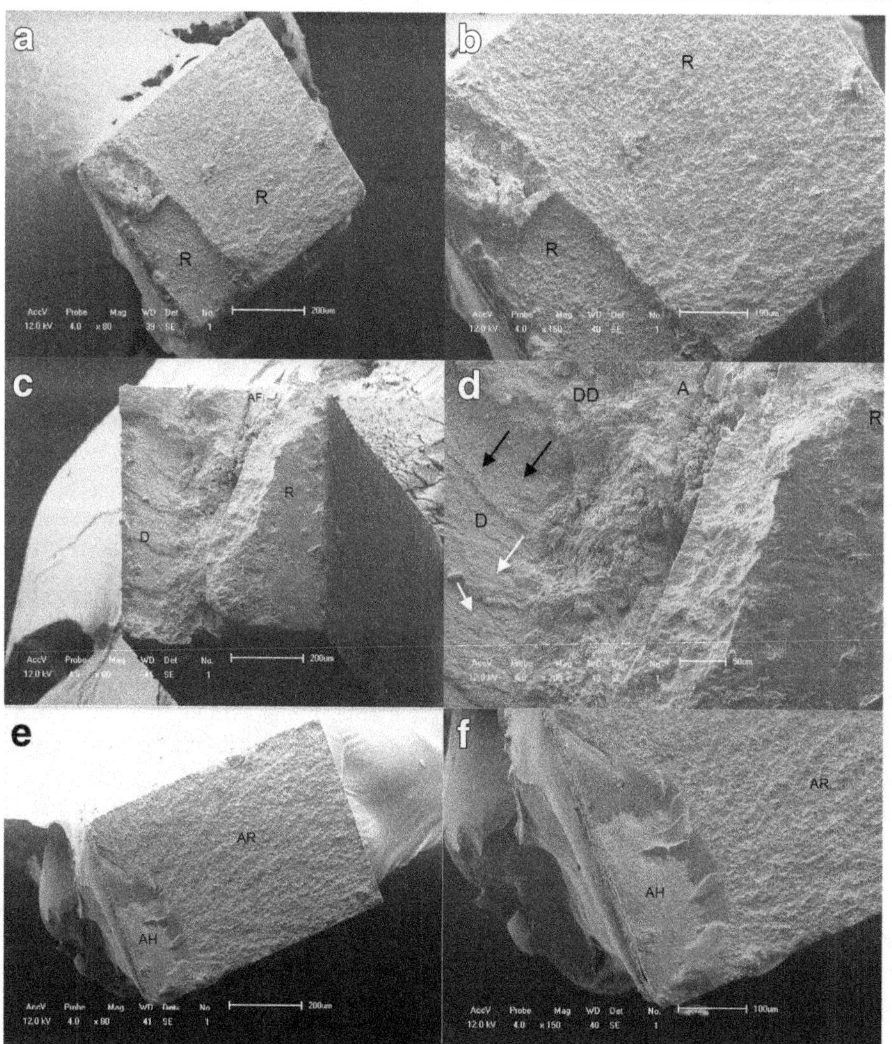

Fig. 5 Representative scanning electron micrographs of the fractured specimens. **a** and **b** Scanning electron photomicrographs of the cohesive failure of resin composite. **c** and **d** Mixed fractures. **c** Part of the fracture occurred inside the adhesive layer, probably just under the hybrid layer, because parts of the dentinal tubules are exposed (D-adhesive fracture) and parts are covered by the adhesive layer (A-cohesive fracture) with resin on top of a small adhesive area (R). **d** A mixed fracture shows deep dentin (DD), a thin adhesive film (AF) on dentin, and the presence of opened dentin tubules (white arrows) and fractured resin tags still attached (black arrows). **e** and **f** Adhesive failure: cohesive failure in the bonding resin and/or in the hybrid layer. **e** The fracture that occurred both between the adhesive layer and resin (AR) and under the hybrid layer (AH)

C. albicans has high collagenolytic activity and can adhere to both intact or denaturated exposed dentin collagen [47].

A longitudinal study in children evaluated the antimicrobial efficacy of a dental varnish with 2.5% Brazilian red propolis against *Streptococcus mutans* compared with chlorhexidine 1% and fluoride 5%. Propolis varnish showed consistent reduction in *S. mutans* for up to 6 months in high-risk caries-free children. At day 180, propolis produced significantly lower *S. mutans* levels than fluoride and chlorhexidine [48]. According to research by Bueno-Silva et al. [38], using in vivo animal model studies, flavonoids such as vestitol and neovestitol can inhibit the incidence and severity of dental caries by a downregulation mechanism. Vestitol and neovestitol inhibit the expression of the virulence factor by inhibiting the activity of the enzymes glucosyltransferases D and B, reducing the accumulation of biofilm on the surface of the tooth, and avoiding the formation of caries and dental demineralization. A similar mechanism of caries inhibition has also been demonstrated by Koo et al. [49] using apigenin as an anti-biofilm agent thus avoiding the formation of caries. In this work, apigenin, flavonol, and flavones were active mainly on defective production of the enzymes glucosyltransferases B and C, affecting the pathogenic potential of dental plaque [49]. A potent inhibitory effect on the activity of streptococcal gucosyltransferase enzymes (glucosyltransferases B, C,

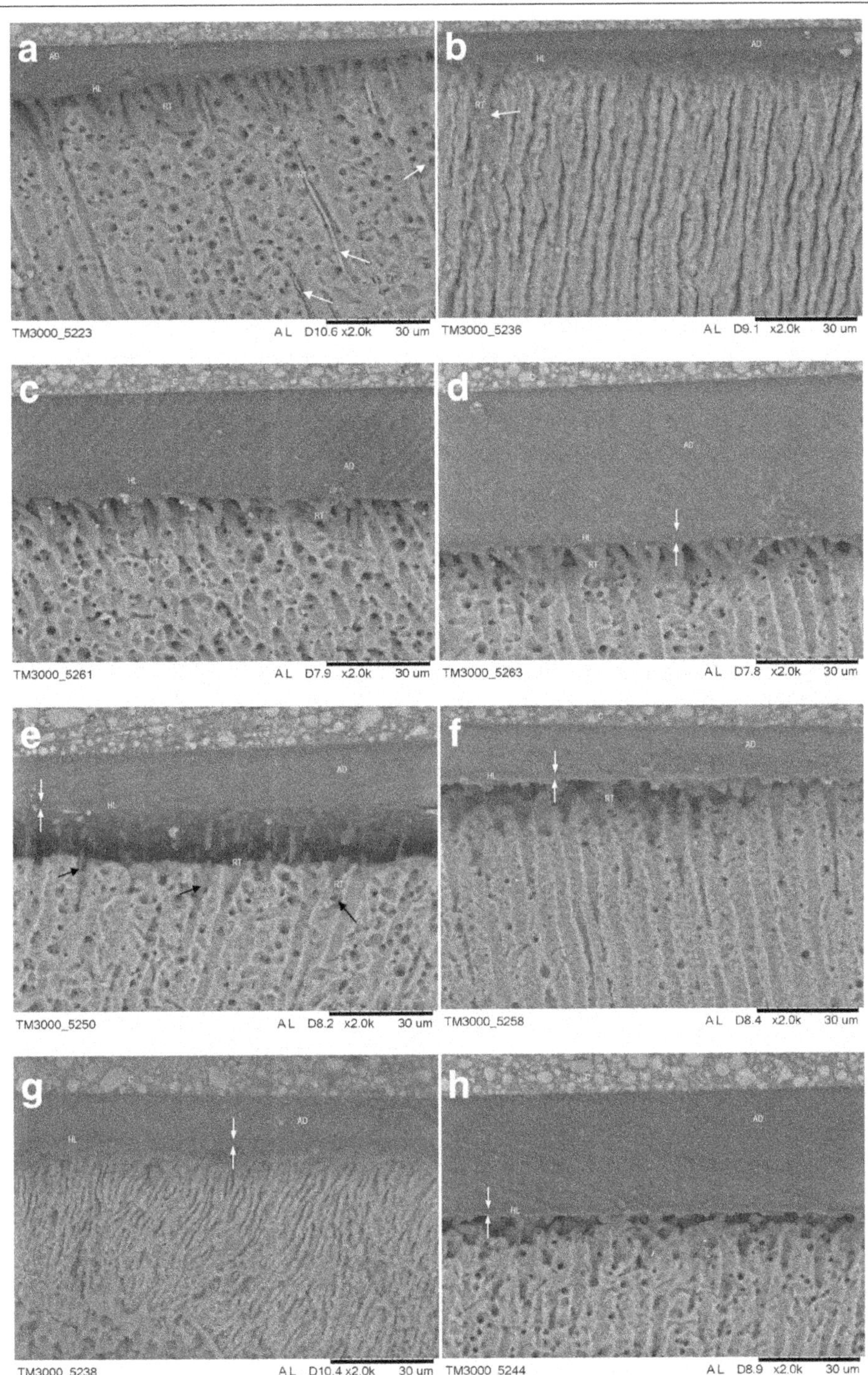

Fig. 6 Scanning electron micrographs show the bonded interface of the experimental and control groups. Resin tag quantity and quality match the bond strength results (MPa). White arrows point toward the hybrid layer. C, composite resin; HL, hybrid layer; RT, resin tags; AD, adhesive resin. A uniform hybrid layer with long well-formed resin tags was observed in the control (**a**) and CHX (**b**) groups. RP3 specimens before etching (**c**) and after etching (**d**) show a thin hybrid layer, and relatively shorter resin tags were identified compared with the control group. Representative SEM images of the resin-dentin interface from the RP6 group applied before etching (**e**) and after etching (**f**) show that a very thin hybrid layer was created (white arrows). Short resin tags were identified inside the dentin tubules (E, black arrows). Hardly any hybrid layer could be observed in RP1 specimens. Lack of well-formed resin tags was observed regardless of whether dentin treatment with micellar nanocomposites loaded with EARP was done before (**g**) or after etching (**h**). Only a few very short resin tags can be seen

and D) was compared in an ethanolic extract of Minas Gerais-Brazil propolis and an ethanolic extract from Rio Grande do Sul-Brazil. However, the inhibitory effect on the glucosyltransferase enzymes (B, C, and D) depends on the geographic origin of the propolis [50].

Propolis can be a promising substance for cavity cleaning due to its anti-inflammatory activity [51] and mainly because it is effective against the most of bacteria involved with dental caries process (7,43,48). However, studies have shown different results, which may have been a result of the chemical variability of propolis, the concentration of propolis in the extract, and the solvent used for extraction. Furthermore, the inconsistent results may have been caused by variations in the susceptibility test, culture media, and the time of incubation. The findings of these studies and the present study support the idea that the antibacterial activity depends not only on the origin of the propolis but also on the extract and solvent used [2, 49, 52–55].

Cavity disinfectants are applied before placing the restorative material to reduce or eliminate bacteria from dentin that remains after tooth preparation. Chlorhexidine is a cationic solution with a wide range of antimicrobial activity and is widely used as a cavity disinfectant [56]. The bactericidal effect of the drug is due to the cationic molecule binding to extra-bacterial complexes and negatively charged bacterial cell walls, thereby changing the osmotic balance of the cells. At low concentrations, low molecular weight substances leak out, specifically potassium and phosphorus, with a subsequent bacteriostatic effect. At higher concentrations, CHX has a bactericidal effect as a result of precipitation and/or coagulation of the cytoplasm of bacterial cells followed by cell death [57].

In the present study, we used a 2% CHX solution, which is the gold standard for cavity disinfection in dentistry, because of its long-lasting bactericidal effect on dentin; 0.12% CHX was used for the antimicrobial tests. However, Bidar et al. [58] demonstrated that CHX was effective against *Streptococcus mutans* and *Candida albicans* without significant differences among the different concentrations of CHX used (2, 0.2, and 0.12%).

The partial removal of carious dentin from deep caries lesions leads to significantly improved preservation of pulpal vitality at 5-year follow-up in adults, irrespective of age, supporting the approach of avoiding pulp exposure. This study did not include evaluation of dentin remineralization, but the results of studies [59] suggest that cavity sealing contributes to the remineralization process in inner carious dentin.

The dentin-pulp complex is an important factor in dentin tissue repair. The response of odontoblasts to the inflammatory reaction induced by a carious lesion is the production of tertiary dentin. Partial removal of caries from deep caries lesions followed by cavity sealing promotes a substantial reduction in bacteria, reorganization of the dentin collagen network, narrowing of the dentinal tubules, changes in the tactile consistency (hardness) of dentin and in its mineral content with a significantly higher percentage of calcium and phosphorus and evidence of apatite mineralization [59].

Remineralization of the affected dentin can occur even without any remineralizing material. This strongly suggests that the most important factor is not the material, but the sealing of the cavity, thereby reducing or eliminating the supply of substrate for any remaining microorganisms. We performed dentin pretreatment with micellar nanocomposites loaded with EARP followed by an adhesive restorative procedure. Dentin bonding agents do not induce dentin repair. Although microleakage in composite restorations after antimicrobial treatments can occur [60], some studies showed success after partial removal of carious dentin and cavity sealing with adhesive restorations [25, 58], even after partial caries removal from the pulpal wall followed by adhesive restoration in a single session [61, 62].

This study used the CIE L*a*b * method, which allows numerical color analysis of an object. The CIE L*a*b* system, determined by the Commission International of L'eclaire (CIE) [35] through the CIELAB color space, defines color based on three coordinates: L*, a*, and b*. The L* coordinate (brightness) refers to the level from light to dark, i.e., this coordinate extends from black ($L = 0$) to white ($L = 100$); a* and b* values represent the two color axes. The a* coordinate refers to a scale from green to red and varies from -90 to $+70$, with negative values approaching green and positive values for reddish colors; the b* coordinate varies from -80 to $+100$ from blue to yellow with negative values indicating a shift to blue and positive values indicating a shift to yellow. By comparing the initial color reading with the final color reading, it is possible to get the value of ΔE, which quantifies the total change in color, but does not qualify it, because it is not possible to indicate on which axis (brightness, red-green, or yellow-blue) the color changes have occurred [36].

To achieve an acceptable aesthetic, the color of dental restorations should match the appearance of the corresponding tissues. The results of this study indicate that the use of micellar nanocomposites loaded with EARP at concentrations of 0.3, 0.6, and 1% did not change the color at the dentin/resin interface in a way that was clinically unacceptable, in agreement with others studies that show clinically acceptable values for color changes in dental restorations [63, 64].

The human eye perceives brightness (L*) more clearly as a result of the higher amount of rod-type cells (responsible for black and white sight) than cone cells (responsible for colored sight) [65]. The color difference between two objects, represented by the ΔE value, is considered to be acceptable or not acceptable. However, the ΔE values corresponding to this classification are still controversial. Paravina et al. [63] found that when ΔE is higher than 3.7, the color difference is easily visible. A value between 3.7 and 1.0 is clinically acceptable and values smaller than 1.0 are not clinically visible. But the study by Douglas et al. [64] reported different data from a survey of dental practice; these authors found that clinicians perceived color changes if $\Delta E \geq 2.6$, but replacement of a restoration because of color changes was only indicated for ΔE values higher than 5.5.

The bond strength tests did not show a significant difference between the positive control (CHX) and the negative control (NT). These data are consistent with other studies that have reported the absence of damage to the bond strength of the dentin/resin interface after application of 2% CHX as a cavity disinfectant [66, 67]. Carrilho et al. [68] showed that significant amounts of CHX were retained in dentin independently of the dose of CHX applied (0.2, 2%) or the time (from 30 min to 8 weeks). The substantivity of CHX to dentin probably has an important role in the inhibition of collagen proteases in dentin and in the stability of CHX-treated resin/dentin interfaces [68, 69].

The RP3 and RP6 groups showed microtensile bond strength statistically similar to the control groups and the mean values in MPa were close to those found by Ayar [70] in restorations using the same adhesive system and the same composite resin.

On the other hand, micellar nanocomposites loaded with EARP at a concentration of 1.0% had an adverse effect on the adhesive process, invalidating its use in adhesive restorations. The hybrid layer is a complex composite structure with morphology and properties that are highly sensitive to both the demineralization process and the specific characteristics of the bonding adhesive system [71]. Because of the minimal thickness of the hybrid layer in the RP1 group, it was barely visible, and the shape of the resin tags suggested possible failure in the infiltration of demineralized dentin by the adhesive resin. That was not expected because nanosized drug delivery systems are suitable for improving the bioavailability of poorly water-soluble drugs [23], and in this study, micellar nanocomposites loaded with EARP at concentration of 1% with a particles size of ~ 70 nm in acetone were used, which could flow easily into the dentin tubules. Chen et al. [9] showed that applying 10% propolis ethanolic extract to dentin leads to deposition of resins and waxes from propolis on the dentin surface and into the dentinal tubules. It can block the entrance to the dentin tubules and cover the dentin surface, interfering with the proper formation of the hybrid layer and resin tags. Although the concentration used in this study was 10 times lower than that used by Chen et al. [9], dentin hybridization was compromised followed by reduced dentin-resin bonding.

Polymeric micelles serve as nanoscopic drug carriers [72] and consist of a core and shell structure; the inner core is the hydrophobic part of the block copolymer, which encapsulates the poorly water-soluble drug, whereas the outer shell or corona of the hydrophilic block of the copolymer protects the drug from the aqueous environment, keeping them stable. The core can sometimes be made up of a water-soluble polymer that is rendered hydrophobic by the chemical conjugation of the water-insoluble drug [73, 74].

For this study, polymeric micelles were prepared from PCL and Pluronic F108 copolymer, biocompatible and biodegradable block copolymers that may remain intact for long duration under sink conditions and may also slowly release drugs. The failure noticed in the RP1 group may be associated with the higher concentration of micellar nanocomposite and the consequent increase in the viscosity.

Donor-acceptor interactions between a solid surface and an organic liquid lead to the creation of surface charge and counter ions in the liquid [75]. Zeta potential, a scientific term for the electrokinetic potential in colloidal systems [76] and nano-medicines, and the particle size exert a major effect on the various properties of nano-drug delivery systems [77] and can be an indicator of stability. High electric charge (+ 30 mV), positive or negative, on the surface of the nanoparticles prevents aggregation of the nanoparticles because of the strong repellent forces among the particles [78, 79]. The highest concentration of micellar nanocomposites loaded with EARP (RP1 group) may have been responsible for a reduction in the zeta potential of the micellar PCL/Pluronic nanocomposite and led to the formation of nanoclusters, which would increase the viscosity and act as physical blockers contributing to less penetration of the adhesive system into the dentin tubules.

Conclusion

Micellar nanocomposites loaded with EARP at concentrations of 0.3 and 0.6% applied as a cavity cleanser do not compromise the aesthetics or microtensile bond strength of the dentin/resin interface. The EARP is rich in flavonoids and isoflavonoids and both EARP and MNRP showed antimicrobial activity for the main agents causing dental caries (*Streptococcus mutans* and *Lactobacillus acidophilus)* and for *Candida albicans.*

Abbreviations

ANOVA: Analysis of variance; CHX: Chlorhexidine gluconate; EARP: Ethyl acetate extract of Brazilian red propolis; MIC: Minimal inhibitory concentration; MNRP: Micellar nanocomposites loaded with EARP; NT: No treatment; PCL: Poly-ε-caprolactone; SEM: Scanning electron microscopy;

UPLC-DAD: Ultra-performance liquid chromatography coupled with a diode array detector; μTBS: Microtensile bond strength

Acknowledgments

The authors thank CESMAC, UFAL, CNPq and FINEP for their financial support (CT-INFRA) for the acquisition of some equipment and laboratory facilities.

Authors' contributions

Conceived and designed the experiments: DCCA, ICCMP, TGN, RUK. Performed the experiments: DCCA, ICCMP, TGN, GVCOC, TSSD, LMN, JMSO, CBS, MLASL, NBS, IDBJ, PBE, EJSF, CBD, RUK. Analyzed the data: DCCA, ICCMP, TGN, RUK, JMSO, CBS, MLASL, NBS, IDBJ, PBE, EJSF, CBD. Contributed reagents/materials/analysis tools: DCCA, ICCMP, TGN, NBS, IDBJ, PBE, EJSF, CBD, RUK. Wrote the paper: DCCA, ICCMP, TGN, GVCOC, TSSD, LMN, RUK, JMSO, CBS, MLASL, NBS, IDBJ, PBE, EJSF, CBD. All authors read and approved the final version of the paper.

Competing interests

The authors of this manuscript certify that they have no proprietary, financial, or other personal interest of any nature in any product, service, and/or company presented in this article. The authors declare that they have no competing interest.

Author details

[1]Postgraduate Program in Health Research, Cesmac University Center, Rua Cônego Machado, 825, Farol, Maceió, Alagoas, Brazil. [2]Department of Restorative Dentistry, Faculty of Dentistry, Federal University of Alagoas, Campus AC Simões, Av. Lourival Melo Mota, S/N, Tabuleiro do Martins, Maceió, Alagoas, Brazil. [3]Laboratory of Quality Control of Drugs and Medicines, Postgraduate Program in Pharmaceutical Sciences, School of Nursing and Pharmacy, Federal University of Alagoas, Campus A. C, Simões, Maceió, Alagoas, Brazil. [4]Laboratory of Applied Electrochemistry, Institute of Chemistry and Biotechnology, Federal University of Alagoas, Campus A. C, Simões, Maceió, Alagoas, Brazil. [5]Department of Cariology, Faculty of Dentistry, Federal University of Alagoas, Campus AC Simões, Av. Lourival Melo Mota, S/N, Tabuleiro do Martins, Maceió, Alagoas, Brazil. [6]Department of Dental Materials and Prosthodontics, Faculty of Dentistry, Universidade Estadual Paulista Júlio de Mesquita Filho-UNESP, Araraquara, São Paulo, Brazil. [7]Faculty of Veterinary Medicine, Federal University of Alagoas, Campus Arapiraca, Unit of Viçosa, Viçosa, Alagoas, Brazil. [8]Laboratory of Bacteriology. Institute of Biological and Health Sciences, Federal University of Alagoas, Campus A. C, Simões, Maceió, Alagoas, Brazil.

References

1. Toreti VC, Sato HH, Pastore GM, Park YK. Recent progress of propolis for its biological and chemical compositions and its botanical origin. Evid Based Complement Alternat Med. 2013;697390 https://doi.org/10.1155/2013/697390.
2. Mendonça ICG, Porto ICCMP, Nascimento TG, Souza NS, Oliveira JMS, Arruda RES, et al. Brazilian red propolis: phytochemical screening, antioxidant activity and effect against cancer cells. BMC Complement Altern Med. 2015;15:357. https://doi.org/10.1186/s12906-015-0888-9.
3. Asawahame C, Sutjarittangtham K, Eitssayeam S, Tragoolpua Y, Sirithunyalug B, Sirithunyalug J. Antibacterial activity and inhibition of adherence of *Streptococcus mutans* by propolis electrospun fibers. AAPS Pharm Sci Tech. 2015;16:182–91.
4. Parolia A, Kundabala M, Rao NN, Acharya SR, Grawal P, Mohan M, et al. A comparative histological analysis of human pulp following direct pulp capping with Propolis, mineral trioxide aggregate and Dycal. Aust Dent J. 2010;55:59–64.
5. Parolia A, Kundabala M. Nonsurgical re-treatment of failed surgical endodontic therapy using propolis as an intra-canal medicament: a case report. Res J Med Sci. 2010;4:292–7. https://doi.org/10.3923/rjmsci.2010.292.297.
6. Malhotra N, Rao SP, Acharya S, Vasudev B. Comparative in vitro evaluation of efficacy of mouth rinses against *Streptococcus mutans, Lactobacilli* and *Candida albicans*. Oral Health Prev Dent. 2011;9:261–8.
7. Anauate Netto C, Marcucci MC, Paulino N, Anido-Anido A, Amore R, de Mendonça S, et al. Effects of typified propolis on mutans streptococci and lactobacilli: a randomized clinical trial. Braz Dent Sci. 2013;16:31–6.
8. Casaroto AR, Hidalgo MM, Sell AM, Franco SL, Cuman RK, Moreschi E, et al. Study of the effectiveness of propolis extract as a storage medium for avulsed teeth. Dent Traumatol. 2010;2:323–31.
9. Chen CL, Parolia A, Pau A, Porto ICCM. Comparative evaluation of the effectiveness of desensitizing agents in dentine tubule occlusion using scanning electron microscopy. Aust Dent J. 2015;60:65–72.
10. Pereira EMR, da Silva JLDC, Silva FF, De Luca MP, Ferreira EF, Lorentz TCM, et al. Clinical evidence of the efficacy of a mouthwash containing propolis for the control of plaque and gingivitis: a phase II study. Evid Based Complement Alternat Med. 2011;750249 https://doi.org/10.1155/2011/750249.
11. Silva BB, Rosalen PL, Cury JA, Ikegaki M, Souza VC, Esteves A, et al. Chemical composition and botanical origin of red propolis, a new type of Brazilian propolis. Evid Based Complement Alternat Med. 2007;5:313–6.
12. Machado CS, Mokochinski JB, Lira TOD, de Oliveira FDCE, Cardoso MV, Ferreira RG, et al. Comparative study of chemical composition and biological activity of yellow, green, brown, and red Brazilian propolis. Evid Based Complement Alternat Med. 2016;2016:6057650. https://doi.org/10.1155/2016/6057650.
13. Rufatto LC, dos Santos DA, Marinho F, Henriques JAP, Ely MR, Moura S. Red propolis: chemical composition and pharmacological activity. Asian Pac J Trop Biomed. 2017;7:591–8.
14. Alencar SM, Oldoni TLC, Castro ML, Cabral ISR, Costa Neto CM, Cury JA, et al. Chemical composition and biological activity of a new type of Brazilian propolis: red propolis. J Ethnopharmacol. 2007;113:278–83.
15. Awale S, Li F, Onozuka H, Esumi H, Tezuka Y, Kadota S. Constituents of Brazilian red propolis and their preferential cytotoxic activity against human pancreatic PANC-1 cancer cell line in nutrient-deprived condition. Bioorg Med Chem. 2008;16:181–9.
16. Righi AA, Alves TR, Negri G, Marques LM, Breyer H, Salatino A. Brazilian red propolis: unreported substances, antioxidant and antimicrobial activities. J Sci Food Agric. 2011;91:2363–70.
17. Bertolini PF, Biodi Filho O, Pomilio A, Pinheiro SL, Carvalho MS. Antimicrobial capacity of Aloe vera and propolis dentifrice against *Streptococcus mutans* strains in toothbrushes: an in vitro study. J Appl Oral Sci. 2012;20:32–7.
18. Bueno-Silva B, Alencar SM, Koo H, Ikegaki M, Silva GV, Napimonga MH, et al. Anti-inflammatory and antimicrobial evaluation of neovestitol and vestitol isolated from Brazilian red propolis. J Agric Food Chem. 2013;61:4546–50. https://doi.org/10.1021/jf305468f.
19. Hegde KS, Bhat SS, Rao A, Sain S. Effect of Propolis on *Streptococcus mutans* counts: an in vivo study. Int J Clin Pediatr Dent. 2013;6:22–5.
20. Bueno-Silva B, Marsola A, Ikegaki M, Alencar SM, Rosalen PL. The effect of seasons on Brazilian red propolis and its botanical source: chemical composition and antibacterial activity. Nat Prod Res. 2017;31:1318–24. https://doi.org/10.1080/14786419.2016.1239088.
21. Munhoz VM, Longhini R, Souza JRP, Zequi JAC, Leite Mello EVS, Lopes GC, et al. Extraction of flavonoids from *Tagetes patula*: process optimization and screening for biological activity. Rev Bras Farmacogn. 2014;24:576–83.
22. Ahangari Z, Ghassemi A, Shamszadeh S, Naseri M. The effects of propolis on discoloration of teeth. J Dent School. 2013;31:33–41.
23. Wang Y, Miao X, Sun L, Song J, Bi C, Yang X, et al. Effects of nanosuspension formulations on transport, pharmacokinetics, in vivo targeting and efficacy for poorly water-soluble drugs. Curr Pharm Des. 2014; 20:454–73.
24. Karpinski TM, Szkaradkiewicz AK. Microbiology of dental caries. J Biol Earth Sci. 2013;3:M21–4.
25. Maltz M, Henz SL, de Oliveira EF, Jardim JJ. Conventional caries removal and sealed caries in permanent teeth: a microbiological evaluation. J Dent. 2012; 40:776–82.
26. Bjørndal L, Fransson H, Bruun G, Markvart M, Kjældgaard M, Näsman P, et al. Randomized clinical trials on deep carious lesions: 5-year follow-up. J Dent Res. 2017;96:747–53.
27. Chibinski AC, Wambier L, Reis A, Wambier DS. Clinical, mineral and ultrastructural changes in carious dentin of primary molars after restoration. Int Dent J. 2016;66:150–7. https://doi.org/10.1111/idj.12219.

28. Kidd E, Fejerskov O, Nyvad B. Infected dentine revisited. Dent Update. 2015; 42:802 6. 808-9
29. Ricketts D, Lamont T, Innes NP, Kidd E, Clarkson JE. Operative caries management in adults and children. Cochrane Database Syst Rev. 2013;28: CD003808. https://doi.org/10.1002/14651858.CD003808.pub3.
30. Araújo NC, Soares MUSC, da Silva MMN, Gerbi MEMM, Braz R. Considerations of partial caries removal. Int J Dent. 2010;9:202–9.
31. Nascimento TG, da Silva PF, Azevedo LF, da Rocha LG, de Moraes Porto IC, Lima e Moura TF, et al. Polymeric nanoparticles of Brazilian red propolis extract: preparation, characterization, antioxidant activity and leishmanicidal activity. Nanoscale Res Lett. 2016;11:301. https://doi.org/10.1186/s11671-016-1517-3.
32. Clinical and Laboratory Standards Institute. M07-A9. In: In methods for dilution antimicrobial susceptibility tests for Bacteria that grow aerobically; approved standard — ninth edition; 2012.
33. Lima BA, Berlinck RGS, Gonçalves RB, Kamiya RU. Halistanol sulfate a and Rodriguesines a and B are antimicrobial and antibiofilm agents against the cariogenic bacterium Streptococcus mutans. Braz J Pharmacogn. 2014;24: 651–9.
34. Arendrup MC, Cuenca-Estrella M, Lass-Flör C, Hope W, EUCAST-AFST. EUCAST technical note on the EUCAST definitive document EDef 7.2: method for the determination of broth dilution minimum inhibitory concentrations of antifungal agents for yeasts EDef 7.2 (EUCAST-AFST). Clin Microbiol Infect. 2012;18:E246-7.
35. Commission Internationale de L'Eclairage (CIE). Recommendations on uniform color spaces, color-difference equations, psychometric color terms. Supplement no. 2 of publication CIE no. 15 (E-1.3.1). Paris: Bureau Central de la CIE; 1978.
36. ISO Colorimetry - Part 4: CIE 1976 L*a*b* Colour Space. ISO 11664–4. 2008.
37. Conover WJ. Practical nonparametric statistics. 3rd ed. New York: Wiley; 1999.
38. Bueno-Silva B, Koo H, Falsetta ML, Alencar SM, Ikegaki M, Rosalen PL. Effect of Neovestitol-vestitol containing Brazilian red propolis on biofilm accumulation *in vitro* and dental caries development *in vivo*. Biofouling. 2013;29:1233–42. https://doi.org/10.1080/08927014.2013.834050.
39. Saavedra N, Barrientos L, Herrera CL, Alvear M, Montenegro G, Salazar LA. Effect of Chilean propolis on cariogenic bacteria *Lactobacillus fermentum*. Cienc Inv Agr. 2011;38:117–25.
40. Duarte S, Rosalen PL, Hayacibara MF, Cury JA, Bowen WH, Marquis RE, et al. The influence of a novel propolis on *mutans streptococci* biofilms and caries development in rats. Arch Oral Biol. 2006;51:15–22.
41. Ishida VFC, Negri G, Salatino A, Bandeira MFCL. A new type of Brazilian propolis: prenylated benzophenones in propolis from Amazon and effects against cariogenic bacteria. Food Chem. 2011;125:966–72. https://doi.org/10.1016/j.foodchem.2010.09.089.
42. Neelakantan P, Rao CV, Indramohan J. Bacteriology of deep carious lesions underneath amalgam restorations with different pulp-capping materials - an in vivo analysis. J Appl Oral Sci. 2012;20:139–45.
43. Oldoni TLC, Cabral ISR, d'Arcea MABR, Rosalen PL, Ikegaki M, Nascimento AM, et al. Isolation and analysis of bioactive isoflavonoids and chalcone from a new type of Brazilian propolis. Sep Purif Technol. 2011;77:208–13.
44. Ghasempour M, Sefidgar SAA, Eyzadian H, Gharakhani S. Prevalence of *Candida albicans* in dental plaque and caries lesion of early childhood caries (ECC) according to sampling site. Caspian J Intern Med. 2011;2:304–8.
45. Klinke T, Kneist S, de Soet JJ, Kuhlisch E, Mauersberger S, Forster A, et al. Acid production by oral strains of *Candida albicans* and lactobacilli. Caries Res. 2009;43:83–91.
46. Ten Cate JM, Klis FM, Pereira-Cenci T, Crielaard W, de Groot PW. Molecular and cellular mechanisms that lead to *Candida* biofilm formation. J Dent Res. 2009;88:105–15.
47. de Carvalho FG, Parisotto TM, Hebling J, Spolidorio LC, Spolidorio DMP. Presence of *Candida* spp. in infants oral cavity and its association with early childhood caries. Braz J Oral Sci. 2007;6:1249–53.
48. Valadas LAR, Rodrigues Neto EM, Lotif MAL, Fonseca SGC, Chagas FO, Fechine FV, et al. Evaluation of propolis dental varnish against *Streptococcus mutans* in children. Dent Mater. 2017;33:e80–1. doi.org/10.1016/j.dental.2017.08.162
49. Koo H, Hayacibara MF, Schobel BD, Cury JA, Rosalen PL, Park YK, et al. Inhibition of *Streptococcus mutans* biofilm accumulation and polysaccharide production by apigenin and tt-farnesol. J Antimicrob Chemother. 2003;52: 782–9. https://doi.org/10.1128/AAC.46.5.1302-1309.2002.
50. Koo H, Smith VAM, Bowen WH, Rosalen PL, Cury JA, Park YK. Effects of *Apis mellifera* propolis on the activities of streptococcal glucosyltransferases in solution and adsorbed onto saliva-coated hydroxyapatite. Caries Res. 2000; 34:418–26.
51. Corrêa FR, Schanuel FS, Moura-Nunes N, Monte-Alto-Costa A, Daleprane JB. Brazilian red propolis improves cutaneous wound healing suppressing inflammation-associated transcription factor NFκB. Biomed Pharmacother. 2017;86:162–17.
52. Cabral ISR, Oldoni TLC, Prado A, Bezerra RMN, Alencar SM, Ikegaki M, et al. Phenolic composition, antibacterial and antioxidant activities of Brazilian red propolis. Quím Nova. 2009;32:1523–7. doi.org/10.1590/S0100-40422009000600031
53. Neves MVM, da Silva TMS, Lima EO, Cunha EVL, Oliveira EJ. Isoflavone formononetin from red propolis acts as a fungicide against *Candida* sp. Braz J Microbiol. 2016;47:159–66. doi.org/10.1016/j.bjm.2015.11.009
54. Almeida ETC, Silva MCD, Oliveira JMS, Kamiya RU, Arruda RES, Vieira DA, et al. Chemical and microbiological characterization of tinctures and microcapsules loaded with Brazilian red propolis extract. J Pharm Anal. 2017;7:280–7. doi.org/10.1016/j.jpha.2017.03.004
55. López BG-C, Schmidt EM, Eberlin MN, Sawaya ACHF. Phytochemical markers of different types of red propolis. Food Chem. 2014;146:174–80. doi.org/10.1016/j.foodchem.2013.09.063
56. Gomes BP, Vianna ME, Zaia AA, Almeida JF, Souza-Filho FJ, Ferraz CC. Chlorhexidine in endodontics. Braz Dent J. 2013;24:89–102. https://doi.org/10.1590/0103-6440201302188.
57. Cheung HY, Wong MMK, Cheung SH, Liang LY, Lam YW, Chiu SK. Differential actions of chlorhexidine on the cell wall of *Bacillus subtilis* and *Escherichia coli*. PLoS One. 2012;7:e36659. doi.org/10.1371/journal.pone.0036659
58. Bidar M, Naderinasab M, Talati A, Ghazvini K, Asgari S, Hadizadeh B, et al. The effects of different concentrations of chlorhexidine gluconate on the antimicrobial properties of mineral trioxide aggregate and calcium enrich mixture. Dent Res J. 2012;9:466–71.
59. Tjäderhane L, Carrilho MR, Breschi L, Tay FR, Pashley DH. Dentin basic structure and composition—an overview. Endod Topics. 2009;20:3–29.
60. Hameed H, Babu BP, Sagir VM, Chiriyath KJ, Mathias J, Shaji AP. Microleakage in resin composite restoration following antimicrobial pre-treatments with 2% chlorhexidine and clearfil protect bond. J Int Oral Health. 2015;7:71–6.
61. Maltz M, Koppe B, Jardim JJ, Alves LS, de Paula LM, Yamaguti PM, et al. Partial caries removal in deep caries lesions: a 5-year multicenter randomized controlled trial. Clin Oral Investig. 2018;22:1337–43. https://doi.org/10.1007/s00784-017-2221-0.
62. De Medeiros Serpa EB, Clementino MA, Granville-Garcia AF, Rosenblatt A. The effect of atraumatic restorative treatment on adhesive restorations for dental caries in deciduous molars. J Indian Soc Pedod Prev Dent. 2017;35:167–73.
63. Paravina GR, Ghinea R, Herrera LJ, Bona AD, Igiel C, Linninger M, et al. Color difference thresholds in dentistry. J Esthet Restor Dent. 2015;27:S1–9.
64. Douglas RD, Steinhauer TJ, Wee AG. Intraoral determination of the tolerance of dentists for perceptibility and acceptability of shade mismatch. J Prosthet Dent. 2007;97:200–8.
65. Grimes WN, Graves LR, Summers MT. Rieke F. A simple retinal mechanism contributes to perceptual interactions between rod- and cone-mediated responses in primates. elife. 2015;4:e08033. https://doi.org/10.7554/eLife.08033.
66. Aykut-Yetkiner A, Candan U, Ersin N, Eronat C, Belli S, Özcan M. Effect of 2% chlorhexidine gluconate cavity disinfectant on microtensile bond strength of tooth-coloured restorative materials to sound and caries-affected dentin. J Adhes Sci Technol. 2015;29:1–9.
67. Chang YE, Shin DH. Effect of chlorhexidine application methods on microtensile bond strength to dentin in class I cavities. Oper Dent. 2010;35: 618–23.
68. Carrilho MR, Carvalho RM, Sousa EN, Nicolau J, Breschi L, Mazzoni A, et al. Substantivity of chlorhexidine to human dentin. Dent Mater. 2010;26:779–85. https://doi.org/10.1016/j.dental.2010.04.002.
69. Umer D, Yiu CK, Burrow MF, Niu LN, Tay FR. Effect of a novel quaternary ammonium silane on dentin protease activities. J Dent. 2017;58:19–27. https://doi.org/10.1016/j.jdent.2017.01.001.
70. Ayar MK. Effect of simplified ethanol-wet bonding on microtensile bond strengths of dentin adhesive agents with different solvents. J Dent Sci. 2015; 10:270–4.

71. Katz JL, Bumrerraj S, Dreyfuss J, Wang Y, Spencer P. Micromechanics of the dentin/adhesive interface. J Biomed Mater Res (Appl Biomater). 2001;58: 366–71.
72. Pelaz B, Alexiou C, Alvarez-Puebla RA, Alves F, Andrews AM, Ashraf S, et al. Diverse applications of nanomedicine. ACS Nano. 2017;11:2313–81. https://doi.org/10.1021/acsnano.6b06040.
73. Torchilin V. Structure and design of polymeric surfactant-based drug delivery systems. J Control Release. 2001;73:137–72.
74. Lu Y, Park K. Polymeric micelles and alternative nanonized delivery vehicles for poorly soluble drugs. Int J Pharm. 2013;453:198–214. https://doi.org/10.1016/j.ijpharm.2012.08.042.
75. Jing D, Pan Y, Li D, Zhao X, Bhushan B. Effect of surface charge on the nanofriction and its velocity dependence in an electrolyte based on lateral force microscopy. Langmuir. 2017;33:1792–8. https://doi.org/10.1021/acs.langmuir.6b04332.
76. Honary S, Zahir F. Effect of zeta potential on the properties of nano-drug delivery systems - a review (part 1). Trop J Pharm Res. 2013;12:255–64.
77. Honary S, Zahir F. Effect of zeta potential on the properties of nano-drug delivery systems - a review (part 2). Trop J Pharm Res. 2013;12:265–73.
78. Vijayakumar S. In vitro stability studies on gold nanoparticles with different stabilizing agents. Int J Curr Sci. 2014;11:E84–93.
79. Kedar U, Phutane P, Shidhaye S, Kadam V. Advances in polymeric micelles for drug delivery and tumor targeting. Nanomed-Nanotechnol. Biol Med. 2010;6:714–29.

Permissions

All chapters in this book were first published in CAM, by BioMed Central; hereby published with permission under the Creative Commons Attribution License or equivalent. Every chapter published in this book has been scrutinized by our experts. Their significance has been extensively debated. The topics covered herein carry significant findings which will fuel the growth of the discipline. They may even be implemented as practical applications or may be referred to as a beginning point for another development.

The contributors of this book come from diverse backgrounds, making this book a truly international effort. This book will bring forth new frontiers with its revolutionizing research information and detailed analysis of the nascent developments around the world.

We would like to thank all the contributing authors for lending their expertise to make the book truly unique. They have played a crucial role in the development of this book. Without their invaluable contributions this book wouldn't have been possible. They have made vital efforts to compile up to date information on the varied aspects of this subject to make this book a valuable addition to the collection of many professionals and students.

This book was conceptualized with the vision of imparting up-to-date information and advanced data in this field. To ensure the same, a matchless editorial board was set up. Every individual on the board went through rigorous rounds of assessment to prove their worth. After which they invested a large part of their time researching and compiling the most relevant data for our readers.

The editorial board has been involved in producing this book since its inception. They have spent rigorous hours researching and exploring the diverse topics which have resulted in the successful publishing of this book. They have passed on their knowledge of decades through this book. To expedite this challenging task, the publisher supported the team at every step. A small team of assistant editors was also appointed to further simplify the editing procedure and attain best results for the readers.

Apart from the editorial board, the designing team has also invested a significant amount of their time in understanding the subject and creating the most relevant covers. They scrutinized every image to scout for the most suitable representation of the subject and create an appropriate cover for the book.

The publishing team has been an ardent support to the editorial, designing and production team. Their endless efforts to recruit the best for this project, has resulted in the accomplishment of this book. They are a veteran in the field of academics and their pool of knowledge is as vast as their experience in printing. Their expertise and guidance has proved useful at every step. Their uncompromising quality standards have made this book an exceptional effort. Their encouragement from time to time has been an inspiration for everyone.

The publisher and the editorial board hope that this book will prove to be a valuable piece of knowledge for researchers, students, practitioners and scholars across the globe.

List of Contributors

Claudia B. Pratesi
Interdisciplinary Laboratory of Biosciences and Celiac Disease Research Center, School of Medicine, University of Brasilia, Asa Norte - CEP 70910900, Brasilia, DF, Brazil.
Post-graduate Program in Health Sciences, Faculty of Health Sciences, University of Brasilia, Brasilia, DF, Brazil

Marilen Queiroz de Souza, Isabella Márcia Soares Nogueira Teotônio, Fernanda Coutinho de Almeida and Riccardo Pratesi
Interdisciplinary Laboratory of Biosciences and Celiac Disease Research Center, School of Medicine, University of Brasilia, Asa Norte - CEP 70910900, Brasilia, DF, Brazil.
Post-graduate Program in Medical Sciences, School of Medicine, University of Brasilia, Brasilia, DF, Brazil

Gabriella Simões Heyn and Priscilla Souza Alves
Department of Pharmacy, Faculty of Health Sciences, University of Brasilia, Brasilia, DF, Brazil.

Luiz Antônio Soares Romeiro
Department of Pharmacy, Faculty of Health Sciences, University of Brasilia, Brasilia, DF, Brazil
Post-graduate Program in Pharmaceutical Sciences, Faculty of Health Sciences, University of Brasilia, Brasilia, DF, Brazil

Yanna Karla de Medeiros Nóbrega
Department of Pharmacy, Faculty of Health Sciences, University of Brasilia, Brasilia, DF, Brazil
Post-graduate Program in Health Sciences, Faculty of Health Sciences, University of Brasilia, Brasilia, DF, Brazil
Post-graduate Program in Medical Sciences, School of Medicine, University of Brasilia, Brasilia, DF, Brazil

Hettiarachchige Dona Sachindra Melshandi Perera, Jayanetti Koralalage Ramani Radhika Samarasekera and Hasitha Dhananjaya Weeratunga
Industrial Technology Institute (ITI), 363, Bauddhaloka Mawatha, Colombo 07, Sri Lanka

Shiroma Mangalika Handunnetti and Ovitigala Vithanage Don Sisira Jagathpriya Weerasena
Institute of Biochemistry, Molecular Biology and Biotechnology, University of Colombo, 90, Cumaratunga Munidasa Mawatha, Colombo 03, Sri Lanka

Almas Jabeen
Dr. Panjwani Center for Molecular Medicine and Drug Research, International Center for Chemical and Biological Sciences, University of Karachi, Karachi 75270, Pakistan

Muhammad Iqbal Choudhary
H. E. J. Research Institute of Chemistry, International Center for Chemical and Biological Sciences, University of Karachi, Karachi 75270, Pakistan

Larisa Ariadne Justine Barnes
Faculty of Pharmacy, The University of Sydney, Camperdown, NSW 2006, Australia
University Centre for Rural Health, The University of Sydney, Lismore, NSW 2480, Australia

Lesley Barclay
University Centre for Rural Health, The University of Sydney, Lismore, NSW 2480, Australia
Sydney School of Public Health, The University of Sydney, Edward Ford Building (A27), Camperdown, NSW 2006, Australia

Kirsten McCaffery
Sydney School of Public Health, Sydney Medical School, The University of Sydney, Rm 128B, Edward Ford Building A27, Camperdown, NSW 2006, Australia

Parisa Aslani
Faculty of Pharmacy, The University of Sydney, Rm N502, Pharmacy & Bank Building (A15), Science Rd, Camperdown, NSW 2006, Australia

Kristina Sivertsen
Department for drugs - and addiction treatment and A-larm Norway, Hospital of Southern Norway, Kristiansand, Norway

Marko Lukic
Department of Community Medicine, Faculty of Health Sciences, UiT The Arctic University of Norway, Tromsø, Norway

Agnete E. Kristoffersen
National Research Center in Complementary and Alternative Medicine (NAFKAM), Department of Community Medicine, Faculty of Health Sciences, UiT The Arctic University of Norway, Tromsø, Norway

Anuradha Sharma and Gurcharan Kaur
Department of Biotechnology, Medical Biotechnology lab, Guru Nanak Dev University, Amritsar, Punjab 143005, India

Shengping Yang and Michael D. Tomison
Department of Pathology, Texas Tech University Health Sciences Center, Lubbock, Texas, USA

Chwan-Li Shen
Department of Pathology, Texas Tech University Health Sciences Center, Lubbock, Texas, USA
Laura W. Bush Institute for Women's Health, Texas Tech University Health Sciences Center, Lubbock, Texas, USA
Department of Laboratory Sciences and Primary Care, Texas Tech University Health Sciences Center, Lubbock, Texas, USA

Shu Wang, Mehrnaz Abbasi, Lei Hao, Sheyenne Scott and Md Shahjalal Khan
Department of Nutritional Sciences, Texas Tech University, Lubbock, TX, USA.

Amanda W. Romero
Clinical Research Institute, Texas Tech University Health Sciences Center, Lubbock, Texas, USA

Carol K. Felton
Department of Obstetrics and Gynecology, Texas Tech University Health Sciences Center, Lubbock, TX, USA

Huanbiao Mo
Department of Nutrition, Georgia State University, Atlanta, GA, USA

Loïc Bareyre, Nicolas Coste and Emmanuel Coudeyre
Service de Médecine Physique et de Réadaptation, CHU de Clermont Ferrand, INRA, Université Clermont Auvergne, Clermont Ferrand, France

Chloe Gay
Service de Médecine Physique et de Réadaptation, CHU de Clermont Ferrand, INRA, Université Clermont Auvergne, Clermont Ferrand, France
Physical and Rehabilitation Medecine Department, University of Clermont Ferrand, Clermont Auvergne University, France, CHU Hôpital Nord, 61 Rue de Châteaugay - BP 30056, 63118 Clermont Ferrand, Cébazat, France

Candy Guiguet-Auclair
Service de Santé Publique, CHU de Clermont Ferrand, PEPRADE, Université Clermont Auvergne, Clermont Ferrand, France

Bruno Pereira
Délégation Recherche Clinique et Innovation, CHU de Clermont Ferrand, Université Clermont Auvergne, Clermont Ferrand, France

Anna Goldstein
Délégation Recherche Clinique et Innovation, CHU de Clermont Ferrand, Clermont Ferrand, France

Chun-li Lu, Xue-han Liu, Xiao Wang and Xue Bai
Centre for Evidence-Based Chinese Medicine, Beijing University of Chinese Medicine, Beijing 100029, China

Jian-ping Liu
Centre for Evidence-Based Chinese Medicine, Beijing University of Chinese Medicine, Beijing 100029, China
The National Research Center in Complementary and Alternative Medicine (NAFKAM), Department of Community Medicine, Faculty of Health Science, UiT, The Arctic University of Norway, 9037 Tromsø, Norway

Trine Stub, Agnete E. Kristoffersen, Arne Johan Norheim, Vinjar Fonnebo, Frauke Musial and Terje Araek
The National Research Center in Complementary and Alternative Medicine (NAFKAM), Department of Community Medicine, Faculty of Health Science, UiT, The Arctic University of Norway, 9037 Tromsø, Norway

Shi-bing Liang
School of Basic Medicine, Shanxi University of Chinese Medicine, Taiyuan 030000, China
Centre for Evidence-Based Chinese Medicine, Beijing University of Chinese Medicine, Beijing 100029, China

Yan-bin Wu
School of Pharmacy, Fujian University of Traditional Chinese Medicine, No. 1 Qiuyang Road, Shangjie Town, Minhou County, Fuzhou 350122, People's Republic of China

Yi Shen and Qi Zhang
School of Pharmacy, Fujian University of Traditional Chinese Medicine, No. 1 Qiuyang Road, Shangjie Town, Minhou County, Fuzhou 350122, People's Republic of China
School of Pharmacy, Zhejiang University of Traditional Chinese Medicine, Gaoke Road, Fuyang District, Hangzhou 310053, People's Republic of China

Qiao-yan Zhang
School of Pharmacy, Fujian University of Traditional Chinese Medicine, No. 1 Qiuyang Road, Shangjie Town, Minhou County, Fuzhou 350122, People's Republic of China
School of Pharmacy, Zhejiang University of Traditional Chinese Medicine, Gaoke Road, Fuyang District, Hangzhou 310053, People's Republic of China
School of Pharmacy, Second Military Medical University, No. 325 Guohe Road, Yangpu District, Shanghai 200433, People's Republic of China

Yu-qiong He, Ting Han, Jian-hua Zhang, Hai-liang Xin and Yun-peng Qi
School of Pharmacy, Second Military Medical University, No. 325 Guohe Road, Yangpu District, Shanghai 200433, People's Republic of China

Liang Zhao
Department of Pharmacy, Eastern Hepatobiliary Surgery Hospital, Second Military Medical University, No. 225 Changhai Road, Yangpu District, Shanghai 200438, People's Republic of China

Hsien-yeh Hsu
Department of Biotechnology and Laboratory Science in Medicine, National Yang-Ming University, No. 155, Section 2, Li Nong Street, Beitou District, Taipei 112-21, People's Republic of China

Hong-tao Song and Bing Lin
Fuzhou General Hospital of Nanjing Military Region, No. 156, West Second Ring North Road, Gulou District, Fuzhou 350025, People's Republic of China

Anchalee Prasansuklab and Atsadang Theerasri
Program in Clinical Biochemistry and Molecular Medicine, Department of Clinical Chemistry, Faculty of Allied Health Sciences, Chulalongkorn University, Bangkok 10330, Thailand

Matthew Payne and Alison T. Ung
School of Mathematical and Physical Sciences, Faculty of Science, The University of Technology Sydney, Sydney, NSW 2007, Australia

Tewin Tencomnao
Age-Related Inflammation and Degeneration Research Unit, Department of Clinical Chemistry, Faculty of Allied Health Sciences, Chulalongkorn University, Bangkok 10330, Thailand

Wen-Haur Chao, Ming-Yi Lai, Hwai-Tzong Pan, Huei-Wen Shiu and Mi-Mi Chen
Institute of Pharmacology, School of Medicine, National Yang-Ming University, Taipei, Taiwan

Hsiao-Ming Chao
Institute of Pharmacology, School of Medicine, National Yang-Ming University, Taipei, Taiwan
Department of Ophthalmology, Cheng Hsin General Hospital, Taipei, Taiwan
Department of Ophthalmology, Taipei Medical University-Shuang Ho Hospital, New Taipei City, Taiwan
Department of Chinese Medicine, School of Chinese Medicine, China Medical University, Taichung, Taiwan

Guixing Ren
College of Pharmacy and Biological Engineering, Chengdu University, Chengdu 610000, People's Republic of China
Institute of Crop Sciences, Chinese Academy of Agricultural Sciences, No.80 XUEYUAN South Road, Handian District, Beijing 100081, People's Republic of China

Peng Xue
Social Risk Prediction and Management, School of Public Health and Management, Weifang Medical University, No.7166 Baotong West Street Weicheng District, Weifang 261053, People's Republic of China
Institute of Crop Sciences, Chinese Academy of Agricultural Sciences, No.80 XUEYUAN South Road, Handian District, Beijing 100081, People's Republic of China

Gang Zhao
Key Laboratory of Coarse Cereal Processing, Ministry of Agriculture, No.2025 Chengluo Road, Longquanyi District, Chengdu 610106, People's Republic of China

Xiaoyan Sun
Institute of Crop Sciences, Chinese Academy of Agricultural Sciences, No.80 XUEYUAN South Road, Handian District, Beijing 100081, People's Republic of China

Ju Ah Lee
Department of Korean Internal Medicine, College of Korean Medicine, Gachon University, Incheon, Republic of Korea

Yui Sasaki and Seong-Gyu Ko
Institute of Safety and Effectiveness Evaluation for Korean Medicine, Department of Preventive Medicine, College of Korean Medicine, Kyung Hee University, Seoul, Republic of Korea

Ichiro Arai and Yun Kung Nam
Department of Pharmaceutical Sciences, Nihon Pharmaceutical University, Saitama, Japan

Ho-Yeon Go
Department of Internal Medicine, College of Korean Medicine, Semyung University, Jecheon, Republic of Korea

Sunju Park
Department of Preventive Medicine, College of Korean Medicine, Daejeon University, Daejeon, Republic of Korea

Keiko Yukawa
Department of Health Policy and Technology Assessment, National Institute of Public Health, Saitama, Japan

Yoshiharu Motoo
Department of Medical Oncology, Kanazawa Medical University, Ishikawa, Japan

Kiichiro Tsutani
Faculty of Health Sciences, Tokyo Ariake University of Medical and Health Sciences, Tokyo, Japan

Myeong Soo Lee
Clinical Medicine Division, Korea Institute of Oriental Medicine, 1672 Yuseong-daero, Yuseong-gu, Daejeon 34054, Republic of Korea

Kambiz Afshar and Jutta Bleidorn
Institute for General Practice, Hannover Medical School, Carl-Neuberg-Str. 1, 30625 Hannover, Germany

Nina Fleischmann and Eva Hummers-Pradier
Department of General Practice, University Medical Center Göttingen, Humboldtallee 38, 37073 Göttingen, Germany

Guido Schmiemann
Department for Health Services Research, Institute for Public Health and Nursing Research, University of Bremen, Bremen, Germany

Tim Friede
Department of Medical Statistics, University Medical Center Göttingen, Humboldtallee 32, 37073 Göttingen, Germany

Karl Wegscheider
Department of Medical Biometry and Epidemiology, University Medical Center Hamburg-Eppendorf, Martinistr, 52, 20246 Hamburg, Germany

Michael Moore
Primary Care and Population Science, University of Southampton Faculty of Medicine, Aldermoor Health Centre, Southampton SO16 5ST, UK

Ildikó Gágyor
Department of General Practice Universitätsklinikum Wurzburg, Josef-Schneider-Str. 2/D7, 97080 Würzburg, Germany

Atta Abbas Naqvi
Department of Pharmacy Practice, College of Clinical Pharmacy, Imam Abdulrahman Bin Faisal University, Dammam 31441, Saudi Arabia

Rizwan Ahmad
Natural Products and Alternative Medicines, College of Clinical Pharmacy, Imam Abdulrahman Bin Faisal University, Dammam 31441, Saudi Arabia

Abdullah Abdul Wahid Elewi, Ayman Hussain AlAwa and Moayed Jafar Alasiri
College of Clinical Pharmacy, Imam Abdulrahman Bin Faisal University, Dammam 31441, Saudi Arabia

Dayse Chaves Cardoso de Almeida, Gabriela Vasconcelos Calheiros de Oliveira Costa, Tayná Stéphanie Sampaio Donato and Letícia Moreira Nunes
Postgraduate Program in Health Research, Cesmac University Center, Rua Cônego Machado, 825, Farol, Maceió, Alagoas, Brazil

Isabel Cristina Celerino de Moraes Porto
Postgraduate Program in Health Research, Cesmac University Center, Rua Cônego Machado, 825, Farol, Maceió, Alagoas, Brazil
Department of Restorative Dentistry, Faculty of Dentistry, Federal University of Alagoas, Campus AC Simões, Av. Lourival Melo Mota, S/N, Tabuleiro do Martins, Maceió, Alagoas, Brazil
Laboratory of Quality Control of Drugs and Medicines, Postgraduate Program in Pharmaceutical Sciences, School of Nursing and Pharmacy, Federal University of Alagoas, Campus A. C, Simões, Maceió, Alagoas, Brazil

Ticiano Gomes do Nascimento, José Marcos dos Santos Oliveira, Irinaldo Diniz Basílio-Júnior, Camila Braga Dornelas and Eduardo Jorge da Silva Fonseca
Laboratory of Quality Control of Drugs and Medicines, Postgraduate Program in Pharmaceutical Sciences, School of Nursing and Pharmacy, Federal University of Alagoas, Campus A. C, Simões, Maceió, Alagoas, Brazil

Carolina Batista da Silva
Laboratory of Applied Electrochemistry, Institute of Chemistry and Biotechnology, Federal University of Alagoas, Campus A. C, Simões, Maceió, Alagoas, Brazil

Natanael Barbosa dos Santos
Department of Cariology, Faculty of Dentistry, Federal University of Alagoas, Campus AC Simões, Av. Lourival Melo Mota, S/N, Tabuleiro do Martins, Maceió, Alagoas, Brazil

Maria Luísa de Alencar e Silva Leite
Department of Dental Materials and Prosthodontics, Faculty of Dentistry, Universidade Estadual Paulista Júlio de Mesquita Filho-UNESP, Araraquara, São Paulo, Brazil

Pierre Barnabé Escodro
Faculty of Veterinary Medicine, Federal University of Alagoas, Campus Arapiraca, Unit of Viçosa, Viçosa, Alagoas, Brazil

Regianne Umeko Kamiya
Laboratory of Bacteriology.Institute of Biological and Health Sciences, Federal University of Alagoas, Campus A. C, Simões, Maceió, Alagoas, Brazil

Index

R

S

T

V

www.ingramcontent.com/pod-product-compliance
Lightning Source LLC
Chambersburg PA
CBHW082045190326
41458CB00010B/3463

* 9 7 8 1 6 3 2 4 2 8 5 8 5 *